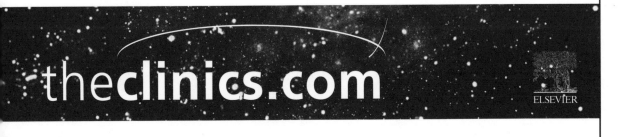

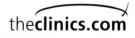

RADIOLOGIC CLINICS
of North America

Pediatric Chest Imaging

DONALD P. FRUSH, MD
Guest Editor

March 2005 • Volume 43 • Number 2

SAUNDERS

An Imprint of Elsevier, Inc.
PHILADELPHIA   LONDON   TORONTO   MONTREAL   SYDNEY   TOKYO

W.B. SAUNDERS COMPANY
A Division of Elsevier Inc.

The Curtis Center • Independence Square West • Philadelphia, Pennsylvania 19106

http://www.theclinics.com

RADIOLOGIC CLINICS OF NORTH AMERICA
March 2005
Editor: Barton Dudlick

Volume 43, Number 2
ISSN 0033-8389
ISBN 1-4160-2759-9

Reprints: For copies of 100 or more, of articles in this publication, please contact the Commercial Reprints Department, Elsevier Inc., 360 Park Avenue South, New York, New York 10010-1710. Tel. (212) 633-3813; Fax: (212) 462-1935; e-mail: reprints@elsevier.com.

The ideas and opinions expressed in *Radiologic Clinics of North America* do not necessarily reflect those of the Publisher. The Publisher does not assume any responsibility for any injury and/or damage to persons or property arising out of or related to any use of the material contained in this periodical. The reader is advised to check the appropriate medical literature and the product information currently provided by the manufacturer of each drug to be administered to verify the dosage, the method and duration of administration, or contraindications. It is the responsibility of the treating physician or other health care professional, relying on independent experience and knowledge of the patient, to determine drug dosages and the best treatment for the patient. Mention of any product in this issue should not be construed as endorsement by the contributors, editors, or the Publisher of the product or manufacturers' claims.

Radiologic Clinics of North America (ISSN 0033-8389) is published bimonthly by W.B. Saunders Company. Corporate and editorial offices: 170 S Independence Mall W 300 E, Philadelphia, PA 19106-3399. Accounting and circulation offices: 6277 Sea Harbor Drive, Orlando, FL 32887-4800. Periodicals postage paid at Orlando, FL 32862, and additional mailing offices. Subscription prices are USD 220 per year for US individuals, USD 331 per year for US institutions, USD 110 per year for US students and residents, USD 255 per year for Canadian individuals, USD 405 per year for Canadian institutions, USD 299 per year for international individuals, USD 405 per year for international institutions and USD 150 per year for Canadian and foreign students/residents. To receive student and resident rate, orders must be accompanied by name of affiliated institution, date of term, and the *signature* of program/residency coordinator on institution letterhead. Orders will be billed at individual rate until proof of status is received. Foreign air speed delivery is included in all *Clinics* subscription prices. All prices are subject to change without notice. POSTMASTER: Send address changes to *Radiologic Clinics of North America*, W.B. Saunders Company, Periodicals Fulfillment, Orlando, FL 32887-4800. **Customer Service: 1-800-654-2452 (US). From outside of the US, call 1-407-345-4000.**

Radiologic Clinics of North America also is published in Greek by Paschalidis Medical Publications, Athens, Greece.

Radiologic Clinics of North America is covered in *Index Medicus, EMBASE/Excerpta Medica, Current Contents/Life Sciences, Current Contents/Clinical Medicine, RSNA Index to Imaging Literature, BIOSIS, Science Citation Index,* and *ISI/BIOMED.*

Printed in the United States of America.

GOAL STATEMENT

The goal of the *Radiologic Clinics of North America* is to keep practicing radiologists and radiology residents up to date with current clinical practice in radiology by providing timely articles reviewing the state of the art in patient care.

ACCREDITATION

The *Radiologic Clinics of North America* is planned and implemented in accordance with the Essential Areas and Policies of the Accreditation Council for Continuing Medical Education (ACCME) through the joint sponsorship of the University of Virginia School of Medicine and W. B. Saunders, an Imprint of Elsevier Science, Inc. The University of Virginia School of Medicine is accredited by the ACCME to provide continuing medical education for physicians.

The University of Virginia School of Medicine designates this educational activity for a maximum of 90 category 1 credits per year, 15 category 1 credits per issue, toward the AMA Physician's Recognition Award. Each physician should claim only those credits that he/she actually spent in the activity.

The American Medical Association has determined that physicians not licensed in the US who participate in this CME activity are eligible for AMA PRA category 1 credit. (This was in the last time)

AMA PRA category 1 credit can be earned by reading the text material, taking the examination online at http://www.theclinics.com/home/cme, and completing the evaluation. After taking the test, your will be required to review any and all incorrect answers. Following completion of the test and the evaluation, your credit will be awarded and you may print your certificate.

FACULTY DISCLOSURE

As a provider accredited by the Accreditation Council for Continuing Medical Education (ACCME), the Office of Continuing Medical Education of the University of Virginia School of Medicine must ensure balance, independence, objectivity, and scientific rigor in all its individually sponsored or jointly sponsored educational activities. All authors/editors participating in a sponsored activity are expected to disclose to the readers any significant financial interest or other relationship (1) with the manufacturer(s) of any commercial product(s) and/or provider(s) of commercial services discussed in an educational presentation and (2) with any commercial supporters of the activity (significant financial interest or other relationship can include such things as grants or research support, employee, consultant, stock holder, member of speakers bureau, etc.) The intent of this disclosure is not to prevent authors/editors with a significant financial or other relationship from writing an article, but rather to provide readers with information on which they can make their own judgments. It remains for the readers to determine whether the author's/editor's interest or relationships may influence the article with regard to exposition or conclusion.

The authors/editors listed below have identified no professional or financial affiliations related to their presentation:
Alan S. Brody, MD; Brian D. Coley, MD; Lane F. Donnelly, MD; Barton Dudlick, Acquisitions Editor; Nancy R. Fefferman, MD; Lynn Ansley Fordham, MD; Arie Franco, MD, PhD; Caroline L. Hollingsworth, MD; Frederick R. Long, MD; Manuel P. Meza, MD; Neeta S. Mody, MD; Anne Paterson, MB BS, MRCP, FRCR, FFR RCSI; Lynne P. Pinkney, MD; E. Christine Wallace, MD; and, Sjirk J. Westra, MD.

The author/guest editor listed below has identified the following professional or financial affiliation related to his presentation:
Donald P. Frush, MD has disclosed that he is a medical advisor to GE Healthcare and has also received research support from them.

Disclosure of discussion of non-FDA approved uses for pharmaceutical products and/or medical devices:
The University of Virginia School of Medicine, as an ACCME provider, requires that all authors/editors identify and disclose any "off label" uses for pharmaceutical products and/or for medical devices. The University of Virginia School of Medicine recommends that each reader fully review all the available data on new products or procedures prior to instituting them with patients.

All authors/editors who provided disclosures will not be discussing any off-label uses except:
Lynn Ansley Fordham, MD will discuss the use of gadolinium for esophageal leak.

TO ENROLL

To enroll in the Radiologic Clinics of North America Continuing Medical Education program, call customer service at 1-800-654-2452 or sign up online at *http://www.theclinics.com/home/cme*. The CME program is available to subscribers for an additional annual fee of $195.00.

FORTHCOMING ISSUES

RECENT ISSUES

THE CLINICS ARE NOW AVAILABLE ONLINE!

Access your subscription at:
http://www.theclinics.com

GUEST EDITOR

DONALD P. FRUSH, MD, Professor, Radiology; and Chief, Division of Pediatric Radiology, Department of Radiology, Duke University Health System, Durham, North Carolina

CONTRIBUTORS

ALAN S. BRODY, MD, Chief, Thoracic Imaging, Department of Radiology, Cincinnati Children's Hospital and Medical Center; and Professor, Radiology and Pediatrics, University of Cincinnati College of Medicine, Cincinnati, Ohio

BRIAN D. COLEY, MD, Chief, Section of Ultrasound, Department of Radiology, Columbus Children's Hospital; and Clinical Associate Professor, Radiology and Pediatrics, Ohio State University School of Medicine and Public Health, Columbus, Ohio

LANE F. DONNELLY, MD, Radiologist-in-Chief, Department of Radiology, Cincinnati Children's Hospital Medical Center; and Professor, Radiology and Pediatrics, University of Cincinnati College of Medicine, Cincinnati, Ohio

NANCY R. FEFFERMAN, MD, Section Chief, Division of Pediatric Radiology; and Assistant Professor, Department of Radiology, New York University School of Medicine, New York, New York

LYNN ANSLEY FORDHAM, MD, Associate Professor and Chief, Pediatric Radiology, Department of Radiology, University of North Carolina School of Medicine, Chapel Hill, North Carolina

ARIE FRANCO, MD, PhD, Assistant Professor, Department of Radiology, Children's Hospital of Pittsburgh, Pittsburgh, Pennsylvania

DONALD P. FRUSH, MD, Professor, Radiology; and Chief, Division of Pediatric Radiology, Department of Radiology, Duke University Health System, Durham, North Carolina

CAROLINE L. HOLLINGSWORTH, MD, Assistant Professor, Division of Pediatric Radiology, Department of Radiology, Duke University Health System, Durham, North Carolina

FREDERICK R. LONG, MD, Section Chief, Body CT/MR Imaging, Department of Radiology, Columbus Children's Hospital; and Clinical Associate Professor, Department of Radiology, College of Medicine and Public Health, Ohio State University, Columbus, Ohio

MANUEL P. MEZA, MD, Associate Professor, Department of Radiology, Children's Hospital of Pittsburgh, Pittsburgh, Pennsylvania

NEETA S. MODY, MD, Radiology Resident, Department of Radiology, Western Pennsylvania Hospital, Pittsburgh, Pennsylvania

ANNE PATERSON, MB BS, MRCP, FRCR, FFR RCSI, Consultant Paediatric Radiologist, Radiology Department, Royal Belfast Hospital for Sick Children, Belfast, United Kingdom

LYNNE P. PINKNEY, MD, Assistant Professor, Division of Pediatric Radiology, Department of Radiology, New York University School of Medicine, New York, New York

E. CHRISTINE WALLACE, MD, Chief, Division of Pediatric Radiology, UMassMemorial Medical Center; and Assistant Professor, Radiology, University of Massachusetts, Worcester, Massachusetts

SJIRK J. WESTRA, MD, Associate Professor, Radiology, Harvard Medical School; and Associate Radiologist, Department of Radiology, Massachusetts General Hospital, Boston, Massachusetts

CONTENTS

challenging but adherence to a relatively straightforward step-by-step method, emphasizing patient preparation and technical familiarity, can result in excellent examinations even in the smallest infants and most complex clinical scenarios.

Immunodeficiencies in children may be caused by primary immunodeficiency syndromes or can result from secondary disorders of immune regulation. Thoracic complications in immunocompromised children are frequent and may vary according to the type of the immunodeficiency. Imaging plays a pivotal role in detection and distinction of the variety of sequelae. It is important for the radiologist to understand both the spectrum of pediatric immune disorders, and the mechanisms underlying these disorders.

RADIOLOGIC
CLINICS
of North America

Radiol Clin N Am 43 (2005) xi – xii

Preface

Pediatric Chest Imaging

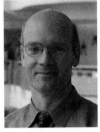

Donald P. Frush, MD
Guest Editor

Children are frightening. Frightening? In nearly all contexts this statement would be indefensible. In medicine, however, children are often frightening. For one thing, clinical evaluation in young children can be more difficult than with adults. In addition, in the acutely ill or injured child, reserve can be limited and appropriate assessment, including imaging evaluation, and subsequent care are critically important in improving outcome. Many care providers are not pediatric specialists by practice, and evaluation and treatment of children is less familiar than with adults. Moreover, the spectrum of disorders that affects the pediatric population can be quite different from disorders more easily recognized in adults. Often there is an extra layer of emotional concern, or anxiety, because a child is involved. Together, these issues reinforce the importance of resources which facilitate the diagnosis and care of the sick or injured child. This is especially relevant to chest disorders, because thoracic abnormalities are common in children, and is also relevant to radiologists, because imaging evaluation of the chest is frequently one of the first (or only) tools used after the clinical assessment.

Presumably, you are reading this because you are an imager, or interested in imaging evaluation, and because you are caring for children in some capacity. Perhaps you are reading this because, like many of us who have contributed to this work, you understand the importance of being familiar with the imaging evaluation of chest disorders in infants and children. Like many of us, you also understand that current information on many topics is difficult to find, and when available, not a comprehensive resource. This issue of *Radiologic Clinics of North America*, then, is compiled to provide a contemporary resource for those interested in imaging evaluation of the pediatric chest.

I am fortunate and thankful to have enlisted an internationally recognized panel of pediatric radiologists who bring an additional expertise in thoracic imaging. Because of the many years of expertise, the work reflects not only knowledge, but wisdom regarding the approach and interpretation of chest imaging that only experience brings. Topics covered include focused evaluation of common clinical scenarios such as pulmonary infection, airway and esophageal disorders, trauma, and chest wall disorders; patterns of presentation, such as interstitial lung disease, and lung and mediastinal masses; imaging techniques including ultrasonography and

radiologic.theclinics.com

CT angiography; as well as special clinical arenas such as chest infection in the immunocompromised child. Together, it is our collective hope that this material will provide you the opportunity to become *familiar and comfortable* with the imaging evaluation of pediatric chest disorders, and in the end, realize that it is not children who are frightening...but, rather, our lack of knowledge of and familiarity with pediatric diseases, imaging techniques, and their interpretation.

Donald P. Frush, MD
Professor, Radiology
Chief, Division of Pediatric Radiology
Department of Radiology
McGovern-Davison Children's Health Center
Duke University Health System
Erwin Road
Box 3808
Durham NC 27710, USA
E-mail address: frush943@mc.duke.edu

RADIOLOGIC
CLINICS
of North America

Radiol Clin N Am 43 (2005) 253–265

Imaging in Immunocompetent Children Who Have Pneumonia

Lane F. Donnelly, MD[a,b,*]

[a]Department of Radiology, Cincinnati Children's Hospital Medical Center, 3333 Burnet Avenue,
Cincinnati, OH 45229–3039, USA
[b]Radiology and Pediatrics, University of Cincinnati College of Medicine, Cincinnati, OH, USA

In 1994, the year that I was a pediatric radiology fellow at Cincinnati Children's Hospital, there was a dramatic increase in the number of children hospitalized with complications related to bacterial pneumonia. This included an increase in the number of purulent lung complications, such as cavitary necrosis, and an increase in the number of empyemas as compared with years past. There was a lot of speculation at the time as to why there had been a sudden increase in the frequency of children with complications related to pneumonia. Some speculated that it was related to an increased frequency of antibiotic-resistant streptococcal pneumonia infections. Others speculated that there had been a strain of influenza A virus that went through the community and was associated with injury to the respiratory mucosa resulting in children who were predisposed to developing complications when they were infected with bacterial pneumonia. In subsequent years, however, there again were increasing numbers of children hospitalized for complications related to pneumonia each year. This trend continues today.

I became involved in several projects reporting on our experience at Cincinnati Children's with the use of CT in these children with pneumonia-related complications [1–5]. Subsequently, I have been involved in writing several review articles on the roles of imaging in children with pneumonia [6,7]. In

preparation for writing this article, I have done a recent literature search and, unfortunately, very little has changed in the past 10 years concerning what is known about the performance of imaging studies in the management of children with pneumonia. Many of the areas of controversy, such as how aggressively parapneumonic effusion should be managed, are still without definitive and agreed on plans of action.

In this article, the roles of imaging in children with pneumonia are discussed. The contents of this article apply to when immunocompetent and previously healthy children develop pneumonia or its complications. The indications for imaging and implication of the findings at imaging are completely different in children who are immunodeficient or have underlying medical conditions, such as sickle cell anemia or cystic fibrosis. A discussion of those children is beyond the scope of this article. The following topics are covered concerning the roles of imaging in the management of pneumonia: evaluation for possible pneumonia, determination of a specific etiologic agent, exclusion of other pathology, evaluation of the child with failure of pneumonia to clear, and evaluation of complications related to pneumonia.

Evaluation for possible pneumonia

Respiratory tract infections are the most common cause of illness in children and one of the most common indications for imaging in children. Chest radiographs are often obtained as part of the evaluation to determine whether or not a child is likely to have bacterial pneumonia. At first, it seems that

* Department of Radiology, Cincinnati Children's Hospital and Medical Center, 3333 Burnet Avenue, Cincinnati, OH 45229-3039.
 E-mail address: Lane.Donnelly@cchmc.org

determining whether a child did or did not have pneumonia is a straightforward issue; however, it is much more complex and difficult [6–11]. First, the signs and symptoms of pneumonia are often much more nonspecific in infants and young children than they are in adults [11,12]. Although children do present with fever and respiratory symptoms, such as cough, wheezing, tachypnea, or retractions, children can often present with non–respiratory-related general symptoms, such as malaise, irritability, headaches, chest pain, or abdominal pain. It is not an uncommon scenario for lower lobe pneumonia to be recognized on the superior aspect of abdominal radiographs being obtained for abdominal pain (Fig. 1). In addition, physical examination is less reliable in children than in adults. Children, related to their small size, have lower tidal volumes and auscultation is more difficult than in adults [8–12]. Moreover, young children may not be able or refuse to cooperate with deep breathing and other aspects of the physical examination. Finally, beyond the chest radiograph, there are no accurate laboratory tests to determine whether or not a child is likely to have pneumonia [8–12]. Such tests as an elevated sedimentation rate or elevated white blood cell count are neither sensitive nor specific. For these reasons, physicians have relied on chest radiography to help determine when a child is likely or unlikely to have an underlying bacterial illness.

Physicians have relied on the results of radiography in the management of children with potential pneumonia. There is evidence that radiography affects management decisions in such cases. There have been a number of articles that have looked into the use of chest radiography in the evaluation of children with the potential for pneumonia [9,13]. Many of these studies were set up similarly [9,13]. Referring physicians were surveyed as to their diagnosis, treatment, and disposition decisions before being given the results of chest radiography and then again after knowing the results of chest radiography. Concerning treatment, it was asked whether they would or would not place a patient on antibiotics or bronchodilators. Concerning disposition, they were asked whether they would admit the child, discharge the child, or what would be their frequency of follow-up for the child. Comparing the pre- versus post chest radiography decisions, there was a change in diagnosis approximately 20% of the time and, more importantly, a change in management decisions in approximately one third of patients [9,13]. There is evidence that referring physicians do alter their management plans based on the information supplied by chest radiography.

Another area of controversy is not only whether it is useful to get chest radiographs, but when it is useful to get chest radiographs. What are the indications to obtain chest radiography in patients suspected of having pneumonia? Although there is some disagreement in this area, most studies support the notion that radiography is a reasonable diagnostic test in children who are febrile and have respiratory symptoms [14,15]. In a recent review of data from the Emergency Department at our institution (E. Melinda Mahabee-Gittens, unpublished data, 2004), approximately 400 patients with suspected pneumonia who underwent radiography were prospectively reviewed for signs and symptoms that were statistically significantly greater associated with the radiographic diagnosis of pneumonia. There was a prevalence of approximately 10% for pneumonia. There was a statistically significant correlation between the following signs and symptoms and the presence of pneumonia: age greater than 12 months, oxygen saturation less than 94%, respiratory rate greater than 60 breaths per minute, nasal flaring, and decreased breath sounds. The presence of these symptoms may be helpful in allowing clinicians to determine when it is appropriate to obtain chest radiography.

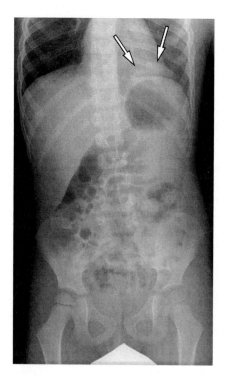

Fig. 1. Left lower lobe pneumonia presenting with abdominal pain in a 4-year-old boy. Radiograph of the abdomen shows opacification (*arrows*) of portion of left lower lobe.

Determination of an etiologic agent

On review of many radiology textbooks, in the portion of the book concerning pneumonia, often the chapters are divided into sections depicting the specific patterns of radiographic appearance for specific bacterial diagnoses. There is often a section on streptococcal pneumonia, a section of staphylococcal pneumonia, and so forth. Pragmatically, the specific bacterial agent responsible is usually not the clinical question expected to be resolved by radiography. The main objective in patients with potential pneumonia is whether the patient is likely to have bacterial pneumonia and should be placed on antibiotics. The question, then, is how accurate is radiography in differentiating viral lower respiratory tract infections from bacterial pneumonia? To address this issue, it is important to discuss several issues including the underlying pathophysiology of both viral and bacterial pneumonia, the classic radiographic patterns of presentation of viral and bacterial pneumonia, and what is known about how well the radiographic findings perform.

Viral disease

Viral infection of the lower respiratory tract predominantly involves the airway mucosal cells [16,17]. The infection leads to inflammation and necrosis resulting in peribronchial edema. The process also results in occlusion of the smaller airways. The occlusion is related to both the peribronchial edema further narrowing the airway and sloughed debris and mucus within the lumen. On radiography, there is a bilateral typically symmetric process of increased peribronchial opacities, hyperinflation, and subsegmental atelectasis (Fig. 2) [16-23].

Increased peribronchial markings are one of the more subjective radiographic findings in pediatric radiology. Residents and other trainees are often frustrated when trying to guess whether the faculty with which they are working will "call" increased peribronchial markings. Certainly, increased peribronchial markings represent a spectrum with ranges from near normal to grossly abnormal. On frontal radiography, it is seen as increased density and indistinctness of the lung markings arising centrally from the hilum (see Fig. 2). Often the hila appear very prominent in size and density on the lateral view. I often use the prominence of the hila on the lateral view to determine whether there are increased peribronchial markings.

In small children, hyperinflation is often much easier to diagnose on the lateral than on the frontal view. On the lateral view, the diaphragm is markedly flattened and the anterior to posterior diameter of the chest often is as large, if not larger, than the superior

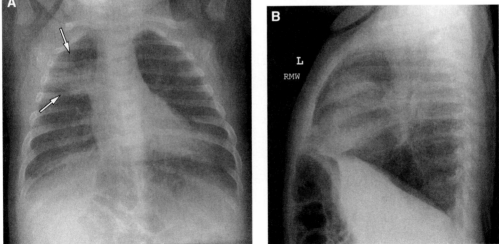

Fig. 2. Viral pneumonia in a 4-month-old boy. (*A*) Frontal radiograph shows hyperinflation, increased peribronchial markings, and focal atelectasis in the right upper lobe as triangular opacity in right upper lobe (*arrows*). (*B*) Lateral radiograph shows flattened hemidiaphrams and increased anterior to posterior diameter of the chest consistent with hyperinflation. The density and prominence of the hila are prominent, a supportive finding of increased peribronchial markings.

to inferior diameter (see Fig. 2). It is important to emphasize the common nature of both air trapping and collapse in association with viral lower respiratory tract infections [16–23]. There are a number of anatomic factors that contribute to the prevalence of air trapping and collapse in children with viral pneumonia. First, in proportion to children's small size, the small bronchials are also proportionately smaller. The amount of peribronchial edema needed to occlude these small vessels is much less in children than in adults. In addition, the collateral pathways, such as the channels of Lambert and pores of Kohn, are poorly developed in young children [16–23]. These collateral pathways for air ventilation do not become mature until about approximately 8 years of age [16–24]. Finally, children have much more abun-

dant mucus production within their bronchial tree than do adults. The combination of these anatomic findings renders children much more susceptible to air trapping and hyperinflation and areas of subsegmental collapse (see Fig. 2) in association with viral illness. Many authors have stated that the overinterpretation of the presence of linear densities consistent with subsegmental atelectasis as suspicious for superimposed bacterial pneumonia is one of the more common errors made in pediatric imaging.

Bacterial pneumonia

In contrast to viral lower respiratory tract infection, bacterial pneumonia tends to be a unilateral

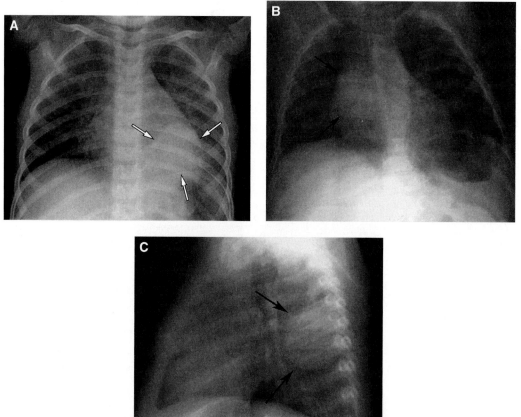

Fig. 3. Round pneumonia. (*A*) Round pneumonia in a 3-year-old boy. Frontal radiograph shows focal round opacity in left lower lobe (*arrows*). (*B,C*) Frontal and lateral radiograph of a well-defined, mass-like round pneumonia in a young child. This could be confused with a posterior mediastinal mass, particularly on the lateral view (*arrows*).

process, segmental to lobar in distribution, and represents true air space opacification (Fig. 3) [16–24]. Air bronchograms are often identified. Pleural effusions are not uncommonly associated with bacterial pneumonia but are rarely associated with viral disease.

How accurate are the classically described radiographic findings in determining whether a child truly does have viral or bacterial or respiratory tract infection? There are a number of factors that might make one think that there are inaccuracies. Infants tend to have predominantly airway infections regardless of the etiology. There is also a subset of children who have initial viral infection, which can denude the respiratory mucosa and predispose to superimposed bacterial pneumonia. Furthermore, in school-aged children, mycoplasma makes up approximately 30% of lower respiratory tract infections and mycoplasma can have a viral or bacterial radiographic pattern on presentation [25–28]. It is also a difficult question to answer. Most children with lower respiratory tract infections never have a specific documented etiology. Most never need an invasive diagnostic procedure. Even in children in whom procedures are performed, a specific infectious agent is not identified because of ongoing treatment with antibiotics.

There have been a number of publications that looked at this issue of predictive radiographic features. In a 1986 publication, authors evaluated the ability of radiographic patterns of infection to predict whether or not a child had bacterial pneumonia based on clinical criteria, such as rapid or short duration of illness, high fever, high white blood cell count, and rapid response to antibiotics [29]. There was no analysis for organisms performed. These authors reported that the radiographic presentation predicted which children meet the clinical criteria for bacterial illness with an accuracy rate of 90% [29]. In response to this publication, a second group published an article in 1988 in which they used the same clinical and radiographic criteria as described in the initial paper and compared clinical criteria as a predictor for microbiology with radiographic criteria as a predictor for microbiology [30]. These authors demonstrated that the clinical criteria had a positive predictive value for bacterial pneumonia of only 18%. Eighty-two percent of the time when the clinical criteria suggested that the patient had bacterial pneumonia, the findings were inaccurate. The negative predictive value for bacterial pneumonia was 81%. The radiographic criteria performed only slightly better. The positive predictive value for bacterial pneumonia was 30% and the negative predictive value for bacterial pneumonia was 92% [30]. This study suggests that the clinical and radiographic criteria substantially overestimate the number of children who have bacterial pneumonia. It is important to understand, however, that only a small percent of children with bacterial pneumonia have the clinical and radiographic findings of viral lower respiratory tract infections. If the goal of obtaining a radiograph is to identify all those children who do not need to be placed on antibiotics while ensuring that those who possibly have bacterial pneumonia do get placed on antibiotics, then the high negative predictive value of radiography in excluding bacterial pneumonia is valuable.

Round pneumonia

When discussing bacterial pneumonia in children, it is worth mentioning round pneumonia. In children less than 8 years of age in whom the collateral pathways of circulation are not well developed, pneumonia can have a very round appearance and mimic a mass (see Fig. 3) [24]. This is referred to as "round pneumonia." In a child with fever and appropriate symptoms, round pneumonia should be the primary working diagnosis when a round mass is seen on chest radiography. Follow-up radiography after antibiotic therapy is warranted to exclude an underlying mass, such as a bronchogenic cyst. Most cases of round pneumonia are related to *Streptococcal pneumoniae* infection [24].

Exclusion of other pathologies

The signs and symptoms of pneumonia in children are often nonspecific, and there are a number of other disease processes that can present with overlapping symptoms. In reviewing chest radiographs in children with suspected pneumonia, one of the roles of the radiologist is to exclude those other potential etiologies producing the symptoms. Reviewing all the potential etiologies that have overlapping symptoms with pneumonia is beyond the scope of this article. Areas that may contain pathology that is initially overlooked include processes that involve the ribs and the airway. It is helpful to go back and look at the ribs and airways a second time whenever interpreting pediatric chest radiographs. Close review of the ribs may demonstrate erosion related to processes, such as neuroblastoma, or rib fractures related to occult child abuse (Fig. 4). Because pathology of the central airways is much less common in adults than in children, disease processes involving the trachea can be overlooked in children. Stridor related to such

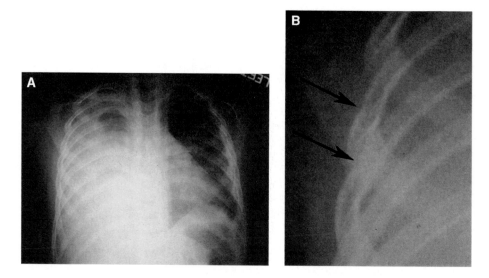

Fig. 4. Large hemothorax caused by child abuse in a 10-month-old boy who presented with tachypnea. (*A*) The right-sided effusion was thought to be a parapneumonic effusion on initial inspection of the frontal radiograph. (*B*) On closer inspection, lateral rib fractures (*arrows*) were evident on the right fourth and fifth ribs.

causes as vascular rings may lead to chest radiography being obtained to exclude pneumonia.

Evaluate failure of pneumonia to clear

It is a common teaching in the management of adults with radiology that the pneumonia should be followed to clearing to exclude an underlying cause of the bronchial obstruction, such as a bronchogenic carcinoma. In children this is not a clinical concern,

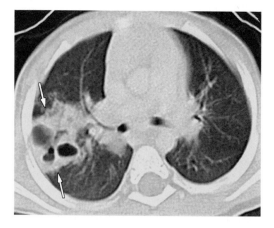

Fig. 5. Congenital cystic adenomatoid malformation in a 2-year-old boy. CT shows multicystic mass (*arrows*) in the right lung. Several cysts contain air-fluid levels.

and follow-up chest radiography should not be obtained routinely. Subsequent radiographs should be reserved for those children who have persistent or recurrent symptoms, or those children who have an underlying condition, such as immunodeficiency, cystic fibrosis, or sickle cell anemia, and considered in those with round pneumonia.

Concerning the temporal resolution of pneumonia on radiography, radiographs are often obtained too early and too often. A pneumonia that is appropriately responding to antibiotics often takes 2 to 4 weeks to resolve radiographically [16–24]. For the persistence of pneumonia radiographically to have more clinical significance, it is important to wait as long as possible before obtaining repeat radiographs. Whenever possible, repeat radiographs should be obtained at no sooner an interval than 2 to 3 weeks.

Failure to clear

There are a number of clinical considerations when a child has failure of pneumonia to clear. This is the presenting finding of an underlying infected developmental lesion. The most common developmental masses that present as persistent or recurrent pneumonia include sequestration or congenital cystic adenomatoid malformation (Fig. 5). Bronchogenic cysts uncommonly present in this fashion (Fig. 6). Other causes of failure to clear that should be entertained in children include bronchial obstruction (most often related to an aspirated foreign body); presenting

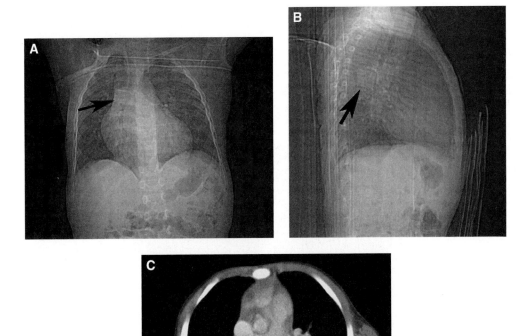

Fig. 6. Bronchogenic cyst in a 4-year-old boy discovered on a chest radiograph obtained for mild symptoms of a respiratory infection. (*A,B*) Frontal and lateral topograms for the CT demonstrate the right hilar mass (*arrows*). (*C*) Intravenous contrast-enhanced axial CT image shows well-defined cyst with fluid density (*arrow*).

findings of gastroesophageal reflux in aspiration; or underlying systemic disorder, such as immunodeficiency [16–23].

Evaluate associated complications

Suppurative complications related to pneumonia can involve the pleura, lung parenchyma, or rarely the pericardium. Pleural complications consist of parapneumonic effusions and their subtypes: transudate effusions, empyema, and inadequately drained effusions. Parenchymal complications include a spectrum of abnormalities, such as cavitary necrosis and lung abscess. Occasionally, patients can also present with purulent pericarditis.

There are primarily two clinical issues in which imaging are often involved. The first question is, does imaging play any role in the decision-making process concerning the primary evaluation or parapneumonia

effusions. The second question is what role imaging plays in the evaluation of the child who has persistent or progressive symptoms of pneumonia despite antibiotic therapy. The following sections address these two questions.

Primary evaluation of parapneumonic effusions

One of the areas in which there is marked controversy and differences of opinion is in regards to the aggressiveness of management of parapneumonic effusions. Therapeutic options of parapneumonic effusion range from observation, antibiotics alone, thoracentesis, chest tube placement, fibrinolytic therapy, video-assisted thoracoscopic surgery and drainage, or surgical thoracotomy and debridement [31–37]. There are marked differences in opinion on how aggressive and what the indications for which aggressive therapy should be implemented. Obviously, in patients with large effusions, lung compression, and shortness of breath, the decision to perform drainage of the fluid should be straightforward.

Historically, parapneumonic effusions are classified into two broad groups: empyema and transudate effusion [38,39]. The gold standard for this classification has been the aspiration and analysis of the fluid. The aggressiveness of therapy has historically been based on this distinction. It is the teaching that those pleural effusions that meet the criteria for empyema benefit from aggressive therapy and without aggressive therapy, there is the potential of increased length of hospitalization and development of fibrothorax [38,39]. Parapneumonic effusions that meet the criteria for transudate effusions are thought to be more optimally managed with less aggressive therapy [38,39].

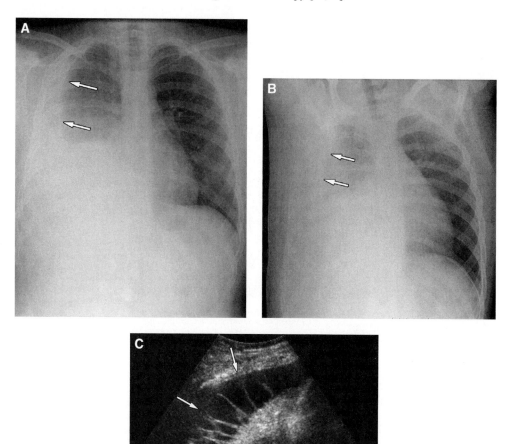

Fig. 7. Complex parapneumonic effusion in a 13-year-old boy. (*A*) Frontal radiograph shows opacification of right lower and right middle lobes with right effusion (*arrows*) extending the length of the hemithorax. (*B*) Radiograph with right side down decubitus positioning shows minimal change. The effusion (*arrows*) is harder to see on this image. The image contributes little to decision making. (*C*) Ultrasound shows the right effusion to contain complex fluid with multiple echogenic septae and debris (*arrows*).

One question that often arises is whether there is any imaging modality that plays a role in helping with decisions concerning the aggressiveness of therapy in the primary evaluation of parapneumonic effusions. The longest-standing imaging method for evaluating whether parapneumonic effusions are complex (empyema) or simple (transudate effusions) is by obtaining chest radiographs with decubitus positioning. If the decubitus radiograph demonstrates that the pleural fluid layers, these effusions are thought to be transudative, and if the decubitus positioned radiograph demonstrates no change in position of the pleural effusion as compared with the upright film, these collections are thought to be complex. In my experience, the findings on decubitus radiographs are often confusing and very rarely are management decisions changed on the basis of obtaining decubitus radiographs (Fig. 7). I think because decubitus radiographs rarely contribute to patient management decisions, they are not worth obtaining.

In the early 1990s there was a lot of enthusiasm that intravenous (IV) contrast-enhanced CT was helpful in separating parapneumonic effusions into empyema and transudative effusion groups (Fig. 8) [40,41]. Such findings as parietal pleural enhancement, parietal pleural thickening greater than 2 mm, extrapleural thickening and increased attenuation of the extrapleural space, and adjacent chest wall edema were all thought to be predictive of the presence of

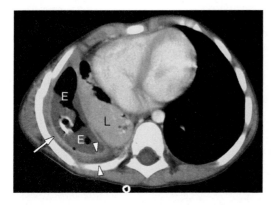

Fig. 8. Parapneumonic effusion in an 11-year-old girl. Intravenous contrast-enhanced CT shows consolidated lung (L) and adjacent pleural collection (E) containing fluid and gas. Some of the gas bubbles are in a nondependent position. There is enhancement of the parietal pleura (*arrow*). There is thickening and increased attenuation of the extrapleural space (between *arrowheads*). There is also asymmetric chest wall edema. These findings have all been reported to suggest empyema over transudative effusion but the results have been shown to be inaccurate in making this distinction in children.

empyema [40,41]. In children, normally the extrapleural space is a nonvisualized area of adipose tissue. With an adjacent inflammatory parapneumonic effusion, the extrapleural space becomes thickened, visualized, and of increased soft tissue attenuation. These conclusions were based on studies that compared empyemas with transudative effusions, such as those secondary to heart failure in adults [40,41]. A study that reviewed a number of parapneumonic effusions in children demonstrated, however, that these findings were inaccurate in determining whether the parapneumonic effusion was an empyema or transudative effusions [1]. In fact, our experience is that ultrasound can demonstrate multiple loculations and debris in parapneumonic effusions, findings that are often not visualized on CT scans obtained in the same patients.

In the late 1990s, there was enthusiasm that ultrasound may be a useful modality in separating parapneumonic effusions into those that need aggressive therapy and those that can be managed conservatively. A study published by Ramnath et al [42] suggested a very simple ultrasound grading system in which parapneumonic effusions were graded as low-grade (anechoic fluid with no septations) or high-grade (presence of echogenic fronds, septations, or loculations) (see Fig. 7). Those patients with high-grade parapneumonic effusions, as demonstrated by ultrasound, and treated with aggressive therapy had a 50% decrease in duration of hospital stay as compared with those who were conservatively managed [42]. In the group of low-grade parapneumonic effusions as determined by ultrasound, there was no change in duration of hospital stay whether the patients were treated aggressively or conservatively. In fact, in the low-grade group, those patients who had thoracentesis alone had a longer hospital stay than those who had no invasive therapy. These authors advocate the use of ultrasound in helping to determine aggressiveness of therapy for parapneumonic effusions [42].

Of the three potential imaging modality choices (decubitus radiographs, CT, and ultrasound) we advocate the use of ultrasound when the issue is determining whether a primary parapneumonic effusion should or should not be aggressively managed.

Evaluation of persistent or progressive symptoms

Another area in which imaging often plays a role is in the evaluation of the child who has failed to respond adequately to antibiotic and other therapy for pneumonia. These patients typically have persistent fever, sepsis, and are often severely ill. Almost all of these patients have some underlying suppurative complication related to their pneumonia [2–7,43,44]. In such patients, chest radiography is the primary imaging modality but is often insensitive to some of the underlying problems that can be present. In the presence of a noncontributory chest radiograph (which is much more common than one might think), IV contrast-enhanced CT is a useful tool. In one study in this scenario, IV contrast-enhanced CT identified an underlying suppurative cause of the persistent illness in 100% of patients [3,43]. This is one of the few indications in pediatric or adult imaging in which a CT is performed primarily to evaluate for lung pathology in which the use of IV contrast material should be routine. It is also the only indication in the evaluation of immunocompetent children with pneumonia for performing a CT scan. The percentage of children with pneumonia who require a CT scan should be the overwhelming minority.

One of the goals of CT is to separate the underlying causes of the persistent illness into those that are related to the pleura and those that are related to lung parenchyma. Most of the pleural causes of persistent illness require interventional or surgical procedures, whereas most of the lung parenchymal complications are managed with conservative monitoring and support.

Pleural complications

By the time a patient with a complication related to pneumonia becomes ill to the point where they are considered to have a progressive illness requiring CT, most often a pleural drainage has already been performed and a chest tube is in place. In these patients, however, residual loculated fluid collections can be a persistent cause of systemic illness, including sepsis [3]. We have found that in such patients, CT is useful in depicting the anatomic location of these fluid collections from a global perspective and is helpful in planning for interventional procedures performed with ultrasound guidance. We have found this much harder to do in the scenario with ultrasound. In addition, CT can be helpful in depicting malpositioned chest tubes.

Lung parenchymal complications

Another cause of persistent systemic illness in patients with complicated pneumonia is when those complications reside within the lung parenchyma. Parenchymal complications include a spectrum of pathologic conditions and a number of associated descriptive terms. Which descriptive term is used to name the process is determined by the imaging appearance, temporal appearance as compared with the timing of the development of pneumonia, and clinical condition of the patient. Used terms include cavitary necrosis, pulmonary abscess, pulmonary gangrene, pneumatocele, and bronchopleural fistula [2–7,44–46].

By far the most common terminology or diagnosis encountered is cavity necrosis. In otherwise healthy immunocompetent patients, lung abscesses are ac-

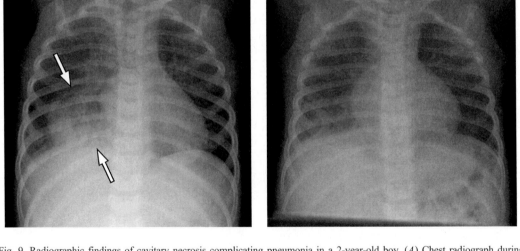

Fig. 9. Radiographic findings of cavitary necrosis complicating pneumonia in a 2-year-old boy. (*A*) Chest radiograph during acute illness shows opacification of right middle and lower lobes. There are multiple air-filled cysts within the opacified lung (*arrows*) consistent with cavitary necrosis. (*B*) Chest radiograph obtained 2 months later shows resolution of cysts and marked decrease in opacity. Linear densities remain.

tually uncommon. A lung abscess is defined as present when there is a fluid or gas and fluid collection within the lung parenchyma with a well-defined border with an enhancing rim [2–7]. The presence of a true lung abscess that requires interventional drainage is again uncommon in otherwise healthy children with complications related to pneumonia.

Cavitary necrosis

Cavitary necrosis is by far the most common parenchymal complication of pneumonia currently encountered in children. It is defined as a dominant area of necrosis with an associated variable number of thin-walled cysts (Figs. 9 and 10). The CT appearance includes decreased contrast enhancement, loss of normal lung architecture, and multiple thin-walled cavities that are filled with either air or fluid and lack an enhancing border (see Fig. 10) [2–7]. Areas of noncomplicated pneumonia and areas of atelectasis diffusely enhance on IV contrast-enhanced CT [2]. The presence of decreased enhancement can be an early finding of impending cavitary ne-

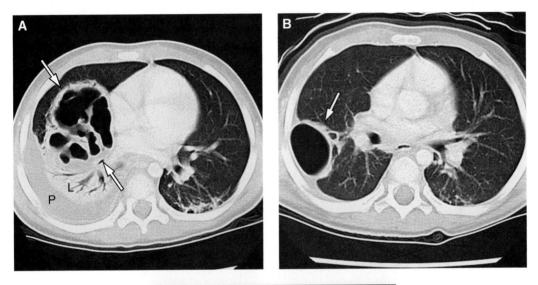

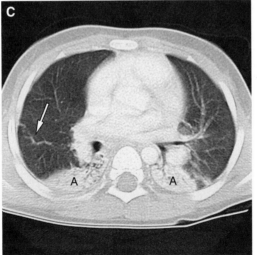

Fig. 10. CT findings of cavitary necrosis complicating pneumonia in a 2-year-old boy (same as in Fig. 9). (*A*) CT at time of acute illness shows large, multiloculated cavity (*arrows*) with adjacent consolidated lung (L). There is also a pleural effusion (P). (*B*) CT 1 month later shows resolution of consolidation and pleural effusion. Most of the cavities have resolved with the exception of a single, large, air-filled cyst (*arrow*). (*C*) CT 4 months following the initial CT shows resolution of cyst with only a linear density remaining (*arrow*). Note areas of atelectasis (A) posteriorly.

crosis. Historically, necrosis and cavitary formation within an area of pneumonia has been associated with staphylococcal pneumonia infection. Currently in children, however, staphylococcal pneumonia is rarely encountered. Overwhelmingly, currently most cases of cavitary necrosis are associated with *S pneumoniae* infection [2–7]. Cavitary necrosis can be identified earlier on CT than chest radiography. It does not become visible on chest radiography until bronchial communication is established and air is introduced into the cavities [4,44]. Although as with other lung parenchymal complications cavitary necrosis is associated with an intense and prolonged illness, cavitary necrosis is not an absolute indication for surgery [4]. This is in contrast to what has been taught in many surgical references for adult disease. Although most patients with cavitary necrosis have an intense and prolonged illness and this information should be communicated to the patient, family, and caring physicians, most patients with cavitary necrosis can be managed successfully with conservative management. Remarkably, in such patients, long-term follow-up chest radiographs at greater than 40 days typically demonstrate normal or near normal-appearing lung parenchyma (see Figs. 9 and 10) [4].

Differentiation of cavitary necrosis from an underlying congenital lesion

One area in which the differential diagnosis can be problematic is when a child with a prolonged lower respiratory system illness has an area of lung consolidation with centralized cystic areas on the initial imaging study obtained. The issue is whether this patient has pneumonia complicated by superimposed cavitary necrosis or has an underlying infected developmental lesion that is presenting with persistent pneumonia. Unless previous imaging is available that demonstrates that the lung parenchyma in that region was previously normal or that pneumonia was present without an underlying cystic area, it may be impossible at that point in time to determine whether an underlying congenital lesion is present or whether the cyst represents cavitary necrosis (see Figs. 4 and 10). This determination may need to be made over time with follow-up imaging. If the surrounding lung consolidation and the cystic areas resolve, the most likely diagnosis is cavity necrosis complicating pneumonia. If the adjacent parenchymal consolidation resolves but a cystic lesion persists over the long term, an underlying congenital malformation, such as a congenital cystic adenomatoid malformation, must be entertained.

Purulent pericarditis

Another complication that can occur occasionally in patients with complicated pneumonia is the presence of purulent pericarditis. Before the advent of antibiotics, purulent pericarditis was the number one killer of children with pneumonia [5]. The presence of pericardial fluid in children who undergo CT for complications of pneumonia is not uncommon [3]. In children, the pericardium can fill with purulent fluid at a rapid rate such that the cardiac silhouette on chest radiography may not be enlarged when symptoms of pericardial tamponade have already developed [5]. Occasionally the symptoms and signs of cardiac tamponade may go unrecognized and a patient who is doing poorly may undergo CT evaluation to evaluate for other complications related to pneumonia. In these situations, the radiologist may be the first to recognize that an effusion is present that may be purulent pericarditis.

Summary

There are a number of clinical scenarios in which imaging is often involved in the diagnosis and management of children with pneumonia. Although there are certainly areas where there are controversies, imaging plays a very important role in many of these management decisions. Because of the high frequency of lower respiratory tract infections in children, it is important to understand the roles of imaging in these clinical scenarios.

References

[1] Donnelly LF, Klosterman LA. CT appearance of parapneumonic effusions in children: findings are not specific for empyema. AJR Am J Roentgenol 1997; 169:179–82.

[2] Donnelly LF, Klosterman LA. Pneumonia in children: decreased parenchymal contrast enhancement - CT sign of intense illness and impending cavitary necrosis. Radiology 1997;205:817–20.

[3] Donnelly LF, Klosterman LA. The yield of CT of children who have complicated pneumonia and non-contributory chest radiography. AJR Am J Roentgenol 1998;170:1627–31.

[4] Donnelly LF, Klosterman LA. Cavitary necrosis complicating pneumonia in children: sequential findings on chest radiography. AJR Am J Roentgenol 1998;171:253–6.

[5] Donnelly LF, Kimball TR, Barr LL. Purulent pericarditis presenting as acute abdomen in children: abdominal imaging findings. Clin Radiol 1999;54: 687–98.

[6] Donnelly LF. Maximizing the usefulness of imaging in children with community-acquired pneumonia. AJR Am J Roentgenol 1999;172:505–12.

[7] Donnelly LF. Practical issues concerning imaging of pulmonary infection in children. J Thorac Imaging 2001;16:238–50.

[8] Condon VR. Pneumonia in children. J Thorac Imaging 1991;6:31–44.

[9] Grossman LK, Caplan SE. Clinical, laboratory, and radiographic information in the diagnosis of pneumonia in children. Ann Emerg Med 1988;17:43–6.

[10] Leventhal JM. Clinical predictors of pneumonia as a guide to ordering chest roentgenograms. Clin Pediatr 1982;21:730–4.

[11] Griscom NT. Pneumonia in children and some of its variants. Radiology 1988;167:297–302.

[12] Peter G. The child with pneumonia: diagnostic and therapeutic considerations. Pediatr Infect Dis J 1988;7: 453–6.

[13] Alario AJ, McCarthy PL, Markowitz R, et al. Usefulness of chest radiographs in children with acute lower respiratory tract disease. J Pediatr 1987;111:187–93.

[14] Heulitt MJ, Ablow RC, Santos CC, et al. Febrile infants less than 3 months old: value of chest radiography. Radiology 1988;167:135–7.

[15] Patterson RJ, Bisset III GS, Kirks DR, et al. Chest radiographs in the evaluation of the febrile infant. AJR Am J Roentgenol 1990;155:833–5.

[16] Aherne W, Bird T, Court DS, et al. Pathological changes in virus infection of the lower respiratory tract in children. J Clin Pathol 1970;23:7–18.

[17] Becroft DMO. Histopathology of fatal adenovirus infection of the respiratory tract in young children. J Clin Pathol 1967;20:561–9.

[18] Wildin SR, Chonmaitree T, Swischuk KE. Roentgenographic features of common pediatric viral respiratory tract infections. Am J Dis Child 1988;142:43–6.

[19] Conte P, Heitzman ER, Markarian B. Viral pneumonia. Radiology 1995;95:267–72.

[20] Osborne D. Radiologic appearance of viral disease of the lower respiratory tract in infants and children. AJR Am J Roentgenol 1978;130:29–33.

[21] Burko H. Considerations in the roentgen diagnosis of pneumonia in children. AJR Am J Roentgenol 1962; 88:555–65.

[22] Kirkpatrick JA. Pneumonia in children as it differs from adult pneumonia. Semin Roentgenol 1980;15:96–103.

[23] Griscom NT, Wohl MB, Kirkpatrick JA. Lower respiratory infections: how infants differ from adults. Radiol Clin North Am 1978;16:367–87.

[24] Rose RE, Ward BH. Spherical pneumonias in children simulating pulmonary and mediastinal masses. Radiology 1973;106:179–82.

[25] Broughton RA. Infections due to *Mycoplasma pneumoniae* in childhood. Pediatr Infect Dis 1986;5:71–85.

[26] Denny FW, Clyde Jr WA. Acute lower respiratory tract infections in nonhospitalized children. J Pediatr 1986; 108:635–46.

[27] Glezen WP, Denny FW. Epidemiology of acute lower respiratory disease in children. N Engl J Med 1973; 288:498–505.

[28] Turner RB, Lande AE, Chase P, et al. Pneumonia in pediatric outpatients: cause and clinical manifestations. J Pediatr 1987;111:194–200.

[29] Swischuk LE, Hayden Jr CK. Viral vs. bacterial pulmonary infections in children (is roentgenographic differentiation possible?). Pediatr Radiol 1986;16: 278–84.

[30] Bettenay FAL, de Campo JF, McCrossin DB. Differentiating bacterial from viral pneumonias in children. Pediatr Radiol 1988;18:453–4.

[31] Lewis RA, Feigin RD. Current issues in the diagnosis and management of pediatric empyema. Semin Pediatr Infect Dis 2002;13:280–8.

[32] Bouros D, Schiza S, Panagou P, et al. Role of streptokinase in the treatment of acute loculated parapneumonic pleural effusions and empyema. Thorax 1994; 49:852–5.

[33] Rosen H, Nadkarni V, Theroux M, et al. Intrapleural streptokinase as adjunctive treatment for persistent empyema in pediatric patients. Chest 1993;103:1190–3.

[34] Moulton JS, Benkert RE, Weisiger KH, et al. Treatment of complicated pleural fluid collections with image-guided drainage and intracavitary urokinase. Chest 1995;108:1252–9.

[35] Kern JA, Rogers BM. Thoracoscopy in the management of empyema in children. J Pediatr Surg 1993;23: 1128–32.

[36] Silen ML, Weber TR. Thoraccoscopic debridement of loculated empyema thoracis in children. Ann Thorac Surg 1995;59:1166–8.

[37] Strovroff M, Teaque G, Heiss KF, et al. Thoracoscopy in the management of pediatric empyema. J Pediatr Surg 1995;30:1211–5.

[38] Light RW. Parapneumonic effusions and empyema. Clin Chest Med 1985;6:55–62.

[39] Light RW. A new classification of parapneumoic effusions and empyema. Chest 1995;108:229–301.

[40] Waite RJ, Carbonneau RJ, Balikian JP, et al. Parietal pleural changes in empyema: appearance at CT. Radiology 1990;175:145–50.

[41] Muller NL. Imaging of the pleura. Radiology 1993; 186:297–309.

[42] Ramnath RR, Heller RM, Ben-Ami T, et al. Implications of early sonographic evaluation of parapneumonic effusions in children with pneumonia. Pediatrics 1998;101:68–71.

[43] Kendrick T, Ling H, Subramaniam R, et al. The value of early CT in complicated childhood pneumonia. Pediatr Radiol 2002;32:16–21.

[44] Hodina M, Hanquinet S, Cotting J, et al. Imaging of cavitary necrosis in complicated childhood pneumonia. Eur Radiol 2002;12:391–6.

[45] Danner PK, McFarland DR, Felson B. Massive pulmonary gangrene. AJR Am J Roentgenol 1968;103: 548–54.

[46] Kissner DG, Lawrence WD, Keshishian M. Pneumococcal lung abscess. Am J Med 1988;84:793–4.

ELSEVIER
SAUNDERS

Radiol Clin N Am 43 (2005) 267–281

RADIOLOGIC
CLINICS
of North America

Imaging Evaluation of Pediatric Chest Trauma

Sjirk J. Westra, MD[a,b,]*, E. Christine Wallace, MD[c,d]

[a]Radiology, Harvard Medical School, Boston, MA, USA
[b]Department of Radiology, Massachusetts General Hospital, 34 Fruit Street, Boston, MA 02114, USA
[c]Division of Pediatric Radiology, UMassMemorial Medical Center, Worcester, MA, USA
[d]Radiology, University of Massachusetts, Worcester, MA, USA

Thoracic injury is a leading cause of death resulting from trauma in children, second only to head injury [1,2]. Blunt injury is approximately six times as common as penetrating injury [1]. Because the physical examination is limited in children with multitrauma, especially when there is loss of consciousness because of head injury, imaging plays an important role in diagnosis. The supine anteroposterior (AP) chest radiograph performed in the trauma room, limited as it may be by technical factors and artifact from overlying immobilization hardware, remains an important tool for the prompt diagnosis of life-threatening conditions such as a tension pneumothorax. With focused sonography the lower chest and pericardial space can be assessed rapidly for the presence of significant hemothorax or hemopericardium, which require urgent aspiration [3]. Once a severely injured child is stabilized hemodynamically, further imaging tests need to be undertaken to identify internal injury. During the past 2 decades, CT has emerged as the most reliable technique to evaluate chest injury in multitrauma patients, not only in adults [4–7], but increasingly in the pediatric population [8,9].

On their 16-detector scanners, the authors use a peak kilovolts (kVp) of 120 to 140 and milliampere-seconds (mAs) adjusted to patient weight and age [10]. More recently, they have implemented auto-matic longitudinal dose adjustment based on the measured attenuation on the scanogram and a preset noise level of 12. Using the shortest available tube rotation time (0.5 seconds) and a table speed of 15 mm/rotation, this protocol allows contiguous slice reconstructions of 5- and 2.5-mm thickness. The 2.5-mm slices are used for generating multiplanar reformatted images from the three-dimensional dataset. All studies preferably are done with CT angiography (ie, use of a power injector, rapid bolus injection, and scan acquisition initiated within 20 seconds after the start of the contrast injection). Chest trauma does not occur in isolation but is often associated with injury to other parts of the body. In fact, the presence of significant chest injury in a multitrauma patient is an indication of the overall severity of the child's injuries [2,11,12]. The demonstration of clinically silent concomitant chest injury in patients with known head, cervical spine, abdominal, and extremity injury substantially affects the prognosis, especially in children [12]. Diagnostic evaluation of injured children should take into account that significant trauma does not respect anatomic boundaries and may lead to multisystem involvement.

On the other hand, one should realize that most pediatric trauma is minor, and children have an amazing capacity to overcome even major injury without residual sequelae. The pediatric body is more flexible, lighter, and proportioned differently than the mature body, leading to unique patterns of injury. Because of their large relative head size, craniofacial injury is more common and can be more severe in young children than in adults, and because

* Corresponding author. Department of Radiology, Massachusetts General Hospital, 34 Fruit Street, Boston, MA 02114.

E-mail address: swestra@partners.org (S.J. Westra).

of ligamentous flexibility major cervical spinal cord injury can occur without radiographic abnormalities [3]. Conversely, extremity injuries from falls are frequently less severe in young children than in adults falling from a similar height, because of children's compact body size and lower weight. Seatbelt injuries and injuries to children ejected from a car restraining device or from airbag deployment often have features that are unique and explainable by maladjustment of these devices to the various pediatric body sizes and proportions. For all these reasons, imaging protocols that were developed in the adult population do not apply optimally to children of all age groups.

Following a discussion of the various imaging manifestations of pediatric chest trauma by anatomic location, the authors discuss their diagnostic approach to the pediatric multitrauma patient with an emphasis on chest imaging.

Chest wall

Rib fractures are less common in children than in adults because of the compliance of the anterior chest wall in children [13]. For this reason, the incidence of an unstable flail chest resulting from multiple adjacent rib fractures, as may be encountered in adult chest trauma patients, is comparatively low in children [12]. In children, the presence of multiple rib fractures signifies a higher-energy impact than in adults [12], because more force is required to break

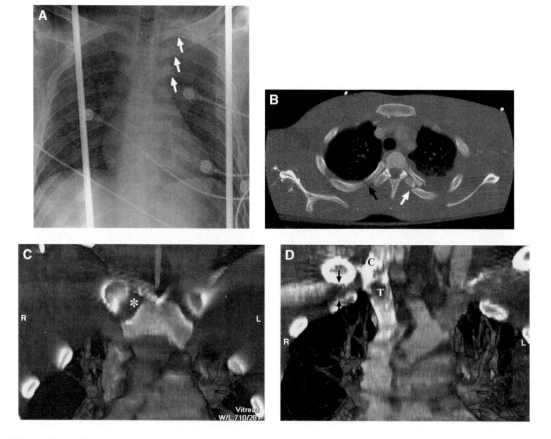

Fig. 1. Chest wall injury in 18-year-old man who has pelvic fractures resulting from a high-impact motor vehicle collision. (A) On frontal chest radiograph, there are displaced fractures of the left second, third, and fourth ribs (arrows). (B) CT shows a left-sided displaced rib fracture (white arrow) and a right-sided nondisplaced rib fracture (black arrow) that was not recognized on the chest radiograph. Note venous collaterals around right scapula caused by venous thrombosis. (C) Volume-rendered coronal image of CT scan demonstrates widening of the right sternoclavicular joint (*), indicative of joint dislocation. (D) Note costoclavicular compression (arrows) of subclavian vein, leading to thrombotic (T) occlusion and collateral flow (C) to the right neck.

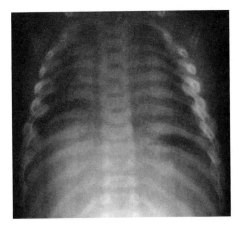

Fig. 2. Child abuse: multiple bilateral nonacute posterior and anterior rib fractures.

the flexible pediatric ribs than to break the more rigid and sometimes osteoporotic ribs of adults. Because of the flexibility of the pediatric chest, significant lung injury (contusions, lacerations) may occur in the absence of any rib fractures. As expected, there is a high association between the occurrence of rib fractures and pneumothorax and hemothorax. Fractures of the upper three ribs signify high-energy impact and are often associated with fractures in the shoulder girdle and vascular injury (Fig. 1) [11].

Acute nondisplaced rib fractures are notoriously difficult to identify on AP chest radiographs and are more reliably imaged with CT (Fig. 1). Detection of isolated rib fractures has little clinical significance (with the exception of child abuse), however, because these fractures do not have specific treatment implications [4,11].

Multiple aligned posterior rib fractures have a well-known association with nonaccidental injury [14] and presumably result from the leveraging motion of the posterior ribs on the transverse processes during AP chest compression (Fig. 2). Acute nondisplaced rib fractures are best detected with skeletal scintigraphy. Because of the delay in clinical presentation that is typical in child abuse, healing fractures with callus are more prevalent than acute nondisplaced fractures, and these are well seen on skeletal surveys, especially when supplemented by oblique views. For these reasons, radiographic skeletal survey in combination with skeletal scintigraphy continues to be the standard of care for the evaluation of suspected child abuse, and CT is generally not indicated in this setting. Recently, a screening fast T2-weighted or inversion-recovery total-body MR imaging examination, performed in conjunction with cranial MR imaging to detect subdural hematomas, has been described [15]. Although considered a sensitive test for acute rib fractures, the

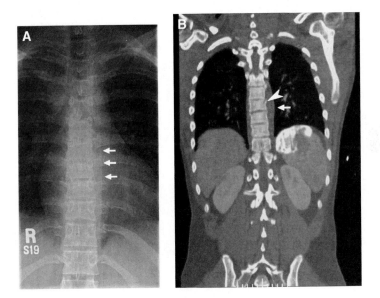

Fig. 3. Subtle thoracic spine fracture in a 15-year-old boy following a bicycle accident with hyperflexion injury. (A) Note widening of the left paraspinal line (arrows) on frontal chest radiograph. No displaced fracture is recognized on this image, but a lateral view (not shown) demonstrated mild loss of height of a mid-thoracic vertebral body. (B) Coronal reformatted image of multidetector row CT confirms left paraspinal hematoma (arrow) and demonstrates subtle fracture in mid-thoracic body (arrowhead). This fracture did not involve the spinal canal and was considered stable.

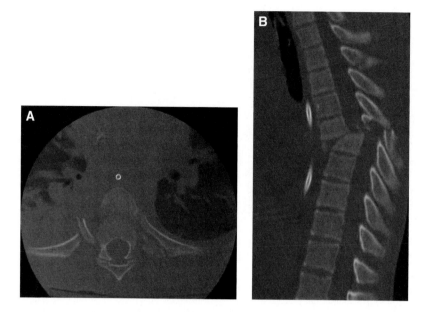

Fig. 4. Severe fracture-dislocation in midthoracic spine in a 17-year-old boy who has sustained major injury in a motorbike accident resulting in paraplegia. (A) Axial and (B) sagittal images of multidetector-row CT show unstable fracture with focal kyphosis and severe impingement of the spinal canal by bone fragments.

clinical utility of fast MR imaging in the setting of suspected child abuse has yet to be established.

An important sign for subtle thoracic spine fractures is widening of paraspinal lines, indicative of a hematoma (Fig. 3). Because of the relative stabilization of the thoracic vertebral column by the rib cage, displaced fractures and dislocations in the thoracic spine are indicative of a high-energy impact (Fig. 4). Most thoracic spine fractures are unstable, and there is a high association with neurologic deficit

because of the relatively large size of the thoracic cord with respect to the spinal canal [7]. Upper thoracic spinal injuries are often poorly demonstrated on AP chest radiographs [16], and CT is the imaging modality of choice both for initial diagnosis and for assessment of complications of surgical immobilization for vertebral trauma.

Fracture of the clavicle can be seen as an isolated injury or can be associated with other injuries involving the shoulder girdle (Fig. 5). Sternal and

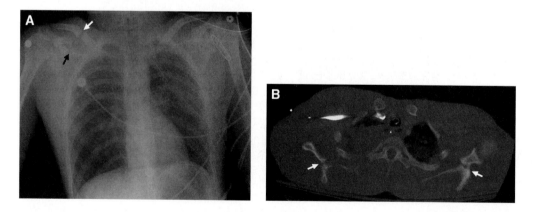

Fig. 5. Right clavicular and bilateral scapular fractures in a 7-year-old boy following a motor vehicle collision. (A) Frontal chest radiograph clearly shows right clavicular fracture (white arrow). (B) Axial CT image demonstrates bilateral minimally displaced fractures in the scapulae (arrows); only the right fracture could be identified—in retrospect—on the frontal chest radiograph (A, black arrow).

scapular fractures (Fig. 5) are more often seen in high-impact motor vehicle accidents involving a shoulder seatbelt [17], and these injuries are associated with a high incidence of vascular and cardiac injury [4,9,11]. In particular, posterior sternoclavicular dislocations often lead to severe injury of the upper thoracic vessels and the trachea [4,9].

Pleura

Pneumothorax can result from penetrating injury to the chest wall, from air leak into the pleural space from an injured lung (laceration), or in association with central air leak from the tracheobronchial tree (pneumomediastinum). High-pressure ventilation in the setting of the adult respiratory distress syndrome (ARDS) can lead to iatrogenic pneumothorax. The presence of a tension pneumothorax, as evidenced by mass effect, constitutes an emergency that requires rapid communication with the treatment team [4,7]. Tension pneumothoraces can be small and may not exhibit any mass effect, especially when occurring bilaterally in a patient receiving positive-pressure ventilation [5,7,11].

Diagnosis of pneumothorax is straightforward on upright chest radiographs, with demonstration of the visceral pleural line outlined by free pleural air in the apex of the chest. Expiration films may enhance the visibility of pneumothoraces. In the multitrauma patient, who is typically in the supine position, pneumothorax is more difficult to diagnose and often can be diagnosed only by indirect signs [9].

Anteromedial pleural air collections are visible on chest radiographs as hyperlucency of the affected hemithorax (Fig. 6), an unduly sharp heart border or the deep-sulcus and double-diaphragm signs [4,7,9] (Fig. 7). Decubitus positioning, as would be optimal to visualize the visceral pleural line, is often not possible because of the need for patient immobilization. The cross-table lateral view is less sensitive to demonstrate small, anteriorly located pleural air collections and often cannot determine laterality. CT is more sensitive than chest radiography for small pneumothoraces [2,8,18], but the clinical significance of small pneumothoraces in patients who are not receiving positive-pressure ventilation support is controversial [12,19].

Hemothorax is a result of venous or arterial bleeding into the pleural cavity. The differential diagnosis includes infusothorax from a misplaced central venous line, reactive effusion secondary to pulmonary parenchymal injury, and traumatic chylothorax. On supine chest radiography, pleural effusions manifest as a veil-like increased density over the involved hemithorax with preserved visibility of pulmonary vascular markings and, in the case of larger amounts of fluid, thickening of the lateral pleural line [4,9]. CT is more sensitive than radiography for demonstrating small effusions (Fig. 7), and Hounsfield density measurements may help confirm their hemorrhagic nature [4,5]. CT is also superior for accurate assessment of chest tube placement and related complications, such as intraparenchymal course and associated pulmonary contusion [5,7]. Active contrast extravasation into the pleural space

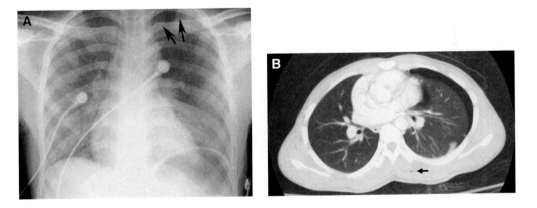

Fig. 6. Pneumothorax secondary to penetrating injury in an 18-year-old man who was stabbed in the left posterior chest. (A) Frontal chest radiograph. Note hyperlucency of upper left hemithorax and sharp outline of left upper mediastinum, consistent with an anteromedial pneumothorax. A small pneumothorax is evident at the apex (arrows). (B) CT confirms left pneumothorax, which required thoracostomy tube placement. Note air in left back musculature (arrow) caused by the stab wound.

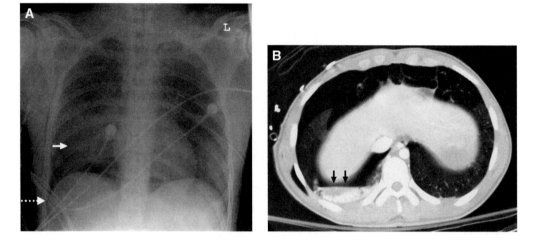

Fig. 7. Hemopneumothorax in a blunt chest injury in an 18-year-old man who has multiorgan trauma (renal contusion, splenic laceration, multiple extremity and mandibular fractures). Bilateral chest tubes were placed in the emergency room as part of resuscitation. (*A*) Frontal chest radiograph demonstrates deep sulcus sign (*dotted arrow*). The free edge of the contused right lung is outlined by pleural air (*white arrow*). (*B*) CT image confirms bilateral pneumothoraces. Air in the right chest wall is related to chest tube placement. Air–fluid level in the right pleural space (*arrows*) indicates the intrapleural hemorrhagic component of the hemopneumothorax.

may occasionally be seen in the case of arterial or major (pulmonary) venous injury [20].

Pulmonary parenchyma

Primary traumatic pulmonary parenchymal lesions include contusion and laceration [4,5,7,21]. Aspiration, fat embolism, intubation-related atelectasis, and superimposed (hospital-acquired) pneumonia

may secondarily affect chest trauma patients and often lead to ARDS.

Pulmonary contusions are commonly found in blunt chest trauma [12] and are caused by the direct impact of adjacent bony structures such as ribs and spine on the lung parenchyma at the time of the injury, leading to focal edema and hemorrhage (Fig. 8). They can be visible on chest radiographs with some delay of up to 6 hours but are more reliably demonstrated on CT as peripherally located

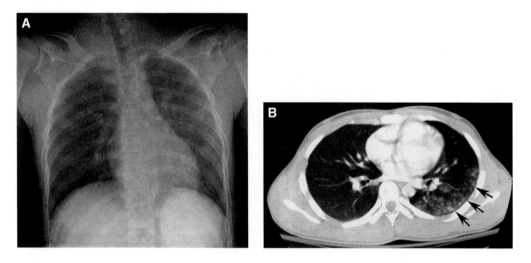

Fig. 8. Pulmonary contusion in a 16-year-old boy who has blunt chest injury following a motor vehicle collision. (*A*) Frontal chest radiograph shows ill-defined alveolar opacities in the left lung. (*B*) CT demonstrates the typical peripheral posterior location of pulmonary contusion with a zone of subpleural lucency (*arrows*).

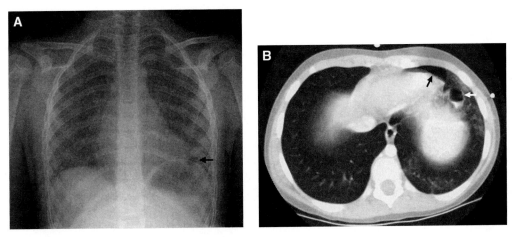

Fig. 9. Pulmonary laceration in an 8-year-old boy who has blunt left upper-abdomen trauma. (*A*) Frontal chest radiograph shows a round lucency in left paracardiac region (*arrow*) and an indistinct left heart border. (*B*) CT confirms lung laceration (*white arrow*) surrounded by areas of contusion. There was also a small anteromedial pneumothorax (*black arrow*) that was not recognized on the chest radiograph but did not require thoracostomy tube placement.

areas of air-space consolidation without air bronchograms. When large, they may cross segmental anatomic boundaries and the interlobar fissures, and they typically exhibit a thin zone of surrounding subpleural lucency. This lucent zone is thought to represent relatively hypovascular lung tissue that was compressed at the moment of the injury and therefore is relatively spared of bleeding [13,22]. Contusions affecting more than one third of the alveolar air space are associated with an increased requirement for mechanical ventilation [23,24], but most resolve without scarring within 7 days. Atelectasis and aspiration pneumonia are differentiated from contusion by their segmental distribution, configuration, and location in the dependent portions of the lung.

Lacerations result from penetrating injuries, such as adjacent displaced rib fractures, or shearing blunt forces to the lung (Fig. 9). Initially, they may be indistinguishable from the surrounding contusion. Because of the disruption of lung tissue, one or more air cavities develop over time and may contain a central density or fluid level because of intrapulmonary hematoma. In the case of large lacerations involving the pleural surface, a bronchopleural fistula may develop. Pulmonary lacerations tend to heal more slowly than contusions, and, especially in chil-

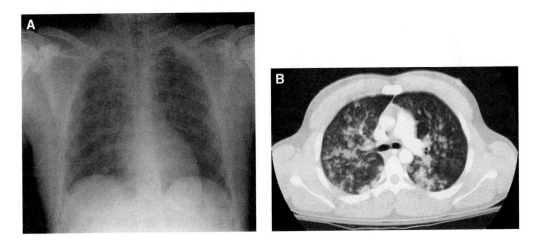

Fig. 10. Probable fat embolism in a 16-year-old boy who has open comminuted tibial fracture. (*A*) Frontal chest radiograph shows bilateral nodular pulmonary opacities. (*B*) CT image demonstrates the widespread perivascular distribution of these opacities, which is more consistent with fat embolism than with contusion or aspiration.

dren, they may leave behind a persistent cavity called a posttraumatic pulmonary pseudocyst.

Fat embolism (Fig. 10) has been described as a cause of geographic ground-glass or diffuse nodular opacity in trauma patients who have sustained major fractures and additionally exhibit petechial skin hemorrhages and neurologic dysfunction [25].

Tracheobronchial tree

Rupture of the major airways is a life-threatening emergency that can be recognized on chest radio-graphs by severe and persistent pneumomediastinum and pneumothoraces in the presence of well-functioning chest tubes [4,5,7,21]. The injury may result from direct involvement by penetrating chest trauma or from a sudden increase in intrathoracic pressure against a closed glottis in blunt chest trauma. The defect typically occurs within 2 cm of the carina, most commonly in the proximal right mainstem bronchus. Particularly in children, a delayed clinical presentation may be encountered [26]. Multidetector-row CT with multiplanar reformatted images and virtual bronchoscopy is an excellent technique to demonstrate the defect and the resulting air leakage

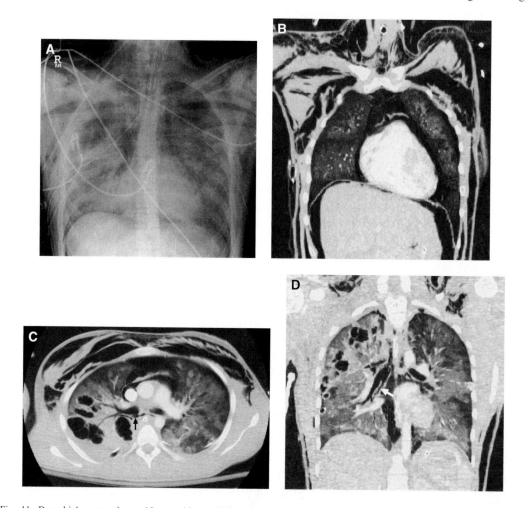

Fig. 11. Bronchial rupture in an 18-year-old man following blunt face and upper-chest trauma. Emergency tracheostomy and bilateral chest tube placement were required for initial stabilization. (A) Frontal chest radiograph shows pneumomediastinum and extensive subcutaneous emphysema. (B) Corresponding coronal reformation of chest CT, obtained because of persistent air leak despite well-functioning chest tubes, demonstrates pneumoperitoneum, pneumomediastinum, subcutaneous air, and left pneumothorax. (C) Axial CT image shows laceration in posterior aspect of right mainstem bronchus (arrow). Note also extensive laceration and surrounding contusion in the right lung. (D) Coronal reconstruction shows interstitial air dissecting medially to the bronchus intermedius (arrow). Bronchial rupture was repaired surgically.

(Fig. 11) [4,5,7,27]. Fiberoptic bronchoscopy is required for confirmation while permitting attempts at endoluminal treatment, such as occlusion of the defect or selective bronchial intubation, which are temporizing measures before final surgical repair.

Mediastinum, heart, and great vessels

Pneumomediastinum is recognized by streaky air collections outlining mediastinal structures such as the thymus (spinnaker-sail or angel-wing signs) or the superior surface of the diaphragm (continuous-diaphragm sign). It can be differentiated from an anteromedial pneumothorax by the bilaterality of its findings and its lack of movement with decubitus positioning. Pneumomediastinum can have benign causes and be self-limiting, or it can be a sign of serious trauma, such as penetrating injury and tracheobronchial and esophageal rupture [7,11]. Rarely, it results from air entering the mediastinum from another anatomic space, such as in penetrating neck or chest wall injury. No matter the cause, pneumomediastinum generally does not require specific treatment, because it decompresses into the soft tissues of the neck and chest wall (Figs. 11 and 12) and occasionally into the peritoneal cavity through existing channels in the diaphragm.

Benign and self-limiting pneumomediastinum can occur with acute increase in alveolar pressure caused by blunt abdominal trauma together with air outflow obstruction (closed glottis at the time of injury), leading to alveolar rupture, with air dissecting into the peribronchial interstitial tissues toward the mediastinum. Such pneumomediastinum is analogous to benign forms of pneumomediastinum occurring in asthmatic patients with severe air trapping or after straining against a closed glottis (eg, when lifting a heavy object). These benign forms of mediastinum generally do not require any follow-up with cross-sectional imaging [28]. A pneumomediastinum that ruptures through the parietal pleura to cause a pneumothorax, however, generally indicates a high-pressure air-leak that warrants further investigation with CT to determine its underlying cause (Fig. 11), especially in patients requiring positive-pressure ventilation and chest tube placement.

Perforation of the esophagus may be caused by penetrating injury from within (a swallowed sharp object) or outside (gunshot wounds with bullet trajectory traversing the posterior mediastinum, as judged from the CT scan) [5]. Unexplained pneumomediastinum and pleural effusions are the most important radiologic signs. If the injury is suspected, an esophagram should be performed, initially with water-soluble contrast material, followed by barium [5,7].

Detection of a mediastinal hematoma (Fig. 13) is extremely important, because it may be a clue to an occult traumatic aortic injury (TAI), which is often clinically silent [6,11,29]. Despite its limitations, a well-penetrated AP chest radiograph obtained in the trauma room is used as the first screening for this condition, which remains quite rare in children but is important because of its potential lethality. Mediastinal measurement criteria published in the adult

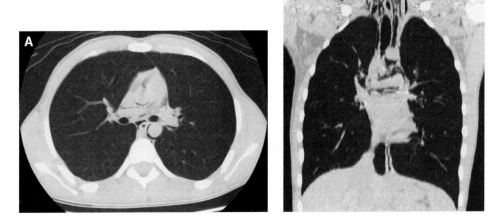

Fig. 12. Benign pneumomediastinum in a 16-year-old boy who has chest pain after blunt injury. (*A*) Axial and (*B*) coronal CT images show small pneumomediastinum. Esophagram (not shown) did not demonstrate any perforation. This pneumomediastinum resolved spontaneously.

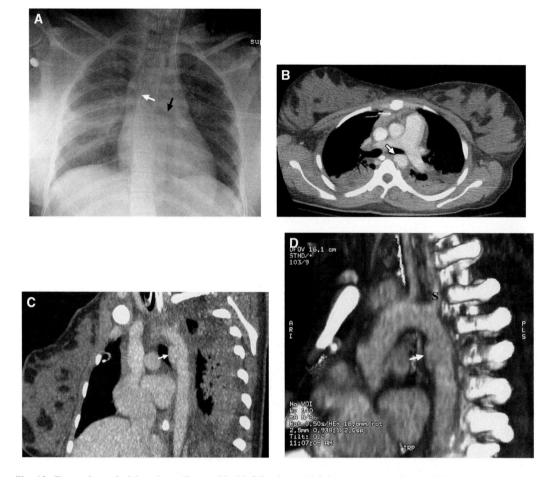

Fig. 13. Traumatic aortic injury in a 17-year-old girl following a high-impact motor vehicle collision. (*A*) Frontal chest radiograph shows a widened mediastinum, obliteration of normal mediastinal contours, rightward displacement of the nasogastric tube (*white arrow*), and downward displacement of the left mainstem bronchus (*black arrow*). (*B*) Axial image and (*C*) oblique-sagittal reconstruction from CT angiogram depict traumatic pseudoaneurysm in proximal descending aorta (*arrows*). (*D*) Volume rendition better shows the relation of the pseudoaneurysm with the left subclavian artery (S), information that was important for the vascular surgeon before successful placement of an endoluminal stent.

literature [12] (mediastinal width greater than 8 cm, mediastinum-to-chest ratio greater than 0.25) have been proven to lack a sufficient predictive value for TAI [4,5,7,11] and do not necessarily apply to children. Of greater value is the combination of a compelling clinical history and the more subtle signs of an abnormal mediastinum (regardless of its size), such as obliterated contour of aortic arch, blurring of the aortopulmonary window, deviation of trachea and nasogastric tube to the right, downward depression of the left mainstem bronchus, widening of the paravertebral and paratracheal stripes, and a left apical pleural cap [11]. Whereas a normal chest radiograph has a high predictive value to rule out TAI, none of the signs is sufficiently specific for diagnosis [9].

Even when a mediastinal hematoma is identified on plain radiography or CT, TAI will be diagnosed in only 10% to 20% of cases; in the remainder, the hematoma is caused by self-limiting bleeding from smaller vessels for which no specific intervention is required. Traditionally, aortography has been used to diagnose TAI, especially in hemodynamically unstable patients. Multidetector-row CT angiography and transesophageal echocardiography have emerged in recent years as tests that are helpful to rule out or demonstrate TAI in patients with an abnormal mediastinum on chest radiography [9,11,12,47].

The most common finding in TAI is a pseudoaneurysm, typically located at the level of the left mainstem bronchus, involving the anterior aspect of the proximal descending aorta, immediately distally to the aortic isthmus. This pseudoaneurysm is not to be confused with the ductus diverticulum ("ductus bump"), a remnant of the ductus arteriosus that can normally be found in this location [9]. The mechanism of TAI is believed to be the ligamentum arteriosum tethering the aorta at the moment of injury, with the resulting shearing forces leading to a tear in the intima and media [4]. The adventitia is the only layer holding the aorta together, accounting for the instability of this pseudoaneurysm and a high mortality (80%–85%). Most affected patients do not reach the hospital alive, and in-hospital mortality 31% to 44% is within the first hours of admission [12]. Because of this early mortality of typical TAI, atypical locations may be encountered more com-

monly in those who survive long enough to be evaluated with CT [9]. Additional signs for atypical TAI (eg, periaortic hematoma, intimal flaps, wall irregularities, abrupt caliber changes, occlusion of major branch vessels, luminal clots, and active contrast extravasation) should be sought [5,7].

Cardiac injury can occur from blunt and penetrating injury [4,30,31], with penetrating trauma more common. A traumatic hemopericardium or pneumopericardium can cause cardiac tamponade requiring urgent decompression. Injuries to the myocardium and valve apparatus are usually investigated with echocardiography [4,30]. Children with penetrating cardiac injury or hemodynamic instability generally require immediate surgical exploration. Those with blunt cardiac injury (contusion) are typically fol-

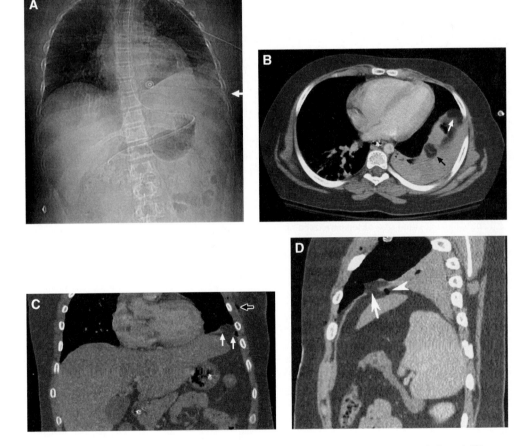

Fig. 14. Diaphragmatic injury in a 14-year-old boy following a stab wound to the left flank. (*A*) Frontal CT scanogram shows abnormal contour of the left hemidiaphragm and air in the soft tissues of the lower chest wall (*arrow*). (*B*) Axial CT image and (*C*) coronal and (*D*) sagittal reconstructions of left hemidiaphragm show herniated mesenteric fat through two separate diaphragmatic defects (*B, white and black arrows; and C and D, white arrows*) that were surgically confirmed. Note also air in the chest wall (*C, black arrow*) and under left hemidiaphragm (*white arrowhead, D*).

lowed up by EKG and echocardiography for development of arrhythmias and cardiac dysfunction. It is important to realize that development of signs of pulmonary edema on follow-up chest radiographs is caused more commonly by fluid overload from aggressive trauma resuscitation than by traumatic myocardial or valvular dysfunction.

Diaphragm

Traumatic rupture of the diaphragm occurs more commonly on the left than on the right because of the protective effect of the liver. It is more frequently associated with penetrating injury to the upper abdomen and lower chest than with blunt chest trauma [32]. Diaphragmatic rupture may also result from serious blunt abdominal injury in children [33]. Because the nonsurgical management of even severe solid abdominal injury has increased in recent years, and there is more reliance on imaging diagnosis, it has become even more imperative not to overlook this important lesion on CT [32]. Initially, diaphragmatic ruptures and hernias are often unrecognized on chest radiography because of associated contusion or atelectasis in the lung bases. Herniation of abdominal viscera may not occur until the patient is no longer receiving positive-pressure ventilation. This herniation may have an acute clinical presentation because of strangulation, but most often it is clinically silent [4,5,7,21,33]. Herniation of aerated abdominal viscera, most frequently the stomach, into the hemithorax is a diagnostic finding that is often associated with contralateral shift of the heart and mediastinum. An anomalous position of a nasogastric tube tip above the left hemidiaphragm indicates herniation of the stomach, which may be confirmed with administration of water-soluble contrast [4]. Diagnosis of diaphragmatic rupture without visceral herniation remains difficult, even with thin-section CT, because of the complex shape of the thin diaphragmatic muscle, the horizontal in-plane orientation of the diaphragmatic dome, and the oft-associated traumatic abnormalities in the lung bases. A number of diagnostic criteria have been proposed using thin-slice CT with multiplanar reformations. Discontinuity of a hemidiaphragm may allow herniation of intra-abdominal mesenteric fat, parenchymal organs, or viscera (Fig. 14). The hourglass (or collar) sign indicates the constriction of partially herniated viscera by the edges of a small diaphragmatic defect. The rim sign indicates a contour deformity of the partially herniated liver, with liver tissue compressed by the margins of the diaphragmatic defect. The dependent-

viscera sign describes the close contact of the herniated stomach or liver with the posterior chest wall, with no diaphragmatic leaflet holding it up against gravity and a lack of normal interposition of aerated posterior lung tissue [4,5,7,32].

Diagnostic algorithms

The arrival of an injured child in the trauma room is an upsetting event for all involved. It is only natural that caregivers are inclined to use the most sensitive and fastest technology available to diagnose all injuries within the shortest possible time frame, and multidetector-row CT seems to fulfill those criteria. As discussed previously, CT has been shown to be more sensitive for the demonstration of rib fractures, pneumothorax, hemothorax, pulmonary contusion and laceration, and diaphragmatic rupture than plain radiography of the chest [34]. Multidetector-row CT is extremely rapid, allowing a complete contiguous scan of head, neck, chest, abdomen, and pelvis to be performed in less than 1 minute, without the need for repositioning the critically injured patient. There is generally no need for repeat imaging, because this modality is not prone to the technical limitations (eg, difficult positioning, views affected by overlying material or stabilization apparatus, and poor exposure parameters) that can affect conventional radiography. In the adult trauma literature, several authors have advocated the liberal use of such a total-body trauma CT protocol [35,36], stating that it is cost effective in all unconscious patients [36].

Although these arguments can be used to justify the routine use of CT in pediatric trauma patients as well, recent reports in the surgical literature have pointed out that findings of chest CT performed for minor trauma rarely influence clinical management [11,12,37]. Clinically and radiographically unexpected findings in the lower thorax, as demonstrated on the upper slices of an abdominal CT scan obtained for blunt abdominal trauma [2,19], rarely require specific intervention such as chest tube placement [19]. The exception is a radiographically occult pneumothorax, which may enlarge following the institution of positive-pressure ventilation [18]. For this reason, the performance of a chest CT is probably warranted only in children whose chest injury is severe enough to require mechanical ventilation.

There are three arguments against the routine use of total-body CT in pediatric trauma imaging. First, there is the important issue of radiation dose in the pediatric age group [38]. In most hospitals in the United States, trauma is a frequent reason for referral for CT imaging. This increased use of imaging, which has only occurred in the past decade, adds substantially to the medical radiation burden and consequently to the cancer induction risk estimates for the entire exposed population [39]. This consideration is especially important in children, who are more radiosensitive and have a longer potential lifespan in which to express radiation-induced tumors [40]. Cognitive impairment from low-dose radiation exposure in infancy has also recently been suggested [41]. Proponents of the use of routine continuous total-body CT have pointed out that some radiation dose can be saved by eliminating overlapping segments from separate acquisitions [42] and by substituting multiplanar reformatted CT images for conventional radiographs of the cervical, thoracic, and lumbar spine [43,44]. When large segments of these scans are not clinically indicated in the first place, however, such modest savings in radiation dose are more than offset by the fact that CT doses are an order of magnitude higher than corresponding conventional examinations [45]. Because the radiation dose of one chest CT can equal that of approximately 250 chest radiographs, CT becomes dose effective only if the information from a particular CT study is expected, a priori, to have a value that is substantially higher that of the corresponding chest radiograph. For example, in the correct clinical setting (high-velocity deceleration trauma mechanism, presence of multiple other significant injuries), a CT angiogram may be required to rule out a traumatic aortic injury in a patient with a borderline abnormal mediastinum on the chest radiograph, because of the potential catastrophic consequence of not diagnosing TAI in a timely manner. Such reasoning can be used to develop appropriateness criteria for the application of CT in other clinical settings as well.

Second, there are considerations of cost effectiveness in the use of expensive imaging resources [46,47], and there is a critical need for developing clinical appropriateness criteria for the application of CT in pediatric trauma patients [47,48]. There is concern that the current medico-legal climate favors defensive medical practices that may lead to overuse of CT, because it is perceived as being the most accurate test for trauma imaging. The fact that many of the injuries demonstrated do not impact patient management or treatment further underscores the need to perform these outcome and cost-effectiveness studies [12,37,49,50].

Third, there is the risk of the possible demonstration of pseudodisease and clinically unimportant findings by overinterpretation of CT findings. Clinicians may perform costly and sometimes invasive additional imaging tests and treatments that can lead to iatrogenic complications and unnecessary expense [51]. Before CT was available, this pseudodisease would have simply remained unnoticed, without adverse effect on patient outcome.

Given these controversies, the authors believe that the initial imaging evaluation of pediatric trauma should consist of the conventional trauma series (lateral in-collar radiograph of the cervical spine, AP radiograph of the pelvis and chest), in conjunction with a careful and rapid triage by an experienced clinician and taking the mechanism and force of injury into account [45]. This approach will determine the need for additional imaging with cross-sectional techniques, such as ultrasound and spiral or multidetector-row CT.

Arguably, all patients with penetrating injury should eventually undergo a CT focused on the area of impact, because the risk of occult internal injury is high in these patients. Unconscious patients and those with suspicion for unstable fractures on the lateral spine radiograph will generally undergo CT of the head and cervical spine, but the decision as to whether to carry the scan down through the rest of the body should be a clinical one. This decision should be influenced by the severity of pelvic and major extremity fractures, as demonstrated on the initial radiographic trauma series, and respiratory failure, hemodynamic instability, and neurologic deficit on clinical examination. Because the simultaneous occurrence of several of these injuries constitutes major multitrauma and suggests a high-energy impact, the performance of a total-body multidetector-row CT may be considered. If a spinal fracture is clinically suspected or demonstrated on the initial radiographic survey, a CT of the relevant area should be performed. The CT should include coronal and sagittal reformatted images.

The specific indications for chest CT in blunt trauma should be guided by the findings of the initial clinical examination and chest radiograph. A spinal fracture or fractures of the upper ribs, shoulder girdle, and sternum will often necessitate a contrast-enhanced CT to look for vascular injury. The indication for the placement of chest tubes is most often clinical or is visible on chest radiographs, but if there is persistent hemorrhagic output from these tubes or progressive pneumomediastinum, a CT is indicated to look for bronchial or vascular injury. Although traumatic aortic injury in children remains rare despite the increased incidence of motor vehicle accidents, a high index of suspicion should be maintained for this condition. In the presence of an abnormal mediastinum on plain radiographs, a CT angiographic study to evaluate for TAI should be performed expeditiously in the hemodynamically stable child. When there are signs of hemodynamic instability, an aortogram should be performed, if possible.

In conclusion, traumatic injury to the chest in children can range from minor to life-threatening. Chest radiography remains the most important imaging modality, supplemented by ultrasound or CT in selected circumstances. The challenge in pediatric trauma imaging is to implement a problem-oriented approach to imaging that addresses the specific mechanism of injury and clinical presentation and that is sufficiently comprehensive to guide treatment decisions, using the least possible radiation dose, time, and expense. This approach requires radiologists to remain actively involved in trauma care, to engage their clinical colleagues in an open dialogue at all times, and to participate in the performance of outcomes studies.

References

[1] Cooper A, Barlow B, DiScala C, et al. Mortality and truncal injury: the pediatric perspective. J Pediatr Surg 1994;29(1):33–8.

[2] Sivit CJ, Taylor GA, Eichelberger MR. Chest injury in children with blunt abdominal trauma: evaluation with CT. Radiology 1989;171(3):815–8.

[3] Vane DW. Imaging of the injured child: important questions answered quickly and correctly. Surg Clin North Am 2002;82:315–23.

[4] Mirvis SE. Diagnostic imaging of acute thoracic injury. Semin Ultrasound CT MR 2004;25(2):156–79.

[5] Rivas LA, Fishman JE, Munera F, et al. Multislice CT in thoracic trauma. Radiol Clin North Am 2003; 41:599–616.

[6] Tello R, Munden RF, Hooton S, et al. Value of spiral CT in hemodynamically stable patients following blunt chest trauma. Comput Med Imaging Graph 1998;22:447–52.

[7] Lomoschitz FM, Eisenhuber E, Linnau KF, et al. Imaging of chest trauma: radiological patterns of injury and diagnostic algorithms. Eur J Radiol 2003; 48:61–70.

[8] Manson D, Babyn PS, Palder S, et al. CT of blunt chest trauma in children. Pediatr Radiol 1993;23(1): 1–5.

[9] Hall A, Johnson K. The imaging of paediatric thoracic trauma. Paediatr Respir Rev 2002;3:241–7.

[10] Donnelly LF, Frush DP. Pediatric multidetector body CT. Radiol Clin North Am 2003;41:637–55.

[11] Chan O, Hiorns M. Chest trauma. Eur J Radiol 1996; 23:23–34.

[12] Furnival RA. Controversies in pediatric thoracic and abdominal trauma. Clin Ped Emerg Med 2001;2:48–62.

[13] Donnelly LF, Frush DP. Abnormalities of the chest wall in pediatric patients. AJR Am J Roentgenol 1999; 173(6):1595–601.

[14] Kleinman PK, Schlesinger AE. Mechanical factors associated with posterior rib fractures: laboratory and case studies. Pediatr Radiol 1997;27(1):87–91.

[15] Kjellin IB, Houriani F, McLeary MS, et al. MR imaging of bony thoracic trauma in child abuse: comparison to radiography. Radiology 2000;217(P):340.

[16] van Beek EJ, Been HD, Ponsen KK, et al. Upper thoracic spinal fractures in trauma patients—a diagnostic pitfall. Injury 2000;31:219–23.

[17] Rozycki GS, Tremblay L, Feliciano DV, et al. A prospective study for the detection of vascular injury in adult and pediatric patients with cervicothoracic seat belt signs. J Trauma 2002;52:618–23.

[18] Bridges KG, Welch G, Silver M, et al. CT detection of occult pneumothorax in multiple trauma patients. J Emerg Med 1993;11:179–86.

[19] Holmes JF, Brant WE, Bogren HG, et al. Prevalence and importance of pneumothoraces visualized on abdominal computed tomographic scan in children with blunt trauma. J Trauma 2001;50(3):516–20.

[20] Taylor GA, Kaufman RA, Sivit CJ. Active hemorrhage in children after thoracoabdominal trauma: clinical and CT features. AJR Am J Roentgenol 1994;162(2): 401–4.

[21] Kang EY, Muller NL. CT in blunt chest trauma: pulmonary, tracheobronchial, and diaphragmatic injuries. Semin Ultrasound CT MR 1996;17(2):114–8.

[22] Donnelly LF, Klosterman LA. Subpleural sparing: a CT finding of lung contusion in children. Radiology 1997;204(2):385–7.

[23] Allen GS, Cox Jr CS. Pulmonary contusion in children: diagnosis and management. South Med J 1998; 91(12):1099–106.

[24] Wagner RB, Crawford Jr WO, Schimpf PP, et al. Quantitation and pattern of parenchymal lung injury in blunt chest trauma. Diagnostic and therapeutic implications. J Comput Tomogr 1988;12:270–81.

[25] Malagari K, Economopoulos N, Stoupis C, et al. High-resolution CT findings in mild pulmonary fat embolism. Chest 2003;123:1196–201.

[26] Ozdulger A, Cetin G, Erkmen Gulhan S, et al. A review of 24 patients with bronchial ruptures: is delay in diagnosis more common in children? Eur J Cardiothorac Surg 2003;23:379–83.

[27] Wan YL, Tsai KT, Yeow KM, et al. CT findings of bronchial transection. Am J Emerg Med 1997;15: 176–7.

[28] Chapdelaine J, Beaunoyer M, Daigneault P, et al. Spontaneous pneumomediastinum: are we overinvestigating? J Pediatr Surg 2004;39(5):681–4.

[29] Spouge AR, Burrows PE, Armstrong D, et al. Traumatic aortic rupture in the pediatric population. Role of plain film, CT and angiography in the diagnosis. Pediatr Radiol 1991;21:324–8.

[30] Bertrand S, Laquay N, El Rassi I, et al. Tricuspid insufficiency after blunt chest trauma in a nine-year-old child. Eur J Cardiothorac Surg 1999;16:587–9.

[31] DeCou JM, Abrams RS, Miller RS, et al. Life-threatening air rifle injuries to the heart in three boys. J Pediatr Surg 2000;35(5):785–7.

[32] Killeen KL, Shanmuganathan K, Mirvis SE. Imaging of traumatic diaphragmatic injuries. Semin Ultrasound CT MR 2002;23(2):184–92.

[33] Ramos CT, Koplewitz BZ, Babyn PS, et al. What have we learned about traumatic diaphragmatic hernias in children? J Pediatr Surg 2000;35(4):601–4.

[34] Shanmuganathan K, Mirvis SE. Imaging diagnosis of nonaortic thoracic injury. Radiol Clin North Am 1999;37:533–51.

[35] Ptak T, Rhea J, Novelline R. Experience with a continuous, single-pass whole-body multi-detector CT protocol for trauma: the three-minute multiple trauma CT scan. Emerg Radiol 2001;8:250–6.

[36] Self ML, Blake AM, Whitley M, et al. The benefit of routine thoracic, abdominal, and pelvic computed tomography to evaluate trauma patients with closed head injuries. Am J Surg 2003;186:609–13.

[37] Jindal A, Velmahos GC, Rofougaran R. Computed tomography for evaluation of mild to moderate pediatric trauma: are we overusing it? World J Surg 2002;26(1):13–6.

[38] Frush DP. Review of radiation issues for computed tomography. Semin Ultrasound CT MR 2004;25(1): 17–24.

[39] Berrington de Gonzalez A, Darby S. Risk of cancer from diagnostic X-rays: estimates for the UK and 14 other countries. Lancet 2004;363:345–51.

[40] Brenner D, Elliston C, Hall E, et al. Estimated risks of radiation-induced fatal cancer from pediatric CT. AJR Am J Roentgenol 2001;176(2):289–96.

[41] Hall P, Adami HO, Trichopoulos D, et al. Effect of low doses of ionising radiation in infancy on cognitive function in adulthood: Swedish population based cohort study. BMJ 2004;328:19–23.

[42] Ptak T, Rhea JT, Novelline RA. Radiation dose is reduced with a single-pass whole-body multi-detector row CT trauma protocol compared with a conventional segmented method: initial experience. Radiology 2003;229(3):902–5.

[43] Sheridan R, Peralta R, Rhea J, et al. Reformatted visceral protocol helical computed tomographic scanning allows conventional radiographs of the thoracic and lumbar spine to be eliminated in the evaluation of blunt trauma patients. J Trauma 2003; 55(4):665–9.

[44] Rhea JT, Sheridan RL, Mullins ME, et al. Can chest and abdominal trauma CT eliminate the need for plain film of the spine? Experience with 329 multiple trauma patients. Emerg Radiol 2001;8:99–104.

[45] Rybicki F, Nawfel RD, Judy PF, et al. Skin and thyroid dosimetry in cervical spine screening: two methods for evaluation and a comparison between a helical CT and radiographic trauma series. AJR Am J Roentgenol 2002;179(4):933–1.

[46] Renton J, Kincaid S, Ehrlich PF. Should helical CT scanning of the thoracic cavity replace the conventional chest X-ray as a primary assessment tool in pediatric trauma? An efficacy and cost analysis. J Pediatr Surg 2003;38(5):793–7.

[47] Holmes JF, Sokolove PE, Brant WE, et al. A clinical decision rule for identifying children with thoracic injuries after blunt torso trauma. Ann Emerg Med 2002;39(5):492–9.

[48] Gittelman MA, Gonzalez-del-Rey J, Brody AS, et al. Clinical predictors for the selective use of chest radiographs in pediatric blunt trauma evaluations. J Trauma 2003;55(4):670–6.

[49] Moss RL, Musemeche CA. Clinical judgment is superior to diagnostic tests in the management of pediatric small bowel injury. J Pediatr Surg 1996; 31(8):1178–81.

[50] Jerby BL, Attorri RJ, Morton Jr D. Blunt intestinal injury in children: the role of the physical examination. J Pediatr Surg 1997;32(4):580–4.

[51] Stanley RJ. Inherent dangers in radiologic screening. AJR Am J Roentgenol 2001;177(5):989–92.

ELSEVIER
SAUNDERS

Radiol Clin N Am 43 (2005) 283 – 302

RADIOLOGIC
CLINICS
of North America

Imaging of the Esophagus in Children

Lynn Ansley Fordham, MD

Pediatric Radiology, Department of Radiology, University of North Carolina School of Medicine,
3325 Old Infirmary Building, CB# 7510, Chapel Hill, NC 27599–7510, USA

The main role of the esophagus is to facilitate passage of food from the mouth to the stomach. A number of conditions can alter esophageal structure or function including congenital anomalies, trauma, infection, and neoplasm. The anatomy, imaging evaluation, and common problems seen in the pediatric thoracic esophagus are reviewed in this article.

Embryology, physiology, and anatomy

The esophagus begins forming during the fourth week of gestation. The primitive foregut gives rise to the esophagus, stomach, proximal duodenum, and trachea. The esophagus begins as a diverticulum, arising from the primitive foregut. This diverticulum elongates and then separates from the trachea because of infolding of the lateral walls of the foregut. The esophagus reaches its normal relative length at approximately 7 weeks. Epithelial proliferation leads to complete or near complete obliteration of the lumen, which then recanalizes at about the tenth week [1–3]. Fibroblast growth factor 2 and p63 seem to be important factors at the cellular level contributing to normal esophageal development [4,5].

The esophagus is composed of three layers: (1) mucosa, (2) submucosa, and (3) muscularis. Unlike the intra-abdominal gastrointestinal tract, the thoracic esophagus does not have a serosal layer. The esophagus is composed of two types of muscle. The upper third is composed of striated muscle and the lower two thirds have smooth muscle. Proper function requires careful coordination of esophageal activity. Peristalsis is initiated with distention of the upper esophagus. Peristalsis is coordinated by the medullary neural reflexes and the vagus nerve in the upper one third. In the lower two thirds of the esophagus the peristalsis depends on intrinsic motor activity, which is modified by vagus nerve activity [6–9]. The esophageal mucosa is composed of squamous epithelium with a transition to glandular epithelium in the distal esophagus [2,8].

The esophagus extends from the level of the hypopharynx at the level of the seventh cervical vertebra down to the stomach at approximately the tenth thoracic vertebral body level. There are upper and lower sphincters at the ends, which prevent retrograde passage of food and fluid. Because of this, the esophagus is narrower at both ends than it is in the middle. The cricopharyngeus muscle is frequently visualized as a transient, nonobstructive posterior filling defect in the proximal esophagus (Fig. 1) [10].

Techniques for imaging the esophagus

The upper gastrointestinal (UGI) series is the most common method for esophageal evaluation. A positive contrast agent, such as barium, is used to opacify the esophagus and fluoroscopic and radiographic images are obtained yielding both functional and structural information. This well-established technique has been modified in recent years as more and more radiology departments move to digital image acquisition. A recent survey found a wide variation in the radiation dose to pediatric patients from fluoroscopy [11]. Beam filtration with addi-

E-mail address: fdh@med.unc.edu

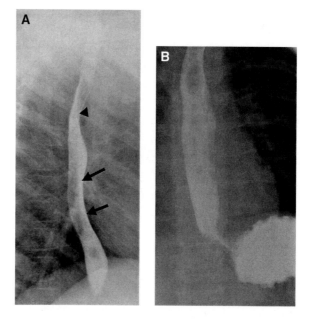

Fig. 1. Normal frontal (*A*) and lateral (*B*) views of the esophagus. Note anterior impression caused by the aorta (*arrowhead*) and left atrium (*arrows*) seen on the lateral view. Normal narrowing at the gastroesophageal junction is seen on both views.

tional layers of aluminum and copper filtration, optimization of the X-ray beam, and use of low-dose pulsed fluoroscopy can decrease the radiation dose significantly [12]. Image acquisition using fluoroscopy capture technology (ie, frame grab) can further decrease the radiation dose by reducing the total number of higher-dose spot film–type exposures. Tight collimation, minimized fluoroscopy time, and optimization of the imaging system also contribute greatly to dose reduction in both analog and digital imaging systems [13,14]. Examinations tailored to the clinical question and careful screening before the performance of any radiologic procedure is also vital in decreasing radiation dose. Analog or digital video recording is also useful because it allows for recording of a single or limited number of swallows with the ability to review images off-line.

Patient immobilization also helps to decrease the radiation dose by decreasing the examination time, and facilitating the use of collimation. At the author's institution an Octostop device (Octostop, Laval, Quebec, Canada) is used to immobilize children up to approximately 3 years of age. This is called a *special car seat* when describing it to the older toddlers and young children. They seem to be less afraid of the special car seat than they are of adult hands reaching under the fluoroscopy tower to position them for the examination. A pillow is placed at the top of the table and the child's caregiver is invited

to rest their elbows on the pillow while leaning in to encourage and comfort the child during the examination. Lead shields are placed on the table to decrease radiation dose to the patient and the radiology team. Gonadal shielding is used routinely for overhead images. Breast shielding may be helpful in older girls [15]. Stickers chosen by the child ahead of time may be placed on the fluoroscopy tower to ease the anxiety of older toddlers and young children. School-aged children are generally interested in seeing themselves on the monitor (*television*) or looking at images painted or projected on the walls and ceiling in the fluoroscopy suite. Barium can be flavored with powdered flavoring agents or syrups to increase its palatability to children or even mixed with milk [16–19]. Barium is generally instilled during voluntary swallowing. If, for a variety of reasons, voluntary swallowing is not achievable, contrast can be instilled through an oral injection by a catheter tip syringe into the cheek pouch, through an enteric feeding tube placed in the mouth threaded through a slit cut into the end of a nipple [20,21], or through an enteric tube placed in the esophagus. When injecting through a tube care should be taken not to overdistend the esophagus or inject too high in the esophagus causing aspiration.

Contrast agents should be carefully selected. In general, a barium suspension is used for most indications. Barium is contraindicated when evaluating the esophagus for possible leak. In these situations a choice is generally made between low-osmolar non-ionic water-soluble contrast agents and high-osmolar ionic water-soluble contrast materials. The former is less likely to lead to pneumonitis if inadvertently aspirated into the lung [22,23]. In the United States low-osmolar water-soluble contrast agents are more expensive than the high-osmolar solutions. At the author's institution dilute iopamidol is used to evaluate for esophageal leak. Oral gadolinium can be used to evaluate for leak in children with iodine sensitivity [24].

In most children, a UGI series is performed rather than just an esophagram. The patient is imaged from the level of the hard palate to the duodenal-jejunal junction to evaluate swallowing, the esophagus, gastric emptying, and small bowel rotation. An isolated esophagram is generally performed in children being followed-up for an esophageal stricture or those being evaluated for an esophageal foreign body. The esophagus is examined in at least two orthogonal imaging planes. Double-contrast examinations can be performed in cooperative older children to look for mucosal abnormalities.

One of the common indications for a UGI is gastroesophageal reflux (GER). The dose of contrast material that is administered and techniques for evaluation of GER vary by department and radiologist. Some radiologists believe that the child should be fed a full feeding volume and then imaged intermittently over a 5-minute period to look for GER. Others give a full feeding volume and rather than 5 minutes of intermittent fluoroscopy, roll the child from side to side, have the child cough or straight leg raise, or drink water or eat food to try to elicit reflux [25–27]. Babies can be given their pacifier, which may either decrease the reflux because the child stops crying or this maneuver may elicit reflux because of the frequent swallowing. Other radiologists have eliminated a formal search for GER in favor of esophageal pH probe testing.

Ultrasound, CT, and MR imaging can all be useful in evaluating the esophagus. Transabdominal ultrasound of the esophagus can be used to evaluate for GER and esophageal varices providing both structural and functional information. Intraluminal ultrasound is currently of limited value in the pediatric population. CT and MR imaging both provide static and multiplanar views of the esophagus. These modalities can be used in a number of indications including evaluation of extrinsic esophageal compression, such as in vascular rings or duplication cysts. CT has superb spatial resolution and may not require sedation, whereas MR imaging has superior

soft tissue contrast and no ionizing radiation. A full description of the techniques for these modalities is beyond the scope of this article.

Approach to esophageal abnormalities

Esophageal pathologies can be organized in a number of ways. For example, esophageal disorders can be grouped into functional or structural alterations. A pattern approach organizes the material by looking at the imaging appearance (eg, filling defect, mass, or narrowing). An etiologic approach divides the disorders into congenital or acquired categories. The etiologic approach is used in this article.

Congenital anomalies

Common congenital anomalies of the esophagus include esophageal atresia (EA) with or without associated tracheoesophageal fistula (TEF), esophageal duplication cysts, and less commonly esophageal stenosis. Rarely, an esophageal bronchus or esophageal diverticulum is seen. Congenital vascular anomalies can also compress the esophagus enough to be symptomatic.

Esophageal atresia

EA is the most significant and most common congenital esophageal malformation. EA occurs in between 1 and 2500 and 4000 live births. It may be isolated or associated with TEF [28,29]. EA is caused by disruption of the normal developmental sequence described previously. The exact etiology is unknown but research on rats that develop EA with TEF following exposure to doxorubicin suggests an abnormality in fibroblast growth factor receptor 2 may lead to TEF formation [5].

There are five different anomalies seen in the spectrum of EA with incomplete formation of the esophagus and abnormal connections between the airway and esophagus (Fig. 2). By far the most common anomaly (90%) is an atresia of the proximal esophagus and continuation of the distal esophagus with a fistulous connection between the airway and the distal esophagus (Fig. 3). The second most common anomaly (3%–9%) is EA without a TEF. Less common (3%) is an intact esophagus with a small fistula (H- or N-type) connection. Other uncommon variants include EA with fistulous connections from both the proximal and distal esoph-

Normal   **EA with distal TEF**   **EA no TEF**

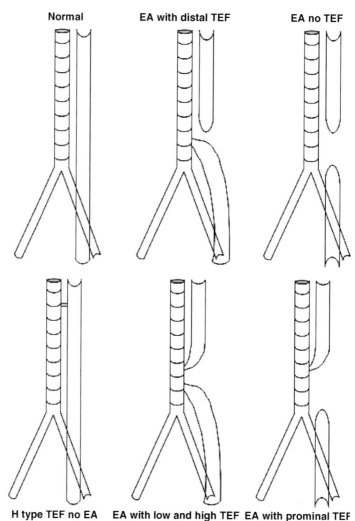

H type TEF no EA   EA with low and high TEF EA with prominal TEF

Fig. 2. Line diagram showing the relationship between the esophagus and trachea in normal children and in different forms of esophageal atresia and tracheoesophageal fistula. The types are drawn in order of decreasing frequency. The mnemonic *low-no-H-double-high* reflects the order of frequency of the various types of esophageal atresia and tracheoesophageal malformations.

ageal (1%) and EA with a proximal TEF (<1%) segment and other very rare variations [29,30]. At birth babies with a connection between their distal esophagus and their airway have air in the gastrointestinal tract. Those with pure EA or an EA with a proximal TEF have a gasless abdomen. Fifty to 70% of children with EA have associated congenital anomalies involving the cardiovascular (35%), genitourinary (20%), gastrointestinal (24%), neurologic (10%), and skeletal (13%) systems [31–37]. The VACTERL (Vertebral anomalies, Anal atresia-malformation, Cardiac anomalies, Tracheal to Esophageal fistula, Renal, and Limb–including ra-

dial ray–anomalies) association is seen in 25% of these patients [31–37].

In children, the diagnosis of EA with possible TEF is made on the basis of clinical grounds. There may also be a history of polyhydramnios. The patient is either unable to tolerate their own secretions with drooling and respiratory distress or the child may present with coughing and choking spells limited to initiation of feeding. The clinical suspicion is confirmed by failure to pass an enteric tube into the stomach. If the diagnosis is in question air can be instilled by the enteric tube to distend the proximal esophagus and demonstrate the dilated proximal

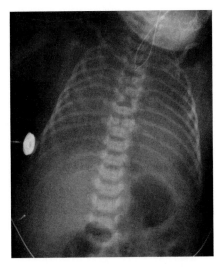

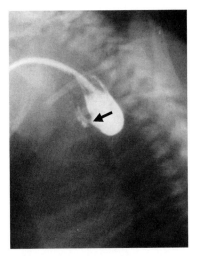

Fig. 3. Infant with prenatal history of polyhydramnios and drooling. Chest radiograph demonstrates an enteric tube coiled within the proximal pouch of the atretic esophagus with air seen in the stomach and proximal bowel indicating a distal or proximal and distal tracheoesophageal fistula. There are parenchymal pulmonary opacities that may be secondary to suboptimal lung inflation or to aspiration. Mid thoracovertebral segmentation anomalies are also seen.

Fig. 4. Infant with esophageal atresia and coughing. A small amount of barium was injected into the esophagus with the patient imaged in the lateral projection. The proximal esophagus is dilated and compresses the trachea. A rare, proximal tracheoesophageal fistula (*arrow*) is demonstrated. Because this child has air in the gastrointestinal tract on the abdominal films, there is also a distal fistula that is not opacified on this study.

esophageal pouch. Liquid contrast material is generally not used because of the potential of aspiration and possible airway compression caused by a dilated fluid-filled esophageal pouch. Barium or water-soluble contrast is used when the patient has EA with a question of a proximal TEF (Fig. 4). The H- or N-type TEF is not associated with EA and a feeding tube passes readily into the stomach. Positive contrast material can then be used to demonstrate the connection that is frequently found near the level of the thoracic inlet (Fig. 5). The H-type fistula may be demonstrated while the patient swallows barium or nonionic water-soluble contrast material. This fistula can be difficult to demonstrate, however, and prone positioning and catheter placement within the esophagus can help bring out subtle connections [38]. CT scanning can demonstrate the findings but is not the primary imaging modality of choice [39,40]. The fistula can be quite proximally located and difficult to differentiate from aspiration of contrast [41].

Surgical repair of the EA depends on the child's anatomy. The approach has changed and the surgical outcomes improved in this population. There are now fewer esophageal replacement surgeries and more primary repairs than in the past [42]. In general, EA with a TEF is approached as a primary repair with an extrapleural approach by a lateral thoracotomy. There

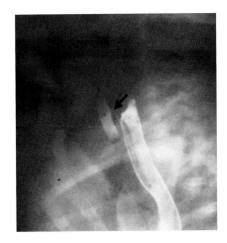

Fig. 5. Infant with respiratory distress during feeding. The patient was given barium and imaged in a lateral projection. A tiny track (*arrow*) is visualized just above the thoracic inlet extending cranial caudally from the esophagus to the trachea. The H-type tracheoesophageal fistula is typically seen at the level of the thoracic inlet. Multiple swallows or even repeated examinations may be necessary to demonstrate the fistula.

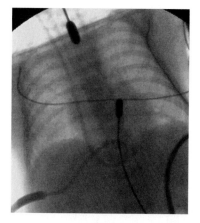

Fig. 6. Two week old with isolated esophageal atresia. This intraoperative spot film demonstrates sounds in the proximal and distal segments of the esophagus during an esophageal lengthening procedure. The child underwent multiple lengthening maneuvers after this one until the esophagus had elongated enough for a primary repair.

are now reports of repair of proximal atresia with distal TEF and H-type fistulae from a thoracoscopic approach [43,44]. This averts the lateral thoracotomy and the associated complications. Occasionally, a patient remains symptomatic after surgery and this suggests a missed double TEF [45]. EA without TEF is generally treated with delayed surgery. In EA with TEF there is a relatively short distance between the proximal and distal esophageal segments allowing for

primary repair. With pure EA there is frequently a long gap between the proximal and distal segments. The gap makes it difficult to establish a primary anastomosis if repair is attempted early. Instead, these children are treated with a gastrostomy tube placement. They then undergo multiple transgastric and transesophageal dilatations and elongation procedures until they can undergo primary anastomosis (Fig. 6) [46]. If primary repair fails, other options for surgical repair include colonic interposition (Fig. 7) or a gastric interposition procedure.

The common primary complication of all of the surgical procedures is esophageal leak, which occurs in approximately 18% of cases [45,47]. Extrapleural fluid seen on chest radiography raises the possibility of an esophageal leak [48]. Stricture and recurrent fistulae may also be identified. Low-osmolar non-ionic water-soluble contrast material is used for the immediate postoperative examinations. Long-term esophageal stenosis is seen in approximately 40% [45] and stenosis is more likely in children who initially had an anastomotic leak [47]. These strictures can be treated with balloon dilatation, often requiring multiple dilations.

At many centers, routine postoperative imaging in these patients is used to exclude an anastomotic leak before feeding the infant. Other institutions base management on clinical assessment because they see little predictive value in the early post-surgical swallow studies [49,50]. Contrast swallow is then reserved for patients where there is a high clinical suspicion for anastomotic leak [51]. When imaging these children, peristalsis is seen in the upper portion of the esophagus. No coordinated peristalsis is seen below the level of the original

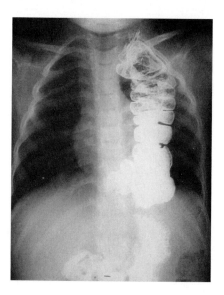

Fig. 7. This child had a failed primary esophageal atresia repair and underwent colonic interposition. Note the haustral markings seen in the intrathoracic colonic loop.

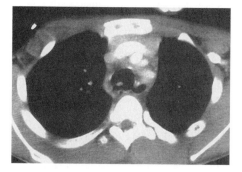

Fig. 8. Teenager with laryngotracheal papillomatosis who developed a posttraumatic tracheoesophageal fistula following laser ablation of tracheal papillomata. Axial CT with intravenous contrast demonstrates continuity between the tracheal and esophageal air columns. This was confirmed with a thoracic esophagram with water-soluble contrast.

anastomosis. The postoperative imaging may also reveal a previously undetected associated congenital esophageal stenosis [52,53]. This congenital distal stricture may be caused by tracheobronchial remnants [54,55]. Balloon dilatation of postoperative strictures is effective with a low rate of complications [56].

The long-term complications of EA repair include esophageal dysmotility, GER, peptic stricture secondary to GER, recurrent anastomotic stricture, tracheomalacia, rib fusion, and scoliosis [29]. GER is seen in 40% to 70% of patients. Antireflux surgery may be required if these children fail medical management of their reflux.

Most TEFs are congenital in origin. Noncongenital TEFs can also be caused by postoperative recurrence of the fistula [57] or acquired secondary to esophageal trauma from endotracheal intubation attempts [58,59], caustic ingestions [60], or erosions from esophageal foreign bodies, such as disk batteries [61], and complications secondary to surgery on the esophagus or trachea (Fig. 8).

Congenital esophageal stenosis and esophageal webs and rings

Congenital esophageal stenosis usually presents as a fixed segment of narrowing in the distal third of the esophagus (Fig. 9). Congenital esophageal stenosis is most commonly secondary to tracheal bronchial tissue and cartilage and may be associated with EA [53,62,63]. This is generally a fixed stenosis and is to be differentiated from peptic strictures related to GER. Successful endoscopic balloon dilatation of congenital esophageal stenosis with tracheobronchial remnants has been reported [64], although others favor a surgical excision and repair [65]. Esophageal stenosis seen in the mid thoracic esophagus is likely fibromuscular in origin [62]. Other distal esophageal anomalies can be seen including esophageal webs, aberrant gastric mucosa, paraesophageal hernia, or a short esophagus [28].

Esophageal duplication cysts

Esophageal duplication cysts are thought to be related to an abnormality in tubulation of the esophagus. Esophageal duplication cysts can also be related to early budding abnormalities and may contain respiratory mucosa. Neuroenteric cysts are malformations that involve the neural elements and the aerodigestive system. Three types of esophageal duplications exist. One type contains respiratory epi-

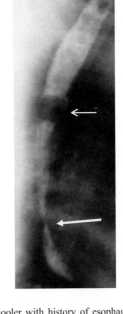

Fig. 9. Preschooler with history of esophageal atresia with tracheoesophageal fistula repair and acute onset of chest pain. There is a filling defect seen proximally (*small arrow*) caused by food impacted above an anastomotic stricture. A second area of narrowing is seen below the first (*large arrow*), which had been present on the earliest imaging studies and was thought to represent a congenital stricture. This cannot be differentiated from a peptic stricture without prior examinations.

thelium, a second type involves a combination of neural and enteric tissue with associated vertebral anomalies, and the third type is true tubular duplication of the esophagus.

Esophageal cysts with respiratory epithelium are a part of the bronchopulmonary foregut malformations. Neuroenteric cysts are related to errors in notochord formation. They are commonly associated with vertebral body anomalies. True tubular duplications of the esophagus are rare. They may be isolated from the gastrointestinal tract or may have a communication. Generally, the evaluation of these entities begins with plain film radiography followed by contrast esophagram (Fig. 10). Duplication cysts are smoothly marginated extrinsic filling defects on UGI. Most do not communicate with the esophagus, although a communicating cyst has been reported [66,67]. Ultrasound, CT, and MR imaging [68,69] can all be helpful in demonstrating the cystic features of the abnormality seen on UGI and demonstrating its position relative to other structures in the chest.

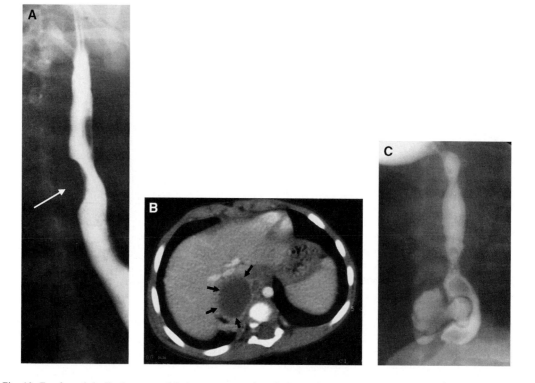

Fig. 10. Esophageal duplication cysts. (*A*) An upper gastrointestinal examination was performed in this toddler for possible gastroesophageal reflux. An ovoid, intramural filling defect was seen along the posterior wall of the esophagus (*arrow*), which proved to be a duplication cyst. (*B*) CT scan in a different patient obtained after intravenous and oral contrast reveals a homogeneous low-density round structure (*arrows*), which shares a common wall with the esophagus. No vertebral body anomalies are seen and the mass is well below the level of the carina, making neurenteric and bronchogenic cysts less likely than an esophageal duplication cyst. (*C*) Upper gastrointestinal series performed in another child demonstrates a complex, tubular-shaped collection of contrast adjacent to the distal esophagus that was also an esophageal duplication cyst.

Vascular rings and slings

Vascular rings, slings, and aberrant vessels can create extrinsic impressions on the esophagus. The main complaints in vascular rings are related to the airway compression. A variety of different malformations can lead to dysphagia and be symptomatic [70,71]. The lateral esophagram is used to evaluate both the airway and the esophagus and differentiate the three types of vascular impressions. An anterior compression on the trachea with a posterior impression on the esophagus is a vascular ring, most often caused by an aberrant subclavian artery. A vessel coursing between the trachea and esophagus is a vascular sling. More specifically, a vascular ring is usually either a double aortic arch or a right aortic arch with an aberrant left subclavian artery and a ductus arteriosus remnant (Fig. 11). A pulmonary sling is a left pulmonary artery that arises from the right pulmonary artery and crosses between the esophagus and trachea to pass back to the left lung.

This vessel might only be demonstrated intermittently on repeated swallows during an UGI. An isolated aberrant subclavian artery does not have any tracheal indentation. It has an obliquely positioned posterior impression on the esophagus, which may be secondary to either a right aortic arch and left aberrant subclavian artery or a left aortic arch and aberrant right subclavian. The side of the aortic arch is determined from the scout radiograph and the anteroposterior esophagram. Cross-sectional imaging with CT or MR imaging is used to define further the anatomy of the complete vascular rings.

Acquired esophageal lesions

Esophageal varices

Esophageal varices are rarely seen in the pediatric population. They are generally associated with under-

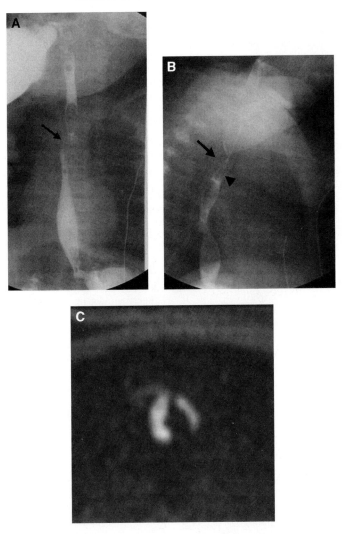

Fig. 11. Toddler with stridor. Chest radiograph (not shown) demonstrated narrowing of the tracheal. (*A*) Frontal projection from a contrast esophagram demonstrates an oblique filling defect on the anteroposterior view (*arrow*). (*B*) There are both anterior (*arrowhead*) and posterior (*arrow*) impressions on the esophagus suggesting a complete vascular ring. (*C*) Postcontrast MR image of the chest reveals a double aortic arch encircling the esophagus and trachea.

lying liver disease. They are occasionally detected on UGI series but are generally seen with ultrasound, CT, or MR imaging during the evaluation of a number of liver diseases or in the post–liver transplant population. The appearance is typically a filling defect or multiple defects of the distal esophagus with a UGI evaluation, or actual delineation of serpiginous vascular structures by CT or MR imaging.

Esophagitis

Except for children with GER, esophagitis is rare in the immunocompetent pediatric patient. Esophagi-

tis can be evaluated with UGI series but is frequently treated without imaging based on findings in the oropharynx. The most common organisms to cause infectious esophagitis in the pediatric population are *Candida albicans*, cytomegalovirus, and herpes simplex virus. All three of these organisms can be seen in the child with AIDS [72]. With *Candida* esophagitis, a shaggy mucosa or cobblestone appearance can be seen caused by barium collections between plaques and areas of necrotic debris. Deep ulcerations can also be seen but are more commonly identified with herpes and cytomegalovirus esophagitis. The imaging findings are relatively nonspe-

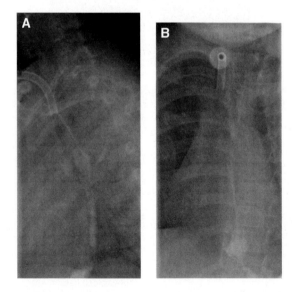

cific and more than one type of infection may be occurring at a time (Fig. 12). Cytomegalovirus is angioinvasive and leads to ischemic necrosis and ulceration because of its invasive nature. It can also cause large ulcers, linear ulcers, nodular thickening, cobblestoning, pseudodiverticula, and strictures. With herpes simplex virus, shallow ulcers are more commonly seen. Esophagitis can also be caused by spread of infection from adjacent mediastinal lymph nodes, such as seen with mycobacterium tuberculosis.

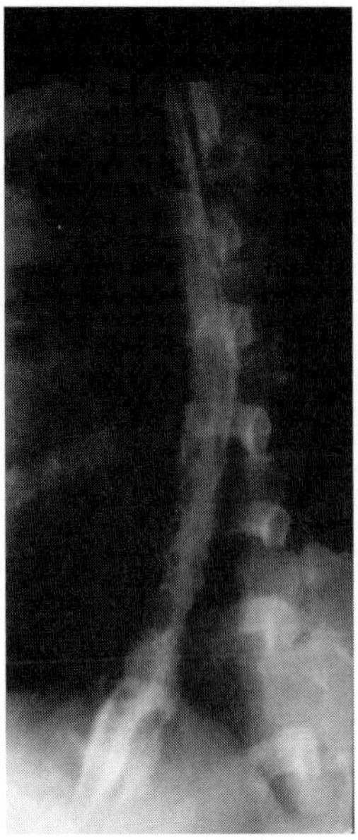

Noninfective esophagitis

Caustic ingestion

Much work has been done to educate parents and caregivers about common household hazards. Unfortunately, tragic accidents still occur with children ingesting caustic substances stored in non–child proof (ie, beverage) containers. Acidic ingestions typically lead to gastric injury. Caustic (lye) ingestions typically affect the esophagus (Fig. 13). The degree of injury is related to the length of contact time with the mucosa. The most affected areas are the middle and lower esophagus. Alkaline agents are also found in granule forms and these may cause stricturing at any level. The initial evaluation is pref-

Fig. 12. Child with chest pain and leukemia. Contrast esophagram demonstrates an irregular esophageal mucosa with numerous ulcerations in this child with *Candida* esophagitis.

Fig. 13. Three-year-old child 3 months after ingestion of a powdered cleaner. Lateral (*A*) and frontal (anteroposterior) (*B*) views demonstrate long segment narrowing and irregularity of the entire length of the esophagus. Liquid agents tend to injure the distal two thirds of the esophagus but the powdered agent ingested injured the mucosa from the mouth to the stomach. A tracheotomy tube is also identified.

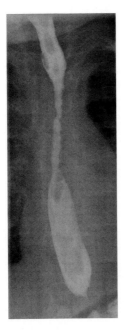

Fig. 14. School-aged child with epidermolysis bullosa and decreased oral intake. Contrast esophagram reveals a long segment very irregular stricture in the mid esophagus. This area was dilated multiple times.

erably performed with low-osmolar nonionic contrast-material because of the possibility of acquired TEF or esophageal perforation. Early findings include epiglottic swelling, mucosal irregularity, esophageal dysmotility, and ulceration. Follow-up studies may demonstrate a fixed stricture, which depending on its severity may require dilatation or surgery.

Epidermolysis bullosa dystrophica

Epidermolysis bullosa dystrophica is a congenital disorder of the squamous epithelium. The skin is quite fragile as is the mucosa throughout the gastrointestinal tract. Minimal trauma in these children can lead to significant desquamation and scarring (Fig. 14). Unfortunately, the process of eating can be enough to damage the esophageal mucosa leading to strictures. The swallow studies should be performed with the patient drinking spontaneously. The children should be treated with great care and placed on padded tables. A feeding tube should not be placed or the patient restrained in any way to prevent possible injury occurring during examination. The esophageal strictures demonstrated are treated with gentle balloon dilatation but they frequently recur. These children are at increased risk for squamous cell carcinoma.

Epidermolysis bullosa is the common name for multiple distinctive congenital skin abnormalities.

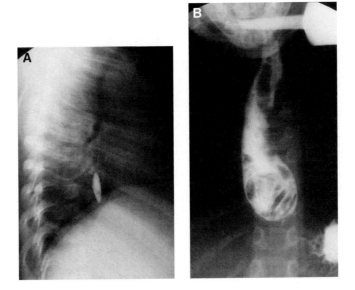

Fig. 15. Toddler refusing to eat. (*A*) Lateral scout radiograph reveals a radiopaque foreign body in the distal esophagus. (*B*) Frontal (anteroposterior) spot film during examination shows that contrast is being administered through a catheter-tip syringe. There are multiple masses outlined by contrast representing nonradiopaque foreign bodies. Endoscopy was performed to remove the foreign bodies. After all the foreign bodies were removed a stricture was identified at the gastroesophageal junction.

294   FORDHAM

Autosomal-dominant epidermolysis bullosa simplex
has skin abnormalities without gastrointestinal manifestations. Autosomal-recessive junctional epidermolysis bullosa is associated with pyloric atresia and
autosomal-recessive and both recessive and dominant varieties of epidermolysis bullosa can lead to
severe esophageal involvement [73–76].

   Other systemic disease can also affect the esophagus. Crohn's disease, Behçet's syndrome, chronic
granulomatous disease, graft-versus-host disease, and
radiation therapy can all lead to esophagitis, including the development of strictures.

Esophageal foreign bodies

   As parents of toddlers know, young children
are drawn to all sorts of dangerous objects. One of
the ways that young children learn is by exploring
through touch and taste. Unfortunately, some of these
small objects that are investigated end up lodged
in the esophagus. Children with esophageal foreign
bodies may present with drooling, inability to swallow solids, chest pain, or even respiratory distress.
Conventional radiography is very helpful in demonstrating radiopaque foreign bodies (Fig. 15). Non-

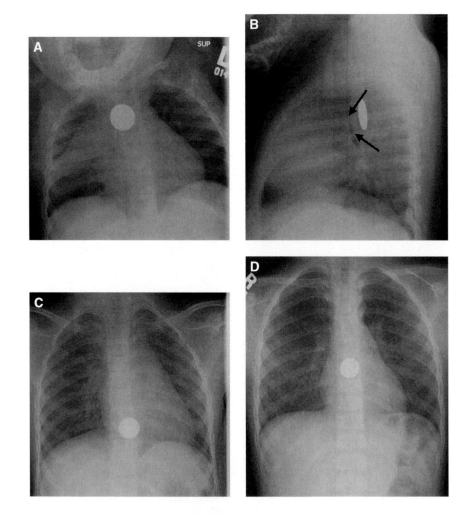

Fig. 16. Multiple examples of chest radiographs demonstrating esophageal coins. (*A,B*) Toddler with respiratory distress. Frontal
(anteroposterior) (*A*) and lateral (*B*) chest views demonstrate a coin lying within the esophagus. There is associated edema
and secondary compression of the airway (*arrows*). The coin is lodged at the level of the aortic arch. (*C*) Frontal view shows that
the coin is at the gastroesophageal junction in a different patient. Frontal (*D*) and lateral (*E*) views show that the coin is lodged at
the level of the left atrium in another child. Frontal (*F*) and lateral (*G*) views show that the coin is lodged above the thoracic inlet
in a different child who has undergone prior cardiac surgery.

radiopaque foreign bodies can be inferred by the patient's clinical symptoms and demonstrated with contrast esophagography.

The initial evaluation of the child should include conventional radiography. Radiopaque foreign bodies represent approximately 60% of all esophageal foreign bodies and most of these objects are coins [77,78]. Nonradiopaque foreign bodies include food, plastic items, and aluminum beverage can tabs [79]. Esophageal foreign bodies frequently lodge at normal areas of relative narrowing or above strictures. For the thoracic course of the esophagus, these areas

of narrowing are the level of the thoracic inlet, the aortic arch or the left main stem bronchus, or just above the gastroesophageal junction. Clinical history may be helpful in determining the length of time a foreign body may be present and help to predict the likelihood of associated complications. Patients with coins in the esophagus who have minimal clinical symptoms have a high chance of passing the coin without further intervention [80]. Pennies minted after 1982 [81,82] and button-type batteries [83,84], however, can rapidly erode the esophageal mucosa and may require an accelerated treatment plan. A

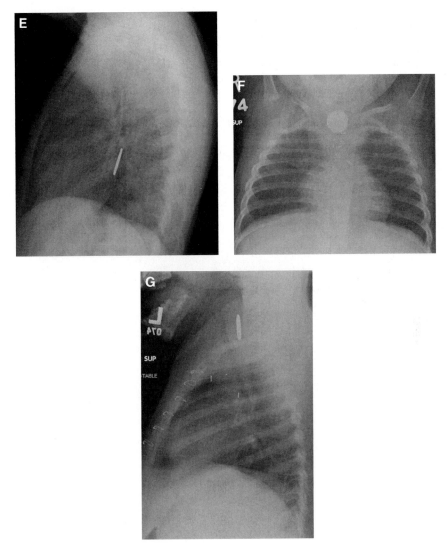

Fig. 16 (*continued*).

lodged foreign body may also be related to an underlying esophageal abnormality, such as a previously unrecognized stricture or vascular ring. Most commonly, no underlying fixed stricture is found [85].

Radiographs are helpful in demonstrating the location of the radiopaque foreign body in craniocaudal and anteroposterior planes. The two-view chest radiograph allows differentiation between foreign bodies in the airway and foreign bodies in the esophagus. A coin in the upper esophagus is en face on the frontal radiograph because of slight compression of the esophagus between the trachea and the spine (Fig. 16). In contrast, a coin in the airway is en face on the lateral because of the c-shaped cartilaginous rings in the trachea. Esophageal foreign bodies can lead to respiratory symptoms because of esophageal and mediastinal edema and secondary compression of the airway.

Foley catheter techniques [77,78] and magnet-tipped nasogastric tube techniques [86,87] have been advocated for the removal of foreign bodies. Although some report high success rates, fatal complications have occurred [88]. Many pediatric radiologists no longer perform foreign body retrieval and these are usually removed during esophagoscopy. A contrast swallow post–foreign body removal can be helpful in demonstrating a posttraumatic pseudodiverticulum or underlying esophageal stricture, if there are complications or suspicious findings during esophagoscopy (Fig. 17) [89].

Esophageal trauma

The most common cause of esophageal-pharyngeal laceration is malposition of an enteric tube [90]. This generally perforates at the level of the pharynx and then tracks along the mediastinum. The best method for detection of this complication is a high level of suspicion and careful evaluation of plain films with each new catheter placement. An esophageal pseudodiverticulum can also be caused by vigorous oral suctioning in the newborn period. Many entities described previously under acquired TEF also qualify as esophageal trauma, and perforation also is a complication of balloon dilation of esophageal strictures (Fig. 18). Esophageal laceration secondary to vomiting is quite rare in childhood but has been reported [91].

Gastroesophageal reflux

GER is a very common clinical problem. All infants have some element of GER and most of these children outgrow this problem. The clinical manifestations can range from simple eructation to vomiting. In children without weight loss or respiratory symptoms GER may be treated with simple reassurance. Thickened feeds and an elevated head position during and after feeding can also be helpful. Children generally outgrow GER by approximately 9 months of

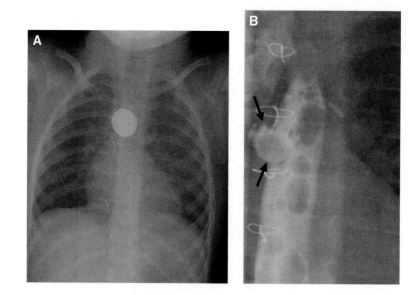

Fig. 17. Toddler with history of cardiac surgery underwent chest radiography to evaluate heart size. (*A*) An esophageal foreign body was detected radiographically and removed endoscopically. (*B*) Following removal, a contrast esophagram demonstrates an extrinsic cavity or pseudodiverticulum (*arrows*).

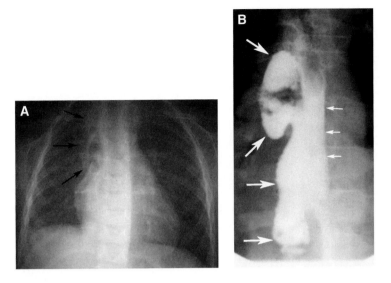

Fig. 18. Esophageal perforation following balloon dilation of an esophageal stricture secondary to esophageal atresia repair in a 3.5-year-old boy with mild chest pain. (*A*) Frontal chest radiograph demonstrates abnormal contour in the right paramediastinal region (*arrows*). Note right-sided rib deformity secondary to the prior thoracotomy. (*B*) Water-soluble contrast esophagram shows large extraesophageal collection of contrast (*large arrows*) extending down to the diaphragm. The native lumen is seen on the left (*small arrows*). A 1- to 2-cm tear was seen at thoracotomy.

age. Decreasing weight gain, weight loss, or multiple bouts of pneumonia signal a more concerning situation and may herald true pathologic GER. There is an increased risk of pathologic GER in children with trisomy 21, cystic fibrosis, and cerebral palsy. GER has been associated with hoarseness or bronchospasm, and treatment for reflux can improve the pulmonary symptoms in children with reactive airways disease [92].

Many normal babies demonstrate GER on UGI examination. This can be graded as insignificant or significant depending on whether the reflux is above or below the aortic arch. Unfortunately, the level of reflux does not correlate well with the clinical picture. At the author's institution, UGI is performed to exclude obstruction (eg, pyloric stenosis) as an etiology for the GER and to document a normally positioned duodenal-jejunal junction. Radionuclide studies have also been used to evaluate for GER. For this examination the child is given radiolabeled milk, formula, or solids, depending on the age-appropriate diet. Immediate and delayed images are obtained. The scintigraphic reflux study can be performed in conjunction with a gastric emptying study. Radionuclide studies are more sensitive than UGI examinations and can be used to quantitate a volume of reflux but lack anatomic detail. Aspiration with increased activity over the lungs is readily identified on nuclear examinations.

Both UGI and radionuclide reflux examinations can be compared with pH probe evaluation for GER. The major advantage for UGI is its anatomic detail and the qualitative information on esophageal function. The major criticism of this examination is the short period of observation. Nuclear scintigraphy is highly sensitive but lacks anatomic detail. The pH probe study occurs over a 24-hour period but does not detect the immediate postprandial reflux because the stomach acid is buffered by the large quantity of recently ingested food [93]. All three studies can be criticized for being nonphysiologic. In the UGI the child is fed barium, which is not the normal feed and is examined restrained in a supine position. The positioning issues also affect nuclear examinations, and compared with pH probe studies, the patient is imaged for a relatively short time. The pH probe examination is less than ideal because of the probe in place in the esophagus for the duration of the examination. When nuclear scintigraphy and pH probe results were directly compared in a study by Vandenplas et al [94], there were 123 episodes of reflux seen in 65 children. Notably, only 6 of the 123 episodes occurred simultaneously. Visualization of high-grade spontaneous reflux on fluoroscopy can be used as a single test for GER eliminating the need for pH probe testing [95]. A prominent cricopharyngeus muscle has been suggested as a sign of GER (Fig. 19) [96].

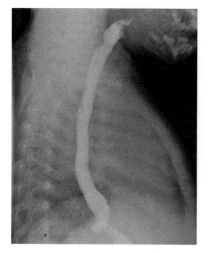

Fig. 19. Toddler with failure to thrive and gastroesophageal reflux seen during an upper gastrointestinal tract examination. A prominent cricopharyngeus muscle is seen in the cervical esophagus and can be a normal variant. Visualization of the cricopharyngeus during a contrast study, however, is also associated with gastroesophageal reflux.

Ultrasonography is becoming increasingly popular in the evaluation of GER [97–100] with results that correlate with pH probe studies. Ultrasound does not use ionizing radiation or an esophageal probe and so in some ways may be more physiologic than the other studies. To perform the examination, the

child is placed supine and given water or an electrolyte solution orally or through a tube in quantities that replicate normal feeding volumes. The gastroesophageal junction is imaged in a longitudinal plane looking for bubbles and fluid passing from the stomach into the esophagus. The study is somewhat time consuming and it can be a challenge in a moving infant. Ultrasound can be used to measure the length of the intra-abdominal esophagus. A decreased length has been correlated with an increase in the severity of GER [101].

Symptomatic GER is initially treated with thickened feedings. If this does not lead to an improvement, pharmacologic management is instituted. If symptoms of GER persist then the patient is referred for surgical management. Many different antireflux procedures have been described. The most common procedure currently is the Nissen fundoplication in which the fundus of the stomach is wrapped 360 degrees around the distal esophagus [102]. The Thal and the Toupet antireflux surgeries are second and third most common, respectively. Surgery can be performed as an open procedure or through a laparoscope [103]. Nissen fundoplication can have complications in both the early and late postoperative period [104]. A normal Nissen wrap creates a consistent filling defect at the gastroesophageal junction. No GER is seen with barium administration. There can be several different types of problems with the wrap. The wrap can be too

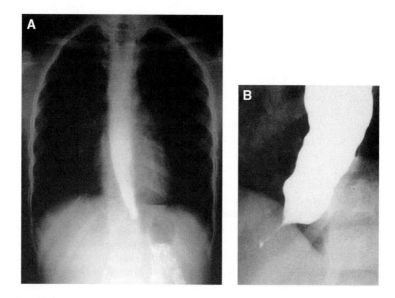

Fig. 20. (A) Erect frontal chest film showing increased retrocardiac tubular density and air fluid level in the upper esophagus. (B) Spot film obtained after a contrast esphagram showing a persistent "bird beak" type narrowing in the distal esophagus in a patient with achalasia.

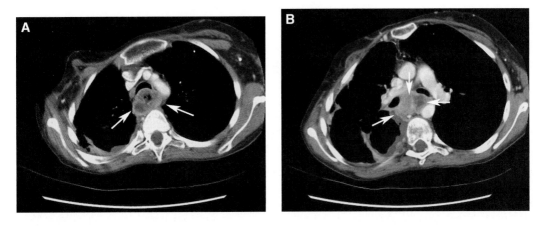

Fig. 21. Radiation-induced esophageal squamous cell carcinoma in a 17-year-old boy with remote history of rhabdomyosarcoma with radiation, development of secondary acute myelogenous leukemia now following bone marrow transplant, with an esophageal stricture secondary to esophagitis. The esophageal cancer was discovered following balloon dilation, perforation, and exploratory thoracotomy. (*A,B*) Axial, intravenous contrast-enhanced CT images in the mid thorax demonstrate the encasing esophageal malignancy (*arrows*).

loose from the outset and allow reflux. The wrap can also loosen over time. The loosening is seen as more and more contrast passes up into the wrap [104]. Hiatal hernias, paraesophageal hernias, and transdiaphragmatic herniation through the esophageal hiatus can all be seen, as can gastric volvulus. The hernia wrap can also slide down over the body of the stomach. A Nissen that is too tight can lead to esophageal obstruction and reflux-like symptoms or even perforation [104].

Achalasia

Achalasia is a rare cause of GER-type symptoms in the pediatric population (Fig. 20). Achalasia is seen in 1% of the general population. Children represent less than 5% of this group but achalasia has been reported in infants as young as 15 days of age. Scleroderma can also lead to GER symptoms or esophageal strictures in children.

Esophageal neoplasms

Esophageal neoplasms are rare in children. Benign lesions include fibrovascular polyps, hairy polyps, granular cell neoplasm [105], other hamartomas, leiomyomas, and diffuse leiomyomatosis. Carcinoma is quite rare in the pediatric population and can be seen with caustic ingestion, achalasia, scleroderma and epidermolysis bullosa, and previous radiation therapy (Fig. 21). Mediastinal neoplasms may lead to an extrinsic esophageal compression but they rarely invade the esophagus.

Summary

There are many differing types of abnormalities seen in the pediatric esophagus ranging from congenital to acquired lesions. GER is a common problem and it can be difficult to differentiate normal amounts of reflux from pathologic amounts. Contrast esophagram and UGI series continue to be the most common radiologic methods for evaluating the esophagus.

References

[1] Bedard MP. Embryology, anatomy, and physiology. In: Kuhn JP, Slovis TL, Haller JO, editors. Caffey's pediatric diagnostic imaging, vol. 1. Philadelphia: Mosby; 2004. p. 105–6.

[2] Berrocal T, Madrid C, Novo S, et al. Congenital anomalies of the tracheobronchial tree, lung, and mediastinum: embryology, radiology, and pathology. Radiographics 2004;24:e17.

[3] Sadler TW. Langman's medical embryology. 5th edition. Baltimore: Williams and Wilkins; 1985. p. 215–8.

[4] Daniely Y, Liao G, Dixon D, et al. Critical role of p63 in the development of a normal esophageal and tracheobronchial epithelium. Am J Physiol Cell Physiol 2004;287:C171.

[5] Spilde TL, Bhatia AM, Mehta SS, et al. Aberrant fibroblast growth factor receptor 2 signalling in esophageal atresia with tracheoesophageal fistula. J Pediatr Surg 2004;39:537.

[6] Jadcherla SR, Shaker R. Esophageal and upper

esophageal sphincter motor function in babies. Am J Med 2001;111(Suppl 8A):64S.

[7] Lang IM, Medda BK, Shaker R. Mechanisms of reflexes induced by esophageal distension. Am J Physiol Gastrointest Liver Physiol 2001;281:G1246.

[8] Robbins SL, Cotran RS, Kumar V. The gastrointestinal tract. Pathologic basis of disease. 3rd edition. Philadelphia: WB Saunders; 1984. p. 797–806.

[9] Schlesinger AE, Parker BR. Normal esophagus. In: Kuhn JP, Slovis TL, Haller JO, editors. Caffey's pediatric diagnostic imaging, vol. 2. Philadelphia: Mosby; 2004. p. 1539–44.

[10] Curtis DJ, Cruess DF, Dachman AH. Normal erect swallowing: normal function and incidence of variations. Invest Radiol 1985;20:717.

[11] Brown PH, Silberberg PJ, Thomas RD, et al. A multihospital survey of radiation exposure and image quality in pediatric fluoroscopy. Pediatr Radiol 2000; 30:236.

[12] Brown PH, Thomas RD, Silberberg PJ, et al. Optimization of a fluoroscope to reduce radiation exposure in pediatric imaging. Pediatr Radiol 2000; 30:229.

[13] Martin CJ, Hunter S. Reduction of patient doses from barium meal and barium enema examinations through changes in equipment factors. Br J Radiol 1994; 67:1196.

[14] Yakoumakis E, Tsalafoutas IA, Sandilos P, et al. Patient doses from barium meal and barium enema examinations and potential for reduction through proper set-up of equipment. Br J Radiol 1999;72:173.

[15] Fordham LA, Brown ED, Washburn D, et al. Efficacy and feasibility of breast shielding during abdominal fluoroscopic examinations. Acad Radiol 1997;4:639.

[16] Auringer ST, Sumner TE. Pediatric upper gastrointestinal tract. Radiol Clin North Am 1994;32:1051.

[17] Coussement AM. Improving acceptance of barium by children by using milk for dilution. Radiology 1992;184:578.

[18] Miller RE. Flavoring barium sulfate. AJR Am J Roentgenol 1966;96:484.

[19] Neaman MP. On flavouring barium sulphate: use of an instant chocolate mixture. J Can Assoc Radiol 1966;17:231.

[20] Poznanski A. A simple device for administering barium to infants. Radiology 1969;93:1106.

[21] Shaw D. Technical note: an aid to barium meal in the infant. Br J Radiol 1995;68:78.

[22] McAlister WH, Askin FB. The effect of some contrast agents in the lung: an experimental study in the rat and dog. AJR Am J Roentgenol 1983;140:245.

[23] McAlister WH, Siegel MJ. Fatal aspirations in infancy during gastrointestinal series. Pediatr Radiol 1984;14:81.

[24] Margulis AR, Auh YH, Gagner M. Oral use of gadopentetate dimeglumine for anastomotic leak in patients with iodine sensitivity. Radiology 2004; 232:937.

[25] Aksglaede K, Funch-Jensen P, Thommesen P. Radiological demonstration of gastroesophageal reflux: diagnostic value of barium and bread studies compared with 24-hour pH monitoring. Acta Radiol 1999;40:652.

[26] Ott DJ. Gastroesophageal reflux: what is the role of barium studies? AJR Am J Roentgenol 1994; 162:627.

[27] Thompson JK, Koehler RE, Richter JE. Detection of gastroesophageal reflux: value of barium studies compared with 24-hr pH monitoring. AJR Am J Roentgenol 1994;162:621.

[28] Leonidas JC, Singh SP, Slovis TL. Congenital anomalies of the gastrointestinal tract. In: Kuhn JP, Slovis TL, Haller JO, editors. Caffey's pediatric diagnostic imaging, vol. 1. Philadelphia: Mosby; 2004. p. 113.

[29] Schlesinger AE, Parker BR. Congenital esophageal malformations. In: Kuhn JP, Slovis TL, Haller JO, editors. Caffey's pediatric diagnostic imaging, vol. 2. Philadelphia: Mosby; 2004. p. 1550–60.

[30] Luo CC, Lin JN, Lien R, et al. A new variant of esophageal atresia with distal tracheo-antral fistula associated with congenital intrathoracic stomach and situs inversus. J Pediatr Surg 2003;38:E25.

[31] Aszodi A, Chaimoff C, Dintsman M. Imperforate anus combined with esophageal atresia and agenesis of the right kidney: a case report. American Journal of Proctology 1974;25:59.

[32] Barnes JC, Smith WL. The VATER Association. Radiology 1978;126:445.

[33] Barry JE, Auldist AW. The Vater association: one end of a spectrum of anomalies. Am J Dis Child 1974;128:769.

[34] Beals RK, Rolfe B. VATER association: a unifying concept of multiple anomalies. J Bone Joint Surg Am 1989;71:948.

[35] Holder TM, Leape LL, Mann Jr CM. Esophageal atresia, tracheoesophageal fistula, and associated anomalies: hyperalimentation as an aid in treatment. J Thorac Cardiovasc Surg 1972;63:838.

[36] Smith DW. The VATER association. Am J Dis Child 1974;128:767.

[37] Tongsong T, Wanapirak C, Piyamongkol W, et al. Prenatal sonographic diagnosis of VATER association. J Clin Ultrasound 1999;27:378.

[38] Stringer DA, Ein SH. Recurrent tracheo-esophageal fistula: a protocol for investigation. Radiology 1984; 151:637.

[39] Johnson JF, Sueoka BL, Mulligan ME, et al. Tracheoesophageal fistula: diagnosis with CT. Pediatr Radiol 1985;15:134.

[40] Tsuchiya T, Mori K, Ichikawa T, et al. Bronchopulmonary foregut malformation diagnosed by three-dimensional CT. Pediatr Radiol 2003;33:887.

[41] Chernoff WG, White AK, Ballagh RH. Tracheoesophageal fistula: a case report. Int J Pediatr Otorhinolaryngol 1993;27:173.

[42] Orford J, Cass DT, Glasson MJ. Advances in the

treatment of oesophageal atresia over three decades: the 1970s and the 1990s. Pediatr Surg Int 2004; 20:402.

[43] Rothenberg SS. Thoracoscopic repair of tracheoesophageal fistula in newborns. J Pediatr Surg 2002;37:869.

[44] Allal H, Montes-Tapia F, Andina G, et al. Thoracoscopic repair of H-type tracheoesophageal fistula in the newborn: a technical case report. J Pediatr Surg 2004;39:1568.

[45] Tsai JY, Berkery L, Wesson DE, et al. Esophageal atresia and tracheoesophageal fistula: surgical experience over two decades. Ann Thorac Surg 1997; 64:778.

[46] Kleinman PK, Waite RJ, Cohen IT, et al. Atretic esophagus: transgastric balloon-assisted hydrostatic dilation. Radiology 1989;171:831.

[47] Chittmittrapap S, Spitz L, Kiely EM, et al. Anastomotic leakage following surgery for esophageal atresia. J Pediatr Surg 1992;27:29.

[48] Donnelly LF, Frush DP, Bisset GS. The appearance and significance of extrapleural fluid after esophageal atresia repair. AJR Am J Roentgenol 1999; 172:231.

[49] Nambirajan L, Rintala RJ, Losty PD, et al. The value of early postoperative oesophagography following repair of oesophageal atresia. Pediatr Surg Int 1998; 13:76.

[50] Yanchar NL, Gordon R, Cooper M, et al. Significance of the clinical course and early upper gastrointestinal studies in predicting complications associated with repair of esophageal atresia. J Pediatr Surg 2001; 36:815.

[51] Patel SB, Ade-Ajayi N, Kiely EM. Oesophageal atresia: a simplified approach to early management. Pediatr Surg Int 2002;18:87.

[52] Newman B, Bender TM. Esophageal atresia/ tracheoesophageal fistula and associated congenital esophageal stenosis. Pediatr Radiol 1997;27:530.

[53] Thomason MA, Gay BB. Esophageal stenosis with esophageal atresia. Pediatr Radiol 1987;17:197.

[54] Nishina T, Tsuchida Y, Saito S. Congenital esophageal stenosis due to tracheobronchial remnants and its associated anomalies. J Pediatr Surg 1981;16:190.

[55] Yeung CK, Spitz L, Brereton RJ, et al. Congenital esophageal stenosis due to tracheobronchial remnants: a rare but important association with esophageal atresia. J Pediatr Surg 1992;27:852.

[56] Said M, Mekki M, Golli M, et al. Balloon dilatation of anastomotic strictures secondary to surgical repair of oesophageal atresia. Br J Radiol 2003;76:26.

[57] Girdany BR, Sieber WK. Tracheoesophageal fistula without esophageal atresia: congenital and recurrent. Pediatrics 1956;18:935.

[58] Marzelle J, Dartevelle P, Khalife J, et al. Surgical management of acquired post-intubation tracheo-oesophageal fistulas: 27 patients. Eur J Cardiothorac Surg 1989;3:499.

[59] Rawlings DJ, Lawrence S, Goldstein JD. Acquired tracheoesophageal fistula in a premature infant. Am J Perinatol 1993;10:164.

[60] Amoury RA, Hrabovsky EE, Leonidas JC, et al. Tracheoesophageal fistual after lye ingestion. J Pediatr Surg 1975;10:273.

[61] Imamoglu M, Cay A, Kosucu P, et al. Acquired tracheo-esophageal fistulas caused by button battery lodged in the esophagus. Pediatr Surg Int 2004; 20:292.

[62] Ramesh JC, Ramanujam TM, Jayaram G. Congenital esophageal stenosis: report of three cases, literature review, and a proposed classification. Pediatr Surg Int 2001;17:188.

[63] Sheridan J, Hyde I. Oesophageal stenosis distal to oesophageal atresia. Clin Radiol 1990;42:274.

[64] Feng FH, Kong MS. Congenital esophageal stenosis treated with endoscopic balloon dilation: report of one case. Acta Paediatr Taiwan 1999;40:351.

[65] Amae S, Nio M, Kamiyama T, et al. Clinical characteristics and management of congenital esophageal stenosis: a report on 14 cases. J Pediatr Surg 2003;38:565.

[66] Dahniya MH, Grexa E, Ashebu S, et al. Communicating oesophageal duplication. Australas Radiol 2004;48:69.

[67] Wootton-Gorges SL, Eckel GM, Poulos ND, et al. Duplication of the cervical esophagus: a case report and review of the literature. Pediatr Radiol 2002; 32:533.

[68] Rafal RB, Markisz JA. Magnetic resonance imaging of an esophageal duplication cyst. Am J Gastroenterol 1991;86:1809.

[69] Rhee RS, Ray CG, Kravetz MH, et al. Cervical esophageal duplication cyst: MR imaging. J Comput Assist Tomogr 1988;12:693.

[70] Adkins Jr RB, Maples MD, Graham BS, et al. Dysphagia associated with an aortic arch anomaly in adults. Am Surg 1986;52:238.

[71] Yap J, Hayward PA, Lincoln C. Right aortic arch with aberrant subclavian arteries: a cause of esophageal compression. Ann Thorac Surg 1999;68:2331.

[72] Stoane J, Haller J, Orentlicher R. The gastrointestinal manifestations of pediatric aids. Radiol Clin North Am 1996;34:779.

[73] Becker MH, Swinyard CA. Epidermolysis bullosa dystrophica in children: radiologic manifestations. Radiology 1968;90:124.

[74] Lin AN, Carter DM. Epidermolysis bullosa. Annu Rev Med 1993;44:189.

[75] Mauro MA, Parker LA, Hartley WS, et al. Epidermolysis bullosa: radiographic findings in 16 cases. AJR Am J Roentgenol 1987;149:925.

[76] Orlando RC, Bozymski EM, Briggaman RA, et al. Epidermolysis bullosa: gastrointestinal manifestations. Ann Intern Med 1974;81:203.

[77] Harned RK, Strain JD, Hay TC, et al. Esophageal foreign bodies: safety and efficacy of Foley catheter extraction of coins. AJR Am J Roentgenol 1997; 168:443.

[78] Macpherson RI, Hill JG, Othersen HB, et al. Esophageal foreign bodies in children: diagnosis, treatment, and complications. AJR Am J Roentgenol 1996;166:919.

[79] Eggli KD, Potter BM, Garcia V, et al. Delayed diagnosis of esophageal perforation by aluminum foreign bodies. Pediatr Radiol 1986;16:511.

[80] Sharieff GQ, Brousseau TJ, Bradshaw JA, et al. Acute esophageal coin ingestions: is immediate removal necessary? Pediatr Radiol 2003;33:859.

[81] Cantu Jr S, Conners GP. The esophageal coin: is it a penny? Am Surg 2002;68:417.

[82] O'Hara SM, Donnelly LF, Chuang E, et al. Gastric retention of zinc-based pennies: radiographic appearance and hazards. Radiology 1999;213:113.

[83] Tibballs J, Wall R, Koottayi SV, et al. Tracheo-oesophageal fistula caused by electrolysis of a button battery impacted in the oesophagus. J Paediatr Child Health 2002;38:201.

[84] Yardeni D, Yardeni H, Coran AG, et al. Severe esophageal damage due to button battery ingestion: can it be prevented? Pediatr Surg Int 2004;20:496.

[85] Lao J, Bostwick HE, Berezin S, et al. Esophageal food impaction in children. Pediatr Emerg Care 2003;19:402.

[86] Berthold LD, Moritz JD, Sonksen S, et al. Esophageal foreign bodies: removal of the new euro coins with a magnet tube. Rofo Fortschr Geb Rontgenstr Neuen Bildgeb 2002;174:1096.

[87] Himadi GM, Fischer GJ. Magnetic removal of foreign bodies from the upper gastrointestinal tract. Radiology 1977;123:226.

[88] Myer CMR. Potential hazards of esophageal foreign body extraction. Pediatr Radiol 1991;21:97.

[89] Dominguez R, Zarabi M, Oh KS, et al. Congenital oesophageal stenosis. Clin Radiol 1985;36:263.

[90] Touloukian RJ, Beardsley GP, Ablow RC, et al. Traumatic perforation of the pharynx in the newborn. Pediatrics 1977;59:1019.

[91] Dubos JP, Bouchez MC, Kacet N, et al. Spontaneous rupture of the esophagus in the newborn. Pediatr Radiol 1986;16:317.

[92] Napierkowski J, Wong RK. Extraesophageal manifestations of GERD. Am J Med Sci 2003;326:285.

[93] Seibert JJ, Byrne WJ, Euler AR, et al. Gastro-esophageal reflux – the acid test: scintigraphy or the pH probe? AJR Am J Roentgenol 1983;140:1087.

[94] Vandenplas Y, Derde MP, Piepsz A. Evaluation of reflux episodes during simultaneous esophageal pH monitoring and gastroesophageal reflux scintigraphy in children. J Pediatr Gastroenterol Nutr 1992;14:256.

[95] Pan JJ, Levine MS, Redfern RO, et al. Gastro-esophageal reflux: comparison of barium studies with 24-h pH monitoring. Eur J Radiol 2003;47:149.

[96] Brady AP, Stevenson GW, Somers S, et al. Premature contraction of the cricopharyngeus: a new sign of gastroesophageal reflux disease. Abdom Imaging 1995;20:225.

[97] Esposito F, Lombardi R, Grasso AC, et al. Transabdominal sonography of the normal gastroesophageal junction in children. J Clin Ultrasound 2001;29:326.

[98] Gomes H, Menanteau B. Gastro-esophageal reflux: comparative study between sonography and pH monitoring. Pediatr Radiol 1991;21:168.

[99] Riccabona M, Maurer U, Lackner H, et al. The role of sonography in the evaluation of gastro-oesophageal reflux: correlation to pH-metry. Eur J Pediatr 1992;151:655.

[100] Westra SJ, Derkx HH, Taminiau JA. Symptomatic gastroesophageal reflux: diagnosis with ultrasound. J Pediatr Gastroenterol Nutr 1994;19:58.

[101] Koumanidou C, Vakaki M, Pitsoulakis G, et al. Sonographic measurement of the abdominal esophagus length in infancy: a diagnostic tool for gastroesophageal reflux. AJR Am J Roentgenol 2004;183:801.

[102] Fonkalsrud EW, Ashcraft KW, Coran AG, et al. Surgical treatment of gastroesophageal reflux in children: a combined hospital study of 7467 patients. Pediatrics 1998;101:419.

[103] Frantzides CT, Richards C. A study of 362 consecutive laparoscopic Nissen fundoplications. Surgery 1998;124:651.

[104] Trinh TD, Benson JE. Fluoroscopic diagnosis of complications after Nissen antireflux fundoplication in children. AJR Am J Roentgenol 1997;169:1023.

[105] Buratti S, Savides TJ, Newbury RO, et al. Granular cell tumor of the esophagus: report of a pediatric case and literature review. J Pediatr Gastroenterol Nutr 2004;38:97.

ELSEVIER
SAUNDERS

Radiol Clin N Am 43 (2005) 303 – 323

RADIOLOGIC
CLINICS
of North America

Imaging Evaluation of Congenital Lung Abnormalities in Infants and Children

Anne Paterson, MB BS, MRCP, FRCR, FFR RCSI

Radiology Department, Royal Belfast Hospital for Sick Children, 180 Falls Road, Belfast BT12 6BE, UK

Congenital lung abnormalities include a wide spectrum of conditions and are an important cause of morbidity and mortality in infants and children. This article discusses focal lung abnormalities (eg, congenital lobar emphysema [CLE], congenital cystic adenomatoid malformation [CCAM], bronchopulmonary foregut malformations [BPFM], pulmonary sequestrations) and the dysmorphic lung (lung-lobar agenesis–hypoplasia complex). Pulmonary arteriovenous malformations (AVMs) are also included. Thus, anomalies affecting the pulmonary parenchyma, its arterial supply, and venous drainage are discussed. Disorders of the airways are described elsewhere in this issue.

Congenital lobar emphysema

Lobar emphysema can either be acquired, or secondary or congenital. CLE refers to progressive overinflation of a pulmonary lobe secondary to air trapping; a ball-valve mechanism allows air into the lobe when there is negative intrathoracic pressure during inspiration, but fails to allow the air out during expiration. Bronchomalacia caused by a deficiency of bronchial cartilage, bronchostenosis, bronchotorsion, obstructive mucosal flaps or mucosal thickening, cartilaginous septa, and bronchial atresia have all been described pathologically in CLE lobectomy specimens [1–5]. In others, no cause is found. Secondary lobar emphysema may result if the bronchus is extrinsically compressed, for example by an enlarged right ventricular outflow tract in patients with congenital heart disease [1,2]. Indeed, there is a reported increase in the incidence of congenital heart disease in association with CLE [2,4]. Lobar overinflation may also occur with an intraluminal obstruction, such as an aspirated foreign body.

Some authors prefer the expression *congenital lobar overinflation* to CLE. This is because microscopically, CLE specimens do not always demonstrate alveolar destruction. Rather, the alveoli are overdistended but intact [4,6,7]. In a pathologic variant of CLE known as the *polyalveolar lobe*, the alveoli are normal in size or small, but are increased in number threefold to fivefold [8]. The airways are normal. When the alveoli distend with air, the lobe overinflates because of the sheer number of air spaces.

Clinically, most infants with CLE present within the first 6 months of life, with symptoms and signs of respiratory distress. The earlier the child presents, the more severe is the involvement. There is a preponderance of male patients. The chest radiograph remains the primary imaging tool. CLE has a predilection for the upper lobes and right middle lobe. The lower lobes are involved in less than 1% of cases. Bilateral or multifocal involvement is rare [3]. The appearance on the chest radiograph depends on timing: if the radiograph is taken in the first 24 hours of life, the involved lobe is seen to be distended and opaque, because of retained fetal lung fluid. This fluid progressively clears by the tracheobronchial system, lymphatic vessels, and capillary network. The lobe increases in size as it distends with air and demonstrates acinar shadowing, a reticular interstitial

E-mail address: annie.paterson@royalhospitals.n-i.nhs.uk

pattern, and finally becomes hyperlucent. The degree of overinflation may cause the overinflated lobe to herniate across the midline. Adjacent lobes are compressed, the ipsilateral hemidiaphragm is depressed, and rib spacing is increased. With severe overdistention of a lobe, contralateral lobar compression results and there is cardiomediastinal shift (Fig. 1). Attenuated lung markings are seen in the overinflated lobe, helping to differentiate it from a pneumothorax. In addition, compression of adjacent lobes pushes them cephalad toward the lung apex or caudad toward the diaphragm. With a pneumothorax, the lung collapses around the hilum. Other differential diagnoses include secondary lobar emphysema; congenital lung cysts (including type I CCAM); pneumatoceles; and the Swyer-James syndrome (unilateral hyperlucent lung). The lateral view shows anterior sternal bowing and posterior displacement of the heart.

CT scans demonstrate which lobes or segments are involved. The affected lobe is overdistended and hypodense, with attenuated vascular markings (Fig. 2). The septa and vascular structures are at the periphery of the distended alveoli [7]. No cysts or soft tissue are seen. CT is useful to exclude secondary causes of lobar overinflation, such as a vascular ring or a mediastinal mass lesion. In addition to the axial

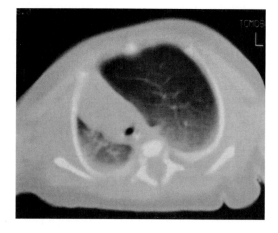

Fig. 2. Congenital lobar emphysema. CT scan of the chest (lung windows) at the level of the thymus, demonstrating overinflation of the left upper lobe with attenuation of the vascular markings. The mediastinal structures are shifted to the right side and the right upper lobe is compressed.

data set, virtual bronchoscopy images may help to define bronchostenosis and exclude an intraluminal foreign body (in an older child). Unsuspected multifocal disease is identified.

Some authors perform ventilation-perfusion scanning on infants with less severe symptoms. This shows a matched defect in the affected lobe when Kr-81m is used for the ventilation studies. Adjacent lobes tend to be both ventilated and perfused, despite appearing compressed and atelectatic on the chest radiograph [1,9].

Traditionally, symptomatic patients with CLE undergo lobectomy. Infants are reported to tolerate lobectomy well, with compensatory growth of the remaining lobes [6,10]. Asymptomatic children or those with only minor symptoms are increasingly being managed conservatively [1,2,6]. Follow-up imaging on this group of children has shown a gradual reduction in size of the involved lobe with time. Serial ventilation-perfusion scans have shown ventilation of the lobe to improve and normalize. The involved lobe, however, may remain underperfused [9].

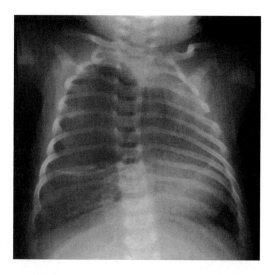

Fig. 1. Congenital lobar emphysema. Chest radiograph of a neonate who developed respiratory distress soon after birth. There is marked overinflation of the right upper lobe, which herniated across the midline. There is compression of the adjacent right middle lobe, contralateral shift of the heart and mediastinum, and widening of the rib spaces on the right side.

Congenital cystic adenomatoid malformation

CCAM is thought to result from a failure of normal bronchoalveolar development early in fetal life. There is communication between the individual cysts within the CCAM and also with the tracheobronchial tree. The classification of Stocker et al [11] has been widely used in both radiologic and pathologic literature.

> Type I CCAMs: contain one or more cysts measuring over 2 cm in diameter, surrounded by multiple smaller cysts. The cysts are lined by ciliated columnar epithelium and their walls contain abundant elastic tissue.
>
> Type II CCAMs: contain cysts measuring up to 2 cm in diameter. These cysts are lined with cuboidal or columnar epithelium and are said to resemble dilated bronchioles.
>
> Type III CCAMs: usually contain cysts less than 0.5 cm in diameter and are lined by cuboidal epithelium.

Type I CCAMs are the most common type seen in radiologic practice, constituting approximately 70% of cases [4]. Type II CCAMs make up around 15% to 20% of cases. Type II CCAMs are associated with other congenital anomalies, including renal agenesis and dysgenesis, cardiac malformations, and pulmonary sequestrations (see later) [5,12–15]. Type III CCAMs are rarely seen postnatally and have a poor prognosis.

CCAMs occur with equal frequency in the upper and lower lobes, but are less often seen in the right middle lobe. Typically, they are unilobar, but segmental CCAMs and lesions involving more than one pulmonary segment or lobe have been reported [6,13,15–17].

In the past, CCAM was usually diagnosed in the early neonatal period, in infants who presented with varying signs of respiratory distress. These days, however, CCAM is increasingly being diagnosed on antenatal ultrasound (US) examinations, where it is seen as an echogenic mass, which may or may not contain cysts [5,17–19]. A CCAM diagnosed in the second trimester of pregnancy, may remain unchanged on subsequent follow-up scans. The lesions, however, can also increase in size and be associated with the development of maternal polyhydramnios or fetal nonimmune hydrops fetalis. The development of nonimmune hydrops fetalis is associated with a poor prognosis [2,5,12,14,18,20]. Antenatal MR imaging may help to evaluate any associated pulmonary hypoplasia and predict the prognosis [20]. Some antenatal CCAMs disappear completely on follow-up US examinations [5,14,18–20]. Such infants may or may not be symptomatic at birth. Older children and adults may also present with a CCAM, usually in the context of recurrent respiratory infections. The

definitive diagnosis of a CCAM is difficult to make in the latter group of patients, because a pathologic specimen from a healing necrotizing pneumonitic process can resemble a CCAM. CCAMs may also be diagnosed incidentally on a chest radiograph.

Postnatally, symptomatic infants with respiratory distress and infants with a previously documented antenatal US anomaly should have a chest radiograph performed. The radiographic findings are variable and correlate with the type of lesion present. Type I CCAMs demonstrate a multicystic lesion, although there can be one dominant cyst (see Fig. 2). Early radiographs may show a water-density mass if the cysts are filled with retained fetal lung fluid; this tends to clear over the first few days of life. In the presence of infection, there may be adjacent alveolar shadowing. Mass effect can cause contralateral mediastinal shift, inversion of the ipsilateral hemidiaphragm, and compression and atelectasis of both ipsilateral and contralateral pulmonary lobes. The involved lobe may herniate across the midline to the opposite side (Fig. 3). As the cysts fill with air, respiratory symptoms can worsen. Type II CCAMs show cysts of a smaller size (Fig. 4), again with the possibility of lesion heterogeneity if some fetal lung fluid is retained. Type III CCAMs tend to be seen as a homogeneous, soft tissue density mass.

The differential diagnosis of a type I or II CCAM in a neonate includes congenital diaphragmatic hernia; a pulmonary sequestration (PS); CLE; and a bronchogenic (or other BPFM) cyst. The visualization of an intact hemidiaphragm and a normal bowel gas pattern in the upper abdomen helps to exclude the former. If the postnatal chest radiograph is reported as normal in an infant with an antenatally diagnosed lung mass (even one that has reportedly disappeared), then it is advisable for these infants to have a CT scan [5,14,19,20], because many have radiographically occult pulmonary abnormalities. CT scans are helpful to document the involved pulmonary segments or lobes and also confirm the diagnosis in symptomatic infants. CT angiography defines the presence of any systemic arterial vessels supplying the involved lung (a hybrid lesion), an important practical point for those infants in whom surgery is being considered. A CCAM appears as a multicystic mass with CT examination. Fluid-filled cysts and air-fluid levels are easily appreciated. In those presenting with recurrent infections (Fig. 5), then differentiation from a necrotizing pneumonia is important. The relatively greater degree of overinflation and the lack of visible air bronchograms favor a CCAM [2,4].

The management of patients with CCAM is controversial. Symptomatic neonates with respiratory

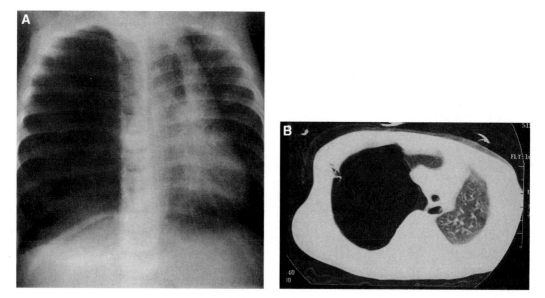

Fig. 3. (*A*) Type I congenital cystic adenomatoid malformation in a 12-month-old boy who presented with shortness of breath. Chest radiograph shows a hyperlucent right hemithorax, with contralateral shift of the heart and mediastinal structures. Sparse lung markings are seen in the right hemithorax. (*From* Donnelly LF. Chest. In: Fundamentals of pediatric radiology. Philadelphia: WB Saunders; 2001. p. 38.) (*B*) CT scan of the chest (lung windows) demonstrates a large cyst filling the right hemithorax. The compressed right middle lobe is seen behind the sternum.

distress usually proceed to surgery. Older children and adults with recurrent pneumonia are also recommended for surgery. The management of those patients with a radiologic CCAM who remain asymptomatic is less clear-cut. Certainly, there is a risk of infection developing in a CCAM and there are also several case reports of malignancy arising in CCAM. Bronchoalveolar carcinoma, pleuropulmonary blastoma, rhabdomyosarcoma, and bronchogenic carcinoma have all been reported [6,15,21–26]. Some authors advocate surgery in these patients, to eradicate the risk of future infection or tumor. Other

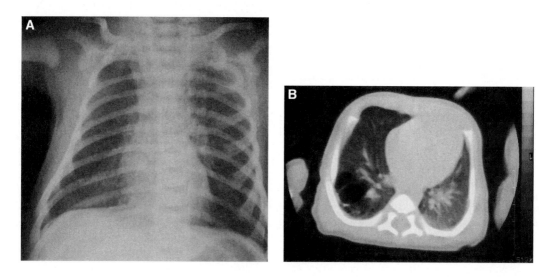

Fig. 4. (*A*) Type II congenital cystic adenomatoid malformation in an asymptomatic neonate (antenatal diagnosis). Chest radiograph shows a hazy opacity in the right lower lobe and upward bowing of the minor fissure. (*B*) CT chest (lung windows) confirms the presence of several small cysts in the right lower lobe. This infant was managed conservatively.

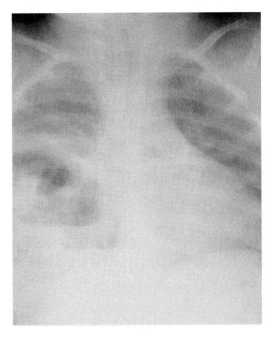

Fig. 5. Chest radiograph of a 2-year-old infant who presented with symptoms and signs suggestive of pneumonia. Multiple air-fluid levels are seen in an infected right lower lobe congenital cystic adenomatoid malformation.

centers prefer to follow such patients expectantly [14,18,20].

Bronchopulmonary foregut malformation

BPFM encompasses a spectrum of developmental abnormalities derived from the embryonic foregut. Duplication cysts arising anywhere from the pharynx to the duodenum, neurenteric cysts, bronchogenic cysts, pulmonary sequestrations, and occasionally CCAMs and CLE are included in this group of lesions. BPFM may or may not communicate with the lumen of the gastrointestinal tract or the airway (Fig. 6). There is no complete unifying embryologic theory to explain their origin.

Esophageal duplication cysts

Esophageal duplication cysts (EDCs) are the second most frequent type of enteric duplication (after ileal) accounting for 15% to 20% of cases [4,27]. Pathologically, they have a well-developed coat of smooth muscle and are lined by epithelium derived from some portion of the alimentary tract. Most lie adjacent to the wall of the esophagus or are intra-

mural, but extraluminal. Gastrointestinal tract duplications may be either spherical or tubular in shape. The latter are much less common, but are more likely to communicate with the lumen of the gastrointestinal tract. Tubular duplications may span more than one segment of the gastrointestinal tract and present as transdiaphragmatic thoracoabdominal masses.

Patients may be asymptomatic, with the cyst being discovered incidentally when they are imaged for some other indication. Alternatively, they may present with acute or subacute symptoms, the nature of which depend on the anatomic location of the cyst, the mass effect it causes, or complications related to the cyst lining. Approximately 60% of EDCs are located in the distal third of the esophagus, 17% are in the middle third, and 23% are at the cervical level [27]. The more distal the location, the more likely the cyst is to be asymptomatic. Cervical EDCs may present as a painless enlarging neck mass or with symptoms of upper airway obstruction. EDCs located in the middle third of the esophagus are more likely to cause airway obstruction leading to cough,

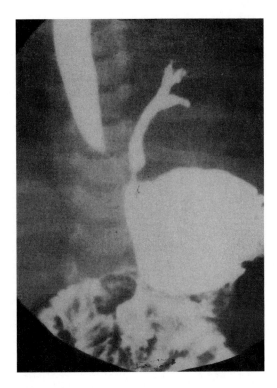

Fig. 6. Bronchopulmonary foregut malformation in a 3-month-old infant who presented with recurrent apneic episodes. Upper gastrointestinal contrast study shows reflux of barium into an aberrant bronchus, which communicates with the left lower lobe.

wheeze, shortness of breath, and recurrent infection. Impingement on the adjacent esophagus can cause dysphagia, vomiting, or feeding intolerance. Over 40% of EDCs are lined by gastric mucosa; this can bleed or ulcerate [4,27–30]. Ulceration may cause the cyst to perforate into the adjacent airway or esophagus causing hemoptysis or hematemesis. Rarely, EDCs may be discovered in remote or ectopic locations, such as the pleural space, tongue, and subcutaneous tissues [27,29]. Vertebral segmentation anomalies, esophageal atresia, and other types of BPFM (mixed lesions) are recognized in association with EDCs [4,27,30].

A mediastinal EDC lies posteriorly on the lateral chest radiograph. The cysts are well-demarcated and usually of soft tissue density. Cervical EDCs may be examined using US, when a cystic lesion lined by an echo-bright mucosal layer is seen [27]. A barium swallow study either shows the esophagus deviated to one side by the cyst or an intramural, extraluminal filling defect (Fig. 7). Tubular EDCs may fill with contrast (Fig. 8). Given that a high percentage of EDCs contain gastric mucosa, technetium-99m pertechnetate scintigraphy is occasionally used to aid in narrowing the differential diagnosis. When scintigraphy is performed, whole-body images should be obtained, because enteric duplications may be multiple (18% of cases) [27] and those in more distant locations may also contain gastric mucosa. CT or MR imaging studies help to define the precise anatomic location of the lesion and allow evaluation of the airway, the pulmonary parenchyma (CT), and the

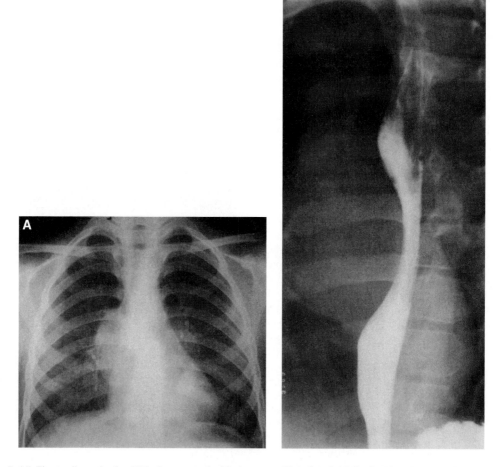

Fig. 7. (*A*) Chest radiograph of a child who presented with shortness of breath and dysphagia. There is a posterior mediastinal mass lesion projecting to the right of the spine. (*B*) Oblique view from an upper gastrointestinal contrast study in the same patient shows the mass narrowing the lumen of the esophagus. At surgery this proved to be a spherical esophageal duplication cyst.

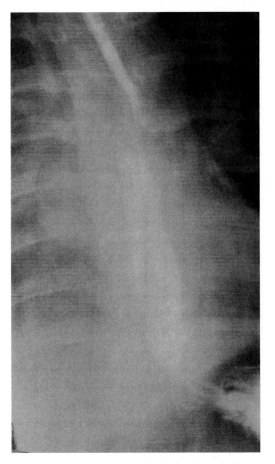

Fig. 8. Fluoro-grab image from an upper gastrointestinal tract contrast study in a 6-month-old infant who presented with recurrent chest infections. There is a tubular esophageal duplication cyst filled with contrast.

spinal canal (MR imaging). The latter is particularly important if vertebral segmentation anomalies have been seen on the frontal chest radiograph. The attenuation or signal of the cyst varies. An uncomplicated EDC is of near water density (ie, $0-20$ HU) on CT, and of low signal intensity on T1- and high signal intensity on T2-weighted images. Hemorrhage into the cyst increases its attenuation on CT images and increases the signal on T1-weighted MR images. Endoscopic US is little used in children at present; when performed, US can confirm continuity of the muscle layers of the esophageal wall and the cyst [4,28].

The differential diagnosis of an EDC depends on its location. In the neck, lymphangiomas, branchial cleft cysts, thyroglossal duct cysts, and atypical abscess are important to distinguish. Posterior and mid-

dle mediastinal lesions, such as neurogenic tumors, anterior meningoceles, and bronchogenic and neurenteric cysts, may have similar imaging appearances in the thorax and more distally.

Most authors agree that EDCs should be surgically resected regardless of whether or not they are symptomatic. There is a high incidence of complications arising in EDCs, including reports of malignant degeneration [29,30]. Both adenocarcinomas and rhabdomyosarcomas have been reported.

Neurenteric cysts

These are the least common subtype of BPFM [28]. They are thought most likely to represent a persistent connection between the spinal canal and primitive foregut [13,31]. Clinically, the patients may present with symptoms relating to the mediastinal component of the cyst or with symptoms suggestive of cord compression. The presence of a posterior mediastinal mass lesion and vertebral segmentation anomalies on the chest radiograph should suggest the diagnosis. MR imaging is the imaging modality of choice to assess the intraspinal component of the lesion before surgical resection (Fig. 9) [13,28].

Bronchogenic cysts

Bronchogenic cysts are thought to arise secondary to abnormal budding of the primitive ventral foregut, early in fetal life. They may be located in the mediastinum or within the pulmonary parenchyma. The former are more common, accounting for around 70% of cases [2,4,5,32]. Rarely, bronchogenic cysts may be found in the neck, pericardium, or abdominal cavity [4,5,32,33]. Uncomplicated bronchogenic cysts do not usually communicate with the tracheobronchial tree. Anatomically, mediastinal type bronchogenic cysts are found in subcarinal, hilar, or right paratracheal locations most commonly. Intrapulmonary masses are more likely to be right-sided.

As with other types of BPFMs, bronchogenic cysts may be an incidental finding on the chest radiograph. Symptomatic infants usually present with respiratory distress. Older children are more likely to present with infected cysts. Spontaneous pneumothorax is a rare presenting symptom of a bronchogenic cyst [34].

The chest radiograph is diagnostic in three out of four cases [2,13]. The cyst is commonly filled with serous or proteinaceous fluid and appears as a well-demarcated soft tissue mass of soft tissue density

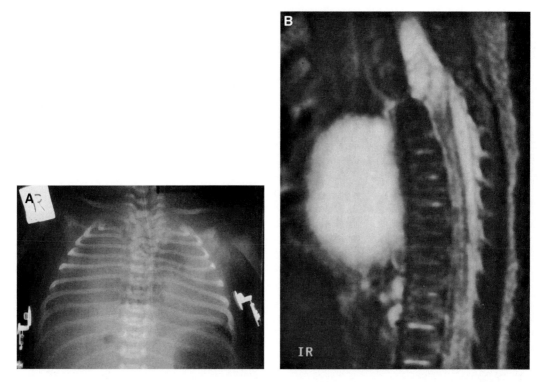

Fig. 9. (*A*) Neurenteric cyst. Chest radiograph of a female neonate who presented with respiratory distress soon after birth. The right hemithorax is opaque and there is contralateral shift of the heart and mediastinal structures. Multiple vertebral segmentation anomalies are seen in the upper thoracic spine. (*B*) Parasagittal T2-weighted fast spin echo MR image shows a high signal mass in the right hemithorax, which communicates with an extradural cystic lesion by one of the anomalous upper thoracic vertebra. There is also an intramedullary component to the lesion. (*From* Paterson A, Sweeney LE. Radiological case of the month. Arch Pediatr 1999;153:645–6. Copyrighted © 1999, American Medical Association; with permission.)

(Fig. 10). Airway compression by the cyst may lead to overinflation of an adjacent lobe if there is air trapping or to lobar atelectasis. Infection of the cyst may lead to surrounding acinar shadowing. An air-fluid level may be present if a complicating tracheobronchial connection develops. Peripheral calcification and layering of fluid with a *milk of calcium* appearance have also been described on plain radiographs [35].

At CT, the precise anatomic location of the cyst can be defined (Fig. 11). The attenuation of uncomplicated cysts varies from water density (0–20 HU) to more solid looking lesions with attenuations of greater than 30 HU [36]. Higher attenuation values are found in bronchogenic cysts complicated by intracyst hemorrhage. Bronchogenic cysts do not enhance following intravenous contrast administration.

Typically, bronchogenic cysts have high signal on T2-weighted MR images. The signal on T1-weighted MR imaging is variable dependent on the protein content of the cyst fluid and whether or not intracyst hemorrhage has occurred [13,32,37,38]. Fluid-fluid levels have also been reported in nonhemorrhagic bronchogenic cysts on MR images [38]. This is postulated to be caused by dependent layering of the proteinaceous contents. Occasionally, bronchogenic cysts may mimic a solid lesion [32,33] with intermediate signal intensity on T1-weighted sequences and intensity lower than that of water on T2-weighted images.

Complications of bronchogenic cysts include infection, hemorrhage, and erosion into adjacent structures. More rarely reported is the development of malignancy within the walls of the cyst; rhabdomyosarcoma, pulmonary blastoma, anaplastic carcinoma, leiomyosarcoma, and adenocarcinoma have all been reported [6,23,29,32,39]. An irregular enhancing wall, a solid nodule, and heterogeneity of the cyst contents should be viewed with suspicion [32,39]. The propensity of bronchogenic cysts to develop

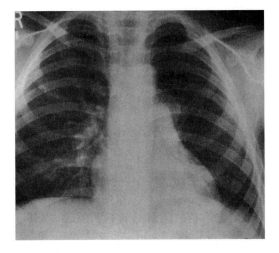

Fig. 10. Bronchogenic cyst. Chest radiograph of a 5-year-old boy who presented with recurrent pneumonias. There is a well-defined, rounded mediastinal mass lesion seen adjacent to the left hilum. Consolidation is present in the left lower lobe behind the heart.

complications supports surgical resection, regardless of the age at presentation.

Pulmonary sequestration

A PS is defined as a segment of lung parenchyma that receives its blood supply from the systemic circulation and that does not communicate with the tracheobronchial tree. Classically, two forms of PS have been described: extralobar (ELPS) and intralobar (ILPS). ELPS is an entirely separate segment of pulmonary tissue that is invested in its own pleural layers. It accounts for 25% of PS and it is typically found in the costophrenic sulcus on the left side. ELPS may also be located in the mediastinum, pericardium, and within or below the diaphragm [2,5,18,40–42]. The abdominal or thoracic aorta usually supplies the arterial vessels, but in some cases (10%–15%) smaller arteries, such as the celiac axis and its branches, the subclavian arteries, and the intercostal arteries, may supply an ELPS [40–42]. In 80% of cases venous drainage is to the systemic circulation [2,40–43], usually by way of the azygous system or inferior vena cava. The remaining cases drain by the pulmonary circulation.

ILPS is a segment of pulmonary tissue that shares the visceral pleural covering of the normal, adjacent lung tissue. ILPS account for 75% of PS [40–42,44] and are usually located in the posterobasal portion of the lower lobes. The arterial supply is typically

from the thoracic or upper abdominal aorta and most drain by way of the pulmonary venous system to the left atrium.

The embryology of both ILPS and ELPS is disputed. Most authors agree that ELPS is a true developmental anomaly that arises from a supernumerary lung bud [18,41,45] from the primitive foregut. This connection may persist, giving rise to a communication with the gastrointestinal tract.

Some authors argue that ILPS are acquired lesions that arise in chronically infected lung segments, with bronchial occlusion and a parasitized systemic arterial supply [2,5,44,45] to support a compromised segment of lung. This theory is supported by the fact that ILPS tend to present later in life and are associated with recurrent pneumonias. ILPS are increasingly being diagnosed in neonates and young infants before the development of pulmonary infections [5,6,14,19, 44,46], however, supporting the assertion that some ILPS are congenital lesions. ILPS may also have a patent communication with the gastrointestinal tract.

ELPS are usually diagnosed in early life. They are associated with other congenital malformations in over 50% of cases, most noticeably congenital diaphragmatic hernias; congenital heart disease; and CCAM type II (hybrid lesions) [2,4–6,18,41–45]. Infants may present with symptoms caused by the associated anomaly, with respiratory distress, or feeding difficulties, or the PS may be an incidental prenatal or postnatal imaging finding. During pregnancy, such complications as polyhydramnios and nonimmune hydrops are recognized. High-output cardiac failure may result from the left-right shunting of blood.

ILPS are more commonly diagnosed in later childhood or even in adults. They may be incidental findings on a chest radiograph or be picked up in an individual who has been treated for recurrent pneu-

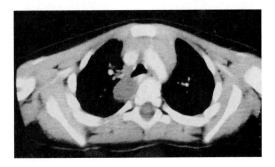

Fig. 11. Bronchogenic cyst. CT chest at the level of the aortic arch, following intravenous contrast material administration. A well-defined, nonenhancing, cystic mass is seen posterior to the origin of the right mainstem bronchus.

monias or hemoptysis. Prenatal diagnosis of ILPS is increasingly recognized and ILPS may be associated with neonatal cardiac failure caused by left-left shunting of blood. Associated congenital anomalies are reported in 6% to 12% of cases with ILPS [44].

Pathologically, an ELPS resembles normal lung tissue, except there is dilatation and tortuosity of the bronchioles, alveolar ducts, and alveoli [41]. ELPS do not contain air unless they communicate with the foregut. ILPSs are covered in thickened pleura that are generally stuck to the adjacent structures. The parenchyma is fibrotic and consolidated and contains small cysts [13,44]. The cysts may be filled with fluid, gelatinous material, or frank pus. Foci of acute pneumonia of fungal infection may be present [44]. Aeration of ILPS can occur by the pores of Kohn, adjacent small bronchi, or a foregut communication [40].

It is difficult to distinguish between an ELPS and an ILPS on plain radiographs alone. ELPS are usually found as well-defined, solid, retrocardiac masses in the cardiophrenic angle. Air bronchograms are absent. They may be found as a subdiaphragmatic or mediastinal mass lesion. Larger lesions can be associated with an opaque ipsilateral hemithorax and a pleural effusion. ILPS tend to be more heterogeneous and less well defined. Focal bronchiectasis, areas of atelectasis, cavitation, and cyst formation may also be recognized within an ILPS. Calcification of either type of PS is unusual.

The main diagnostic feature that must be identified by imaging in either type of PS is the feeding systemic arterial vessels (Figs. 12 and 13). In the past,

conventional angiography was the modality of choice to do this; this is no longer the case. US with color Doppler is a readily available, noninvasive technique, which is particularly useful in the neonate and young infant. Gray-scale imaging can outline the mass adjacent to the hemidiaphragm. It may be seen as a homogeneous, echogenic mass or may be heterogeneous and contain cysts. The arterial supply and possibly the venous drainage can then be shown with color Doppler [41–43,47,48].

CT and MR imaging provide a more global assessment of sequestration and are, in general, recommended for full evaluation. CT images show an ELPS as a homogeneous, well-circumscribed mass of soft tissue attenuation. The mass may enhance brightly with intravenous contrast material. Cystic areas may be seen within the mass. An ILPS may have a more irregular outline and also a more heterogeneous appearance. Cysts and areas of cavitation with air-fluid levels may be seen. Emphysematous changes in the adjacent lung and hypervascularity of the sequestered segment have also been reported [47,49,50]. CT angiography techniques can identify the aberrant systemic arterial supply [13,41,44,49,51,52] and with three-dimensional rendering of multidetector row CT, also the venous drainage [52].

As an alternative to CT, MR imaging may also be used to identify the feeding arterial vessels and further delineate the character of the mass. The mass is usually of high signal on both T1- and T2-weighted images. Any hemorrhage or cystic components are easily identified using standard spin echo sequences. Gradient echo sequences may identify the arterial

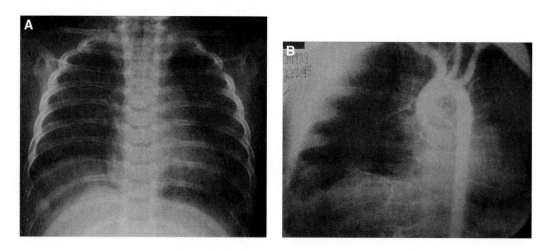

Fig. 12. (*A*) Pulmonary sequestration in an infant girl. Chest radiograph shows a soft tissue mass adjacent to the right hemidiaphragm. (*B*) The arterial supply to the sequestrated segment arises from the descending aorta, as demonstrated on this conventional aortogram.

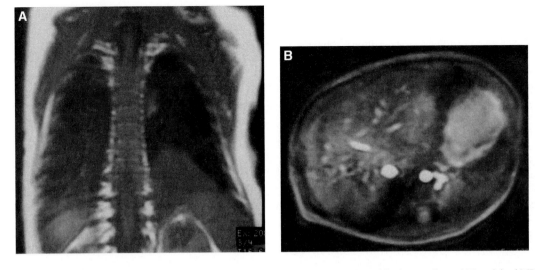

Fig. 13. (*A*) Female neonate with an antenatal diagnosis of a mass adjacent to the left hemidiaphragm. Coronal T1-weighted MR image shows the soft tissue mass lying posteromedially, abutting the left hemidiaphragm. (*B*) Axial gradient echo MR image shows the arterial supply arising from the descending aorta.

supply and two-dimensional time-of-fight MR angiography has also been used [47]. The latter is limited by low spatial resolution and turbulent flow. Breath-hold, contrast-enhanced MR angiography (if necessary under general anesthesia in infants and young children) offers superior images [47,53,54].

Additional imaging studies that may be helpful include an upper gastrointestinal contrast examination, if a communication with the gastrointestinal tract is suspected. Bronchography and conventional arteriography are unnecessary in general with modern noninvasive imaging options.

Antenatally, PS is seen as a well-defined, hyperechoic mass lesion at US; the mass may contain cysts. Doppler US may demonstrate the anomalous vascular supply. More recently, antenatal MR imaging has been used to confirm the diagnosis. Serial antenatal and postnatal imaging in asymptomatic infants has shown gradual shrinkage of these lesions in some cases [18,19,45,55].

Most PS is managed surgically. ELPS are resected. ILPS generally require a segmentectomy or lobectomy, particularly when there is a history of recurrent infection. More recently, embolization of the feeding arterial vessels has been described in the treatment of PS [56].

Hybrid lesions

A PS may coexist with CCAM. ELPS are reported to exist with type II CCAM in up to 50% of cases [57]. PS and CCAM likely represent part of a

spectrum of related congenital lung anomalies [55]. Although the definitive diagnosis of such a hybrid lesion is obviously made by the pathologist, the radiologist needs to be alert to the possibility and to search for an aberrant systemic arterial vessel when imaging suspected cases of CCAM (Fig. 14). The natural history of these lesions depends on the size of the pulmonary mass lesion and the physiologic problems it causes [55].

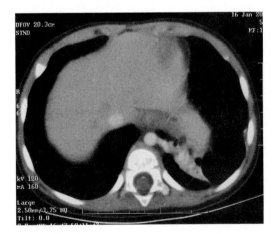

Fig. 14. Hybrid lesion. CT scan at the level of the diaphragm following intravenous contrast material administration. The arterial supply to the left lower lobe mass lesion arises from the descending aorta. The pathology of this segment revealed a type II congenital cystic adenomatoid malformation in a sequestered segment. (Courtesy of Dr. K.A. Duncan, Aberdeen Royal Infirmary, Scotland.)

Isolated systemic arterial supply to normal lung

Although anomalous systemic arterial supply is a recognized feature of PS, CCAM (hybrid lesions), and the scimitar syndrome, the presence of a systemic arterial vessel supplying normal lung tissue is a much rarer occurrence. Patients may be asymptomatic or they may present with heart failure secondary to the left-left shunt, hemoptysis, or for investigation of a vascular murmur. This abnormality is thought to arise because of persistence of an embryologic connection between the aorta and pulmonary parenchyma [58]. The basal segments of the left lower lobe are most commonly involved. Drainage is to the inferior pulmonary vein and they retain a normal tracheobronchial tree.

With chest radiography, the anomalous vessel may be seen as a serpiginous opacity behind the heart; the left pulmonary artery is usually small [58,59]. The diagnosis can be confirmed by CT or MR angiography. The former technique is preferred, because it gives greater detail about the tracheobronchial tree and the pulmonary parenchyma of the involved segment [58,59]. Patients are managed conservatively unless there is left heart overload, in which case segmentectomy or lobectomy may be performed.

Dysmorphic lung

Lung agenesis–hypoplasia complex

Lung agenesis–hypoplasia complex describes arrested development of the whole lung and may be categorized as:

Lung agenesis: total absence of the lung and bronchi; or

Lung aplasia: total absence of the lung with a rudimentary main bronchus; or

Lung hypoplasia: hypoplastic bronchi and an associated variable amount of lung tissue [60–63].

In both lung agenesis and aplasia, the ipsilateral pulmonary artery is absent. Lung hypoplasia is discussed separately.

Unilateral lung agenesis–aplasia occurs with equal frequency on both the right and left sides. There is no sex predilection. Bilateral agenesis–aplasia is obviously fatal [60,62,64]. Around half of all patients with lung agenesis–aplasia have associated congenital anomalies, most frequently radial ray defects and facial or ear abnormalities. These are usually ipsilateral to the pulmonary abnormality [64]. Lung agenesis may also form part of the complex including vertebral (and other osseous) anomalies; cardiovascular defects; anorectal malformations; esophageal atresia and tracheoesophageal fistula; and genitourinary anomalies [62,65]. In these instances it may occur as an alternative to esophageal atresia and tracheoesophageal fistula.

Lung agenesis–aplasia may remain asymptomatic throughout life, particularly when there are no other congenital abnormalities. There is a group of children, however, who present early with respiratory distress and recurrent pulmonary infections. Airway compression by the aortic arch, pulmonary artery, and ductus arteriosus, along with intrinsic tracheobronchial anomalies (tracheal stenosis, tracheobronchial-malacia) may in part be responsible, particularly with right-sided agenesis–aplasia [66]. Spillage of contents from a rudimentary bronchial pouch into the opposite lung may help to disseminate infection [40,43]. Several authors report a worse prognosis for right-sided lesions. This is attributed to greater hemodynamic disturbance, secondary to a more marked shift of the heart and mediastinal great vessels [62].

The frontal chest radiograph classically demonstrates a small, opaque hemithorax, with ipsilateral heart and mediastinal shift, and elevation of the hemidiaphragm on the affected side. The contralateral lung is overinflated and herniated across the midline (Fig. 15). The differential diagnosis for this appear-

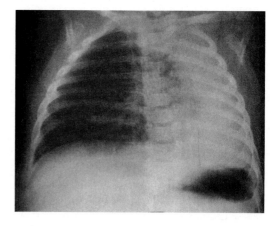

Fig. 15. Left lung agenesis. Chest radiograph shows a small, opaque left hemithorax with ipsilateral shift of the heart and mediastinal structures. There is compensatory overinflation of the right lung, which herniated across the midline.

ance includes whole-lung atelectasis, postpneumonectomy, fibrothorax, and aspiration of a foreign body. The clinical history and physical examination findings help to differentiate. The chest radiograph in congenital lung agenesis–aplasia may demonstrate associated vertebral segmentation anomalies. On the lateral view, the heart and great vessels are displaced posteriorly and there is an increased lucency seen behind the sternum, because of compensatory overinflation and herniation of the contralateral lung.

In the evaluation of a symptomatic child in whom the diagnosis requires confirmation, cross-sectional imaging with CT or MR imaging has superseded bronchography and pulmonary angiography in most patients [60,61,66,67]. Both techniques demonstrate the presence or absence of a rudimentary bronchus, and differentiate between agenesis and aplasia. The difference is clinically unimportant. The degree of mediastinal displacement and the size of the contralateral pulmonary artery are shown. An ipsilateral pleural fluid collection may also be seen [60,61]. Images reformatted in the coronal and oblique planes demonstrate more clearly the bronchial and vascular anatomy. Vascular compression of the trachea and the occasionally reported association with a pulmonary artery sling are important to document [66].

Patients with lung agenesis–aplasia should also be evaluated for the presence of associated abnormalities. Their work-up may include echocardiography and a renal tract US. Gastroesophageal reflux may contribute to the respiratory symptoms with which some children present. Evaluation with a barium swallow study may be helpful [62]. Alternatively, pH probe studies may be beneficial.

Lung hypoplasia

In lung hypoplasia there is a decrease in the number and size of the airways and alveoli. The condition may be unilateral or bilateral, primary or secondary. The latter is more common (Box 1). Infants with pulmonary hypoplasia usually present early in the neonatal period with symptoms of respiratory distress, although the presentation varies depending on the amount of functioning lung parenchyma and any associated abnormalities.

Several factors are required for normal growth and development of the lungs. These include adequate size of the thoracic cage, normal respiratory motion of the fetus, and an appropriate amount of fluid to distend the developing lung [4,68,69]. A decrease in the volume of the affected hemithorax, for example caused by an intrathoracic space-occupying lesion,

leads to compression of the developing ipsilateral lung. If the mass lesion is large enough to cause cardiac and mediastinal shift, then the contralateral lung is also compressed and hypoplastic. An intra-abdominal mass lesion has the same effect. The small, rigid thoracic cage seen in several skeletal dysplasias (many of which are lethal) restricts fetal respiratory motion and leads to bilateral pulmonary hypoplasia. Oligohydramnios leads to reduced fetal respiratory motion with compression of the thoracic cage and a reduction in the volume of lung liquid. Premature rupture of membranes in the second trimester has a reported prevalence of pulmonary hypoplasia of between 9% and 28% [4]. The mechanism responsible for the development of hypoplastic lungs in association with such conditions as trisomy 21 is unknown [68].

The findings on the chest radiograph are variable. With bilateral pulmonary hypoplasia, the lungs are small and poorly aerated. The thorax may have a *bell-shaped* configuration and the hemidiaphragm may be elevated. Skeletal abnormalities in keeping with an underlying dysplasia may be apparent. Pneumothoraces are not uncommon and may develop spontaneously or after the commencement of mechanical ventilation. If hypoplasia is primary, unilateral, and severe, the findings may be indistinguishable from unilateral pulmonary agenesis–aplasia [60,61]. In less severe cases of unilateral hypoplasia, there is ipsilateral cardiomediastinal shift and loss of definition of the cardiac border on the affected side. A retrosternal dense stripe seen on the lateral radiograph may be caused by extrapleural accumulation of alveolar connective tissue [70,71] or, more likely, by the cardiomediastinal shift and rotation [72]. Cross-sectional imaging studies in primary pulmonary hypoplasia demonstrate either a hypoplastic ipsilateral pulmonary artery or a vessel of near normal caliber [60,61]. Secondary unilateral hypoplasia may show the radiographic features of the underlying cause, in addition to the hypoplastic lung. With secondary hypoplasia caused by an intrathoracic mass lesion, the mediastinal shift is contralateral to the abnormal lung.

The antenatal diagnosis of pulmonary hypoplasia is difficult with US. More recently, some authors are using fast-sequence MR imaging to assess fetal lung volumes to predict outcome [4].

Management of infants with pulmonary hypoplasia is both supportive and directed toward the treatment of any underlying abnormalities. Oxygen therapy, mechanical ventilation, and possibly extracorporeal membrane oxygenation may be required. The prognosis depends on the degree of hypo-

Box 1. Conditions associated with pulmonary hypoplasia

Decrease in lung volume
Intrathoracic mass effect
  Diaphragmatic defect
    Congenital diaphragmatic hernia
    Agenesis of diaphragm
  Excess pleural fluid
    Chylothorax
    Nonimmune fetal hydrops
  Large intrathoracic mass
    Thoracic ganglion tumor (eg, neuro-
      blastoma, ganglioneuroma)
    Extralobar pulmonary sequestration
    Congenital cystic
      adenomatoid malformation
  Chronically elevated diaphragm
    Phrenic nerve agenesis
    Membranous
      diaphragm (eventration)
    Abdominal mass or ascites
Thoracic cage abnormalities
  Thoracic dystrophies
    Asphyxiating thoracic dystrophy
    Achondrogenesis
    Thanatophoric dysplasia
    Severe achondroplasia
    Osteogenesis imperfecta
    Ellis-van Creveld syndrome
    Short rib–polydactyly syndrome
    Metatrophic dwarfism
  Muscular disease
    Congenital myotonic dystrophy
    Arthrogryposis congenita
Oligohydramnios
With renal disease
  Bilateral renal agenesis
    (Potter's) syndrome
  Bilateral dysplastic kidneys
  Obstructive uropathy
Without renal disease
  Amniotic fluid leak
Decreased pulmonary vascular perfusion
Cardiovascular
  Tetralogy of Fallot
  Ebstein's anomaly
  Hypoplastic right heart

Pulmonary vascular anomalies
  Pulmonary artery agenesis
  Scimitar syndrome
Miscellaneous
Chromosomal abnormalities
  Trisomy 13
  Trisomy 18
  Trisomy 21
Central nervous system anomalies
Rhesus isoimmunization of the fetus

From Keslar P, Newman B, Oh KS. Radiographic manifestations of anomalies of the lung. Radiol Clin North Am 1991;29: 255–70.

plasia and the severity of any associated congenital anomalies.

Absence of a pulmonary artery

Unilateral congenital absence of the pulmonary artery is a rare malformation. It may occur in isolation but is more typically seen in association with other cardiovascular abnormalities [73–75]. Patients generally present with symptoms and signs secondary to their underlying cardiac malformation, but those with isolated absence of the pulmonary artery are also symptomatic: recurrent pneumonia, limited exercise tolerance, and hemoptysis are not uncommon. Pulmonary hypertension is a recognized complication.

It is usually only the proximal section of the vessel that is absent. The more peripheral pulmonary arterial tree may be near normal in size [40,73–75]. This is explained by the different embryologic origins of the proximal and distal pulmonary artery branches. In childhood, a collateral circulation from the bronchial and intercostal arteries, and directly from the aorta to the lower lobes, develops [71,73–75]. In infants a patent ductus arteriosus on the same side as the absent artery maintains lung perfusion until the collateral network develops [75].

The chest radiograph shows a hypoplastic lung on the same side as the absent pulmonary artery (Fig. 16). The hilar shadow is small or absent. Peripherally, the ipsilateral lung is oligemic but there is a reticular network of vascular markings, which reflect the collateral arterial supply. Ipsilateral rib notching may be seen in the older patient, in whom

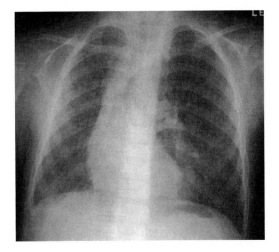

Fig. 16. Hypoplastic right lung secondary to an absent right pulmonary artery. Chest radiograph shows the small right hemithorax with reduced right hilar vascular markings. There is compensatory overinflation of the left lung.

prominent collateral supply has developed from the intercostal arteries [40]. The aortic arch is usually on the opposite side to the absent pulmonary artery [73,74].

Echocardiography is recommended to assess the intracardiac anatomy and to look for associated defects. An echocardiogram also confirms the anatomy of the main pulmonary arteries and measures any degree of pulmonary hypertension. CT or MR angiography accurately depicts the hilar anatomy, and delineates the collateral vascular network [73–75]. CT has the added advantage of depicting the lung parenchyma and any associated bronchiectasis, which may be the end result of the recurrent pneumonias. Several authors recommend cardiac catheterization with pulmonary venous wedge angiography to demonstrate the hilar arteries. This is important if revascularization is proposed [74,75]. Embolization of large collateral vessels can also be performed, if recurrent hemoptysis or pulmonary hypertension develops [74].

Lobar agenesis–aplasia complex

The term *lobar agenesis–aplasia complex* encompasses a spectrum of pulmonary malformations including absence or hypoplasia of one or more pulmonary lobes, often with an associated pulmonary venous abnormality [60,61,67].

Hypogenetic lung syndrome

With lobar agenesis–aplasia complex, the right lung is almost always involved and the upper lobe is most commonly affected. The pulmonary venous anatomy is normal. Systemic arterial supply from the thoracic or abdominal aorta is usually present and indeed accompanies most of the malformations included in the lobar agenesis–aplasia spectrum [60,61,67]. An accessory diaphragm (a membrano-muscular diaphragmatic duplication that is attached anteriorly to the diaphragm, and courses posteriorly and superiorly to fuse with the posterior chest wall) [40,61,71] may also be seen with any abnormality of the lobar agenesis–aplasia spectrum. Patients with isolated hypogenetic lung syndrome are usually asymptomatic, although some present with dyspnea on exertion if the degree of pulmonary hypoplasia is severe [40,60,61].

The chest radiograph shows features similar to those of unilateral pulmonary hypoplasia (Fig. 17). CT examinations demonstrate the bronchial anatomy more elegantly: a hyparterial right main bronchus is seen with absence of the right upper lobe, in a pattern that mimics the anatomy of the left main bronchus [40,60,61]. The pulmonary artery supplying the hypogenetic lung is generally hypoplastic [40].

Anomalous unilateral single pulmonary vein

In this variant of the lobar agenesis–aplasia complex, the hypogenetic lung is accompanied by

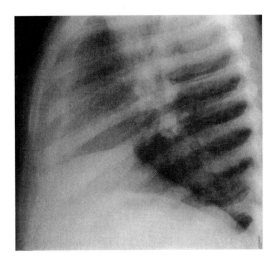

Fig. 17. Lateral chest radiograph of an infant with hypoplasia of the right upper lobe. There is a dense retrosternal stripe visible.

an anomalous, ipsilateral single pulmonary vein draining appropriately to the left atrium. Synonyms for this vein include pulmonary varix and a meandering pulmonary vein [60,61,76]. The tubular shadow caused by the vein is visible on the chest radiograph. Echocardiography, CT, or MR imaging can noninvasively confirm the termination of the vein into the left atrium. There is no left-right shunting with this anomaly, given that pulmonary venous drainage is appropriate.

The levoatriocardinal vein

The levoatriocardinal vein is a rare anomaly. The hypogenetic lung is seen to be drained by an anomalous vein, which branches to drain into both the left atrium and a systemic vein [60]. The course of this anomalous vein may be demonstrated by CT, MR imaging, or conventional angiography.

Congenital pulmonary venolobar syndrome

The association of partial anomalous pulmonary venous return and a hypogenetic lung is perhaps more well-recognized as the scimitar syndrome. The name is derived from the contour of the anomalous vein, which drains part or all of the small lung; it is said to resemble a Turkish scimitar sword. The scimitar vein most commonly empties into the infradiaphragmatic inferior vena cava. The suprahepatic inferior vena cava, hepatic veins, portal veins, azygous vein, coronary sinus, and right atrium may also receive the pulmonary venous drainage from the hypogenetic (almost always right-sided) lung. Single case reports of left-sided scimitar syndrome exist [77]. Associated cardiovascular defects are well described and include most commonly a sinus venosus or secundum atrial septal defect. Many other anomalies of the thorax and its vasculature have been described in the scimitar syndrome. These include vertebral anomalies, abnormal lung lobation, tracheal stenosis and diverticula, and gastrointestinal tract anomalies [4,40,61,77].

Infants tend to present early with scimitar syndrome, particularly when they have coexistent congenital heart disease or systemic arterial supply to the right lung [78]. This group of patients statistically has a higher morbidity and mortality, and is more likely to develop pulmonary hypertension [4,77,78]. Multiple factors contribute to the development of pulmonary hypertension, including the left-right shunts caused by the scimitar vein, septal defect, and the ab-

errant systemic arterial supply. Some patients, however, may remain asymptomatic or present in adult life with mild exertional dyspnea or recurrent lower respiratory tract infections [4,61,77].

The chest radiograph shows features of the hypogenetic lung syndrome, along with the curved density of the scimitar vein (Fig. 18). If the vein is small or retrocardiac, however, it may not be visible on a frontal radiograph. The vein lies posteriorly on the lateral view. Cardiac dextroposition or dextrocardia may be apparent. Doppler studies may show the union of the scimitar and systemic veins. CT and MR imaging allow direct visualization of the anomalous vein, and with angiographic techniques and multiplanar reconstructions, allow the radiologist to detail the arterial and bronchial anatomy. Absence of the normal (right) inferior pulmonary vein is useful supporting evidence for the diagnosis. Velocity-encoded cine–MR imaging has been used to quantify the degree of left-right shunting in the scimitar vein [79]. Conventional angiographic studies may still be requested by some surgeons to delineate the arterial and venous anatomy before surgical repair. This is usually considered in those symptomatic children with coexistent congenital heart disease and left-right shunts of greater than 2:1. Direct reimplantation of the scimitar vein into the left atrium may be feasible in some patients, avoiding cardiopulmonary bypass [80]. Alternatively, intracardiac repairs using atrial baffles may be used [77,80].

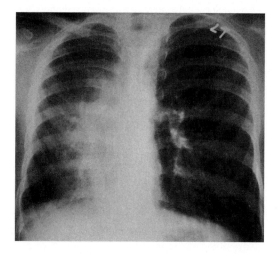

Fig. 18. Congenital pulmonary venolobar syndrome (scimitar syndrome). Chest radiograph of a 10-year-old boy with recurrent chest infections. There is a hypogenetic right lung. The *scimitar vein* is seen as a curved density behind the right heart border.

Horseshoe lung

This is an uncommon malformation that is typically associated with the hypogenetic lung syndrome and all variants of the lobar agenesis–aplasia complex. In horseshoe lung, a portion of the right lower lobe crosses the midline and is fused with the left lower lobe. Anatomically, this isthmus of pulmonary tissue is located posterior to the heart and anterior to the esophagus and descending aorta. The right and left lower lobes may fuse, either with or without intervening layers of visceral pleura. Typically they are sheathed in a continuous layer of parietal pleura, forming a communication between the right and left pleural cavities [81,82]. In most reported cases, the arterial supply to the isthmus is from an anomalous branch of the right pulmonary artery. The bronchi arise from the right bronchial tree [81,82].

The chest radiograph shows features of the hypogenetic lung syndrome. If there is associated congenital venolobar syndrome, the scimitar vein may also be visualized. The isthmus is seen at the medial aspect of the left lung base; it is often lucent because of its relative hypovascularity [81,82]. A subtle linear density representing the left border of the isthmus can also be seen at the left base [81]. If necessary, the diagnosis can be confirmed by CT imaging. The mediastinal discontinuity posterior to the heart is clearly seen. The advent of multidetector row CT has obviated the need for invasive bronchography and angiography, because the airways and vascular supply to the isthmus may be demonstrated using standard postprocessing techniques, typically multiplanar reconstructions and multiplanar reformats; three-dimensional depiction (volume rendering usually); and transparency views [61,83].

Management of these children depends on their symptoms. Asymptomatic patients and those presenting early in life with lower respiratory infections are managed conservatively. Children with coexistent congenital heart disease or recurrent pneumonias may require surgery [81,82].

Pulmonary arteriovenous malformations

A pulmonary AVM is an abnormal anatomic communication between a pulmonary arterial branch and a pulmonary vein. Congenital pulmonary AVMs are thought to occur secondary to failure of development of the pulmonary capillary network, with persistence of primitive arteriovenous communications [84]. A pulmonary AVM is usually fed by a single artery and drained by a single vein, although occasionally multiple feeding and draining vessels may be identified. The lesions may be single or multiple, with up to half of patients with multiple AVMs having a diagnosis of hereditary hemorrhagic telangiectasia or Rendu-Osler-Weber syndrome [84].

Pulmonary AVMs are often asymptomatic in childhood, but they enlarge over time and most patients develop symptoms by the third or forth decade of life. Classical symptoms include dyspnea on exertion and central or peripheral cyanosis. Finger clubbing may be found on physical examination. The degree of right-left shunting and the extent of systemic arterial oxygen desaturation determine the severity of the clinical problems. Polycythemia and pulmonary hypertension can develop. Complications caused by paradoxical central nervous system emboli and lesion rupture (causing hemoptysis or hemothorax) are more common in those with hereditary telangiectasia. The diagnosis is suspected clinically in those symptomatic patients whose hypoxemia is not corrected by supplemental oxygen therapy and whose oxygen saturations fall in the upright position. The latter is explained by the preferential flow of blood to the lung bases, where most pulmonary AVMs are located [84–86].

The chest radiograph may show a well-circumscribed serpiginous or lobulated density (Fig. 19). Calcification in pulmonary AVMs is rare. Rib notching is occasionally seen in older patients, if there is associated systemic arterial supply to the le-

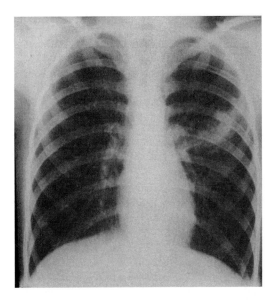

Fig. 19. Pulmonary arteriovenous malformation. Chest radiograph in an 8-year-old girl demonstrates a lobular soft tissue mass in the left upper lobe.

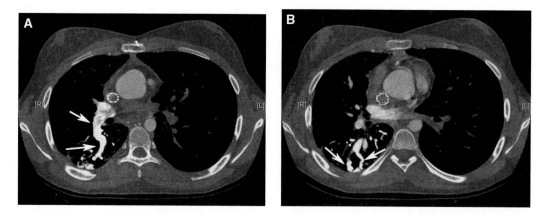

Fig. 20. Twenty-year-old woman status post-Glenn anastomosis. CT angiogram was performed to assess for acquired pulmonary arteriovenous malformations. (*A*) Axial, intravenous contrast-enhanced image demonstrates dense contrast enhancement of an enlarged right lung branch pulmonary artery (*arrows*). (*B*) Enlarged veins (*arrows*) seen slightly more inferiorly to drain from one of several acquired malformations (only one shown). (*From* Frush DP, Herlong JR. Pediatric thoracic CT angiography. Pediatr Radiol 2005;35:11–25; with permission.)

sion [84]. This may be present de novo, or can arise secondary to pulmonary ischemia induced by the shunt [58]. A diffuse reticulonodular pattern on the chest radiograph has been reported in patients with multiple, small lesions [87]. The diagnosis can be confirmed noninvasively using contrast-enhanced CT (Fig. 20), with three-dimensional reformats [58,84, 87,88] or gadolinium-enhanced three-dimensional MR angiography techniques [89]. It is important accurately to map the arterial supply vessels and draining veins before therapy.

Screening asymptomatic relatives of patients with hereditary telangiectasia is important because treatment can avert the serious central nervous system complications, which complicate pulmonary AVMs. Contrast-enhanced echocardiography is the most commonly used imaging technique. If the atrial septum is intact, then the presence of microbubbles in the left atrium following contrast injection into a peripheral vein confirms the presence of a pulmonary AVM [84,86,87,90]. This technique is also helpful to monitor patients following therapy.

The aim of therapy in patients with pulmonary AVMs is to eliminate the right-left shunt and to prevent and treat complications of the condition. Historically, surgical resection of these lesions was performed, although this required bilateral thoracotomies in some patients. Transcatheter balloon or coil closure of pulmonary AVMs is now the preferred method of treatment [85,91]. The techniques are challenging to the radiologist and require initial diagnostic pulmonary (with or without systemic)

angiography to define the lesion. Complications of embolotherapy include pleuritic chest pain, pulmonary infarction, cardiac ischemia, transient confusion, systemic migration of a coil, and cerebrovascular accidents [84,85,87]. Recanalization of pulmonary AVMs is recognized in up to 10% following embolization [84,91], necessitating a repeat procedure.

Summary

The radiologist's role in the investigation of congenital lung abnormalities has changed considerably in recent years. Improved antenatal sonography and the introduction of antenatal MR imaging have led to the identification of a group of asymptomatic children who in the past may not have come to attention and who now require postnatal follow-up. Advances in cross-sectional techniques, however, such as multidetector row CT and CT angiography, with improved MR imaging sequences now mean that invasive diagnostic angiography and bronchography are essentially obviated. Conservative management is increasingly used for children who would have been referred for open surgery in the past.

Infants and children with a suspected congenital lung abnormality should only be imaged following discussion with the radiologist regarding the most appropriate technique; the examination should give the clinical information required, be noninvasive, and use the lowest radiation dose possible.

Acknowledgments

The author thanks Mrs. Barbara Carleton for her help with typing the manuscript.

References

[1] Stigers KB, Woodring JH, Kanga JF. The clinical and imaging spectrum of findings in patients with congenital lobar emphysema. Pediatr Pulmonol 1992; 14:160–70.

[2] Nuchtern JG, Harberg FJ. Congenital lung cysts. Semin Pediatr Surg 1994;3:233–43.

[3] Hugosson C, Rabeeah A, Al-Rawaf A, et al. Congenital bilobar emphysema. Pediatr Radiol 1995;25: 649–51.

[4] Berrocal T, Madrid C, Novo S, et al. Congenital anomalies of the tracheobronchial tree, lung, and mediastinum: embryology, radiology, and pathology. Radiographics 2003;24:e17–62.

[5] Winters WD, Effman EL. Congenital masses of the lung: prenatal and postnatal imaging evaluation. J Thorac Imaging 2001;16:196–206.

[6] Coran AG, Drongowski R. Congenital cystic disease of the tracheobronchial tree in infants and children: experience with 44 consecutive cases. Arch Surg 1994;129:521–7.

[7] Donnelly LF, Frush DP. Localized radiolucent chest lesions in neonates: causes and differentiation. AJR Am J Roentgenol 1999;172:1651–8.

[8] Cleveland RH, Weber B. Retained fetal lung liquid in congenital lobar emphysema: a possible predictor of polyalveolar lobe. Pediatr Radiol 1993;23:291–5.

[9] Kennedy CD, Habibi P, Matthew DJ, et al. Lobar emphysema: long-term imaging follow-up. Radiology 1991;180:189–93.

[10] McBride JT, Wohl ME, Strieder DJ, et al. Lung growth and airway function after lobectomy in infancy for congenital lobar emphysema. J Clin Invest 1980;66: 962–70.

[11] Stocker JT, Madewell JE, Drake RM. Congenital cystic adenomatoid malformation of the lung: classification and morphologic spectrum. Hum Pathol 1977; 8:155–71.

[12] Rosado-de-Christensen ML, Stocker JT. Congenital cystic adenomatoid malformation. Radiographics 1991; 11:865–86.

[13] Haddon MJ, Bowen A'D. Bronchopulmonary and neurenteric forms of foregut anomalies: imaging for diagnosis and management. Radiol Clin North Am 1991;29:241–54.

[14] Pumberger W, Hörmann M, Deutinger J, et al. Longitudinal observation of antenatally detected congenital lung malformations (CLM): natural history, clinical outcome and long-term follow-up. Eur J Cardiothorac Surg 2003;24:703–11.

[15] Papagiannopoulos K, Hughes S, Nicholson AG, et al. Cystic lung lesions in the pediatric and adult population: surgical experience at the Brompton Hospital. Ann Thorac Surg 2002;73:1594–8.

[16] Kim WS, Lee KS, Kim I-O, et al. Congenital cystic adenomatoid malformation of the lung: CT-pathologic correlation. AJR Am J Roentgenol 1997;168:47–53.

[17] Patz Jr EF, Müller NL, Swensen SJ, et al. Congenital cystic adenomatoid malformation in adults: CT findings. J Comput Assist Tomogr 1995;19:361–4.

[18] Pilling D. Fetal lung abnormalities: what do they mean? Clin Radiol 1998;53:789–95.

[19] Winters WD, Effman EL, Nghiem HV, et al. Disappearing fetal lung masses: importance of postnatal imaging studies. Pediatr Radiol 1997;27:535–9.

[20] Sauvat F, Michel J-L, Benachi A, et al. Management of asymptomatic neonatal cystic adenomatoid malformations. J Pediatr Surg 2003;38:548–52.

[21] Wang N-S, Chen M-F, Chen F-F. The glandular component in congenital cystic adenomatoid malformation of the lung. Respirology 1999;4:147–53.

[22] Ueda K, Gruppo R, Unger F, et al. Rhabdomyosarcoma of lung arising in congenital cystic adenomatoid malformation. Cancer 1977;40:383–8.

[23] Murphy JJ, Blair GK, Fraser GC, et al. Rhabdomyosarcoma arising within congenital pulmonary cysts: report of three cases. J Pediatr Surg 1992;27:1364–7.

[24] d'Agostino S, Bonoldi E, Dante S, et al. Embryonal rhabdomyosarcoma of the lung arising in cystic adenomatoid malformation: case report and review of the literature. J Pediatr Surg 1997;32:1381–3.

[25] Benjamin DR, Cahill JL. Bronchioloalveolar carcinoma of the lung and congenital cystic adenomatoid malformation. Am J Clin Pathol 1991;95:889–92.

[26] Senac Jr MO, Wood BP, Isaacs H, et al. Pulmonary blastoma: a rare childhood malignancy. Radiology 1991;179:743–6.

[27] Macpherson RI. Gastrointestinal tract duplications: clinical, pathologic, etiologic, and radiologic considerations. Radiographics 1993;13:1063–80.

[28] Azzie G, Beasley S. Diagnosis and treatment of foregut duplications. Semin Pediatr Surg 2003;12:46–54.

[29] Nobuhara KK, Gorski YC, La Quaglia MP, et al. Bronchogenic cysts and esophageal duplications: common origins and treatment. J Pediatr Surg 1997;32: 1408–13.

[30] Carachi R, Azmy A. Foregut duplications. Pediatr Surg Int 2002;18:371–4.

[31] Brooks BS, Durall ER, El Gammal T, et al. Neuroimaging features of neurenteric cysts: analysis of nine cases and review of the literature. Am J Neuroradiol 1993;14:735–46.

[32] McAdams HP, Kirejczyk WM, Rosado-de-Christenson ML, et al. Bronchogenic cyst: imaging features with clinical and histopathologic correlation. Radiology 2000;217:441–6.

[33] Kim YC, Goo JM, Han JK, et al. Subphrenic bronchogenic cyst mimicking a juxtahepatic solid lesion. Abdom Imaging 2003;28:354–6.

[34] Matzinger MA, Matzinger FR, Sachs HJ. Intrapulmo-

nary bronchogenic cyst: spontaneous pneumothorax as the presenting symptom. AJR Am J Roentgenol 1992; 158:987–8.

[35] Hisatomi E, Miyajima K, Yasumori K, et al. Retroperitoneal bronchogenic cyst: a rare case showing the characteristic imaging feature of milk of calcium. Abdom Imaging 2003;28:716–20.

[36] Mendelson DS, Rose JS, Efremidis SC, et al. Bronchogenic cysts with high CT numbers. AJR Am J Roentgenol 1983;140:463–5.

[37] Nakata H, Egashira K, Watanabe H, et al. MRI of bronchogenic cysts. J Comput Assist Tomogr 1993;17: 267–70.

[38] Lyon RD, McAdams HP. Mediastinal bronchogenic cyst: demonstration of a fluid-fluid level at MR imaging. Radiology 1993;186:427–8.

[39] Ashizawa K, Okimoto T, Shirafuji T, et al. Anterior mediastinal bronchogenic cyst: demonstration of complicating malignancy by CT and MRI. Br J Radiol 2001;74:959–61.

[40] Woodring JH, Howard TA, Kanga JF. Congenital pulmonary venolobar syndrome revisited. Radiographics 1994;14:349–69.

[41] Rosado de Christenson ML, Frazier AA, Stocker JT, et al. Extralobar sequestration: radiologic-pathologic correlation. Radiographics 1993;13:425–41.

[42] Felker RE, Tonkin ILD. Imaging of pulmonary sequestration. AJR Am J Roentgenol 1990;154:241–9.

[43] Kravitz RM. Congenital malformations of the lung. Pediatr Clin North Am 1994;41:453–72.

[44] Frazier AA, Rosado de Christenson ML, Stocker JT, et al. Intralobar sequestration: radiologic-pathologic correlation. Radiographics 1997;17:725–47.

[45] García-Peña P, Lucaya J, Hendry GMA, et al. Spontaneous involution of pulmonary sequestration in children: a report of two cases and review of the literature. Pediatr Radiol 1998;28:266–70.

[46] Laurin S, Hägerstrand I. Intralobar bronchopulmonary sequestration in the newborn: a congenital malformation. Pediatr Radiol 1999;29:174–8.

[47] Ko S-F, Ng S-H, Lee T-Y, et al. Noninvasive imaging of bronchopulmonary sequestration. AJR Am J Roentgenol 2000;175:1005–12.

[48] Hernanz-Schulman M, Stein SM, Neblett WW, et al. Pulmonary sequestration: diagnosis with color Doppler sonography and a new theory of associated hydrothorax. Radiology 1991;180:817–21.

[49] Ikezoe J, Murayama S, Godwin JD, et al. Bronchopulmonary sequestration: CT assessment. Radiology 1990;176:375–9.

[50] Stern EJ, Webb WR, Warnock ML, et al. Bronchopulmonary sequestration: dynamic, ultrafast, high-resolution CT evidence of air trapping. AJR Am J Roentgenol 1991;157:947–9.

[51] Frush DP, Donnelly LF. Pulmonary sequestration spectrum: a new spin with helical CT. AJR Am J Roentgenol 1997;169:679–82.

[52] Lee EY, Siegel MJ, Sierra LM, et al. Evaluation of angioarchitecture of pulmonary sequestration in pediatric patients using 3D MDCT angiography. AJR Am J Roentgenol 2004;183:183–8.

[53] Au WK, Chan JKF, Chan FL. Pulmonary sequestration diagnosed by contrast enhanced three-dimensional MR angiography. Br J Radiol 1999;72:709–11.

[54] Kouchi K, Yoshida H, Matsunaga T, et al. Intralobar bronchopulmonary sequestration evaluated by contrast-enhanced three-dimensional MR angiography. Pediatr Radiol 2000;30:774–5.

[55] Cass DL, Crombleholme TM, Howell LJ, et al. Cystic lung lesions with systemic arterial blood supply: a hybrid of congenital cystic adenomatoid malformation and bronchopulmonary sequestration. J Pediatr Surg 1997;32:986–90.

[56] Curros F, Chigot V, Emond S, et al. Role of embolisation in the treatment of bronchopulmonary sequestration. Pediatr Radiol 2000;30:769–73.

[57] Conran RM, Stocker JT. Extralobar sequestration with frequently associated congenital cystic adenomatoid malformation, type 2: report of 50 cases. Pediatr Dev Pathol 1999;2:454–63.

[58] Do K-H, Goo JM, Im J-G, et al. Systemic arterial supply to the lungs in adults: spiral CT findings. Radiographics 2001;21:387–402.

[59] Miyake H, Hori Y, Takeoka H, et al. Systemic arterial supply to normal basal segments of the left lung: characteristic features on chest radiography and CT. AJR Am J Roentgenol 1998;171:387–92.

[60] Mata JM, Cáceres J, Castañer E, et al. The dysmorphic lung: imaging findings. Postgrad Radiol 2000;20: 3–15.

[61] Mata JM, Cáceres J. The dysmorphic lung: imaging findings. Eur Radiol 1996;6:403–14.

[62] Argent AC, Cremin BJ. Computed tomography in agenesis of the lung in infants. Br J Radiol 1992;65: 221–4.

[63] Chopra K, Sethi GR, Kumar A, et al. Pulmonary agenesis. Indian J Pediatr 1988;25:678–82.

[64] Cunningham ML, Mann N. Pulmonary agenesis: a predictor of ipsilateral malformations. Am J Med Genet 1997;70:391–8.

[65] Knowles S, Thomas RM, Lindenbaum RH, et al. Pulmonary agenesis as part of the VACTERL sequence. Arch Dis Child 1988;63:723–6.

[66] Newman B, Gondor M. MR evaluation of right pulmonary agenesis and vascular airway compression in pediatric patients. AJR Am J Roentgenol 1997; 168:55–8.

[67] Mata JM, Cáceres J, Lucaya J, et al. CT of congenital malformations of the lung. Radiographics 1990;10: 651–74.

[68] Husain AN, Hessel RG. Neonatal pulmonary hypoplasia: an autopsy study of 25 cases. Pediatr Pathol 1993;13:475–84.

[69] Swischuk LE, Richardson CJ, Nichols MM, et al. Primary pulmonary hypoplasia in the neonate. J Pediatr 1979;95:573–7.

[70] Cremin BJ, Bass EM. Retrosternal density: a sign of pulmonary hypoplasia. Pediatr Radiol 1975;3:145–7.

[71] Currarino G, Williams B. Causes of congenital unilateral pulmonary hypoplasia: a study of 33 cases. Pediatr Radiol 1985;15:15–24.

[72] Ang JGP, Proto AV. CT demonstration of congenital pulmonary venolobar syndrome. J Comput Assist Tomogr 1984;8:753–7.

[73] Debatin JF, Moon RE, Spritzer CE, et al. MRI of absent left pulmonary artery. J Comput Assist Tomogr 1996;16:641–5.

[74] Harkel ADJT, Blom NA, Ottenkamp J. Isolated unilateral absence of a pulmonary artery: a case report and review of the literature. Chest 2002;122:1471–7.

[75] Apostolopoulou SC, Kelekis NL, Brountzos EN, et al. "Absent" pulmonary artery in one adult and five pediatric patients: imaging, embryology, and therapeutic implications. AJR Am J Roentgenol 2002;179: 1253–60.

[76] Chilton SJ, Campbell JB. Pulmonary varix in early infancy: case report with 8-year follow-up. Radiology 1978;129:400.

[77] Rutledge JM, Hiatt PW, Vick III GW, et al. A sword for the left hand: an unusual case of left-sided scimitar syndrome. Pediatr Cardiol 2001;22:350–2.

[78] Dupuis C, Charaf LAC, Breviere G-M, et al. Infantile form of the scimitar syndrome with pulmonary hypertension. Am J Cardiol 1993;71:1326–30.

[79] Henk CB, Prokesch R, Grampp S, et al. Scimitar syndrome: MR assessment of hemodynamic significance. J Comput Assist Tomogr 1997;21:628–30.

[80] Brown JW, Ruzmetov M, Minnich DJ, et al. Surgical management of scimitar syndrome: an alternative approach. J Thorac Cardiovasc Surg 2003;125:238–45.

[81] Frank JL, Poole CA, Rosas G. Horseshoe lung: clinical, pathologic, and radiologic features and a new plain film finding. AJR Am J Roentgenol 1986;146:217–26.

[82] Dupuis C, Rémy J, Rémy-Jardin M, et al. The "horseshoe" lung: six new cases. Pediatr Pulmonol 1994;17:124–30.

[83] Goo HW, Kim YH, Ko JK, et al. Horseshoe lung: useful angiographic and bronchographic images using multidetector-row spiral CT in two infants. Pediatr Radiol 2002;32:529–32.

[84] Pick A, Deschamps C, Stanson AW. Pulmonary arteriovenous fistula: presentation, diagnosis, and treatment. World J Surg 1999;23:1118–22.

[85] Dutton JAE, Jackson JE, Hughes JMB, et al. Pulmonary arteriovenous malformations: results of treatment with coil embolization in 53 patients. AJR Am J Roentgenol 1995;165:1119–25.

[86] Kjeldsen AD, Oxhøj H, Andersen PE, et al. Pulmonary arteriovenous malformations: screening procedures and pulmonary angiography in patients with hereditary hemorrhagic telangiectasia. Chest 1999;116: 432–9.

[87] Panicek DM, Heitzman ER, Randall PA, et al. The continuum of pulmonary developmental anomalies. Radiographics 1987;7:747–72.

[88] Remy J, Remy-Jardin M, Giraud F, et al. Angioarchitecture of pulmonary arteriovenous malformation: clinical utility of three-dimensional helical CT. Radiology 1994;191:657–64.

[89] Puvaneswary M. Three-dimensional gadolinium-enhanced magnetic resonance angiography of pulmonary arteriovenous malformation. Australas Radiol 2002;46:189–93.

[90] Nanthakumar K, Graham AT, Robinson TI, et al. Contrast echocardiography for detection of pulmonary arteriovenous malformations. Am Heart J 2001;141: 243–6.

[91] Abushaban L, Uthaman B, Endrys J. Transcatheter coil closure of pulmonary arteriovenous malformations in children. J Interv Cardiol 2004;17:23–6.

ELSEVIER
SAUNDERS

Radiol Clin N Am 43 (2005) 325 – 353

RADIOLOGIC
CLINICS
of North America

Imaging Evaluation of Pediatric Mediastinal Masses

Arie Franco, MD, PhD[a],*, Neeta S. Mody, MD[b], Manuel P. Meza, MD[a]

[a]Department of Radiology, Children's Hospital of Pittsburgh, Pittsburgh, PA 15213, USA
[b]Department of Radiology, Western Pennsylvania Hospital, Pittsburgh, PA 15224, USA

The mediastinum is located in the central portion of the thorax, between the two pleural cavities, the diaphragm and the thoracic inlet [1]. The classification of Fraser et al [2] divides the mediastinum into the traditional anterior, middle, and posterior compartments based on the lateral chest radiograph. There are no fascial planes that separate these compartments, but this division categorizes diseases and masses to their location of origin. The anterior mediastinum is defined as the region posterior to the sternum and anterior to the heart and brachiocephalic vessels and from the thoracic inlet superiorly to the diaphragm inferiorly. It contains the thymus, fat, and lymph nodes. The middle mediastinal compartment is located posterior to the anterior mediastinum and anterior to the posterior mediastinum. This space contains the heart and pericardium, the ascending and transverse aorta, the brachiocephalic vessels, the vena cava, the main pulmonary artery and veins, the trachea, bronchi, and lymph nodes. The posterior mediastinal compartment is located posterior to the heart and trachea and extends posteriorly to the thoracic vertebral margin and includes the paravertebral gutters. It contains the descending thoracic aorta, esophagus, azygos veins, autonomic ganglia and nerves, thoracic duct, lymph nodes, and fat [3].

Mediastinal masses in children are a heterogeneous group of asymptomatic or potentially life-threatening congenital, infectious, or neoplastic lesions that present complex diagnostic and therapeutic dilemmas. Most commonly they are discovered incidentally on chest radiographs. Large mediastinal masses can cause compression of adjacent mediastinal structures. Patients may have airway compression or cardiovascular compromise [4].

Mediastinal masses are usually assigned to a single mediastinal compartment to limit the differential diagnosis. Sometimes they cannot be localized to a single anatomic compartment. The epicenter of the mass and the direction of the mass effect on adjacent structures, such as trachea and great vessels, suggest the site of origin of the mass [5]. Because some normal structures are located within multiple mediastinal regions, a given tumor mass can arise in any compartment (Boxes 1–3). The epicenter of the mass, its effect on adjacent mediastinal organs, and its internal characteristics (calcification, fat, water, and so forth), based on conventional radiographic examination and cross-sectional imaging, can help in establishing a differential diagnosis and clinical planning [5].

Anterior mediastinal masses

Normal thymus

The thymus is a ductless gland located in the upper anterior portion of the mediastinum. It is most active and largest during puberty, after which it shrinks in size and activity in most individuals and is replaced with fat. The thymus consists of two lateral lobes placed in close contact along the midline, situated partly in the thorax, partly in the neck, and extending from the fourth costal cartilage upward, as high as the lower border of the thyroid gland. It is covered by the sternum, and by the origins of the

---

* Corresponding author.
E-mail address: arie.franco@chp.edu (A. Franco).

sternohyoid and sternothyroid muscles. Posteriorly, it rests on the pericardium, and is separated from the aortic arch and great vessels by a layer of fascia. In the neck it lies on the front and sides of the trachea, behind the sternohyoid and sternothyroid. The two lobes generally differ in size; they are occasionally united, so as to form a single mass; and sometimes

---

Box 1. Pediatric anterior mediastinal masses

Thymus
  Normal thymus[a]
  Thymic cyst
  Thymomegaly
  Thymoma
  Thymic hemorrhage

Adenopathy
  Infectious adenopathy[a]
  Lymphoma or leukemia[a]
  Sarcoidosis
  Castleman disease
  Rosai-Dorfman disease

Tumors
  Germ cell tumors (eg, teratoma)[a]
  Thyroid or parathyroid tumors
  Hamartoma
  Vagus-phrenic nerve tumors
  Hemangioma
  Sternal tumors

Infections
  Mediastinitis
  Sternal osteomyelitis or abscess

Vascular abnormalities
  Vascular malformations (eg, lymphatic malformation, venous malformation, mixed malformations)
  Aneurysm

Other
  Histiocytosis
  Morgagni's hernia
  Hematoma
  Extension of middle mediastinal mass

[a] These masses are more common.

Box 2. Pediatric middle mediastinal masses

Extension of anterior mediastinal mass into the middle mediastinum

Adenopathy
  Infectious adenopathy (eg, tuberculosis)[a]
  Metastatic disease[a]
  Lymphoma or leukemia[a]
  Sarcoidosis
  Castleman disease
  Rosai-Dorfman disease

Tumors
  Thyroid or parathyroid tumors
  Vagus-phrenic nerve tumors
  Cardiac tumors
  Hemangioma
  Hamartoma

Infections
  Mediastinitis

Vascular abnormalities
  Vascular malformations (eg, lymphatic malformation, venous malformation, mixed malformations)
  Vascular rings
  Aneurysm

Other
  Bronchopulmonary foregut malformations (ie, esophageal duplication cyst, esophageal duplication cyst, neurenteric cyst)[a]
  Histiocytosis
  Hematoma
  Diaphragmatic rupture
  Pancreatic pseudocyst
  Esophageal hernia
  Achalasia, chalasia
  Pericardiac cysts

[a] These masses are more common.

Box 3. Pediatric posterior mediastinal masses

Ganglion cell tumors
  Neuroblastoma[a]
  Ganglioneuroma[a]
  Ganglioneuroblastoma[a]

Other nervous system tumors
  Nerve sheath tumors
      (schwannoma, neurofibroma)
  Paraganglioma

Adenopathy
  Metastasis
  Infectious adenopathy
  Sarcoidosis
  Castleman disease
  Rosai-Dorfman disease

Tumors
  Osseocartilaginous tumors
  Thoracic duct cyst
  Hemangioma

Infections
  Mediastinitis
  Vertebral osteomyelitis
  Diskitis

Vascular abnormalities
  Vascular malformations (eg, lymphatic
      malformation, venous malforma-
      tion, mixed malformations)
  Aneurysm
  Dilated azygous system

Others
  Hematoma (eg, secondary to fracture)
  Bochdalek's hernia
  Extramedullary hematopoiesis
  Lateral meningocele
  Extension of normal thymus
  Histiocytosis

  [a] These masses are more common.

separated by an intermediate lobe. The thymus is of a pinkish gray color, soft, and lobulated on its surfaces. The thymus appears in the form of two flask-shaped entodermal diverticula, which arise, one on either side, from the third branchial pouch, and extend lateral and backward into the surrounding mesoderm in front of the ventral aorta. The thymus plays an important role in the development of the immune system in early life, and its cells form a part of the body's normal immune system.

The thymus size in healthy infants increases from birth to between 4 and 8 months of age and then decreases. It normally weighs about 15 g at birth and 35 g at puberty. Most of the individual variation can be explained by breast-feeding status and body size and to a lesser extent by illness [6]. Studies demonstrate that the size of the thymus in healthy neonates as measured by sonography is significantly correlated to the weight of the infant. For a given weight of an infant it is possible to predict the normal range of thymic size [7]. Any type of stress can cause decrease in the size of the thymus because of the lymphocytic effect of the steroids. During puberty the gland begins to involute and it is gradually replaced by fat.

The normal thymus appears on chest radiography as a prominent soft tissue density in the anterosuperior mediastinum of infants and toddlers. Thereafter, it is less prominent. The left lobe mimics widening of the superior mediastinum and indentations of the anterolateral edge of a prominent left lobe of the thymus opposite the costal cartilage are often seen, called the thymic wave sign (Fig. 1). The inferior margin of the right lobe of the thymus is flattened

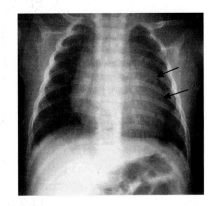

Fig. 1. Thymic wave sign. Three-month-old infant presenting with vomiting. Undulations of the left lobe of the normal thymus (*arrows*) are caused by the adjacent costal cartilage.

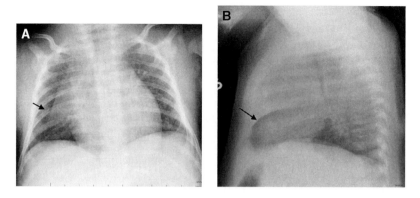

Fig. 2. Thymic sail sign. Four-month-old infant presenting with shortness of breath. Frontal (*A*) and lateral (*B*) radiographs of the chest demonstrate a normal thymus with the sail sign representing flattening of the lower margin of the gland abutting the minor fissure (*arrows*).

at the minor fissure and produces the appearance of the sail sign (Fig. 2). On the lateral radiograph the thymus appears as a soft tissue opacity filling the anterosuperior mediastinum. On both views the thymus is often inseparable from the upper cardiac margin, mimicking cardiomegaly. The thymus has homogeneous smooth appearance on chest radiograph and does not displace mediastinal structures.

On sonography the normal thymus has homogeneous and fine granular echotexture with some echogenic strands. It is mildly hypoechoic relative to the liver, spleen, and thyroid gland. The normal thymus has a smooth, well-defined margin because each lobe is surrounded by a fibrous capsule. Color

Doppler sonography shows that the normal thymus is hypovascular or nearly avascular [8–11]. The thymus also is pliable and moves with respiration and cardiac pulsation.

On noncontrast CT the thymus has higher attenuation than the vessels, but has the same intensity as muscle tissue. During infancy the mean attenuation level of the thymus is 80.8 HU. In teenagers the mean attenuation level of the normal thymus is 56 HU; this is attributable to fatty infiltration. The thymus shows homogeneous enhancement of 20 to 30 HU (Fig. 3) following contrast bolus injection [12]. With MR imaging, the normal thymus has homogeneous signal intensity. T1-weighted images

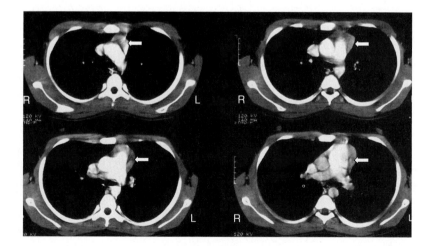

Fig. 3. CT appearance of normal thymus. A 12-year-old boy presenting with chest pain at an outside hospital. The CT was considered suspicious for lymphoma. A series of axial images from an intravenous contrast-enhanced chest CT demonstrate homogeneous enhancement of prominent but normal left thymic lobe (*arrows*).

demonstrate slightly brighter signal than normal muscle. On T2-weighted images, the signal of the normal thymus is much brighter than the signal of the muscle, likewise when fat saturation is used. Inhomogeneous signal of the thymus should be considered pathologic. The thymic tissue revealed homogeneous decrease in intensity on opposed-phase MR images relative to that seen on in-phase images of healthy volunteers and two patients with hyperplastic thymus. Chemical-shift MR imaging may be useful in identifying normal thymic tissue and the hyperplastic thymus in early adulthood [13].

Various radiopharmaceuticals localize in the thymus. Gallium 67 (^{67}Ga) citrate uptake has been shown in as many as 61% of children younger than 2 years of age with lymphoid and nonlymphoid tumors. Thymic ^{67}Ga uptake is most often seen after chemotherapy. This reflects the presence of activated thymic lymphocytes as part of the immunologic response that leads to hyperplasia [14]. [67]Ga uptake may also occur in children stressed by illness [15,16]. Iodine 131 uptake has been shown to occur in hyperplastic thymus that does not contain ectopic thyroid tissue or metastatic foci [17]. The presence of somatostatin receptors in the thymus accounts for the occasional visualization of a normal thymus in children who undergo imaging with indium 111 pentetreotide [18,19].

There is increased uptake of 2-[fluorine 18]-fluoro-2-deoxy-D-glucose (FDG) in the normal thymus gland of patients between the ages of 2 and 13 years [20,21]. Most of the patients studied had positron emission tomography (PET) scans for various oncologic conditions and had no known or suspected thymus abnormality. This uptake assumes an important role when evaluating mediastinal uptake in whole-body PET scans in pediatric oncology patients to avoid false-positive interpretation. Previous treatment with a high dose of radioiodine and chemotherapy may contribute to visualization of a normal thymus with FDG-PET scans [22].

Ectopic thymus

Most cases of ectopic thymus are found at any level of the pathway of normal thymic descent, from the angle of the mandible to the upper anterior mediastinum [23]. Infrequently, because of abnormal migration during fetal development, the thymus extends from its usual anterior mediastinal position into the middle and posterior mediastinum as one contiguous structure [24,25]. Rarely, ectopic thymus is reported to cause airway compression. It was reported that ectopic thymic tissue in infants should be considered in the differential diagnosis of secondary pneumonias and emphysema especially located in the upper lung zones [26].

Cross-sectional imaging in multiple plains may be necessary to define aberrant thymus [27–29]. Although this can be accomplished with CT, MR imaging is preferable [5]. The diagnosis of ectopic mediastinal thymus can be made on the basis of four criteria: (1) signal intensity similar to normally located thymus on MR imaging sequences, (2) homogeneous signal intensity, (3) uniform mild enhancement of contrast, and (4) continuity with normally positioned thymic tissue. The fourth criterion is helpful but is not required, because aberrant thymus sometimes is not attached to anterior mediastinal thymus or is connected by a thin, fibrous band that cannot be seen by imaging techniques. Ectopically located normal tissue may exert mass effect on adjacent structures (Fig. 4). Most commonly, aberrant thymus is identified in a right paratracheal location [30,31]. It has been reported that 10% of children have a "nubbin of what appears to be normal thymus posterior to the superior vena cava" on MR images [32].

Thymic pathology

Thymic disorders are rare in the pediatric population. Hyperplasia of the thymus is the most common process to involve the thymus gland in infants and children. It is, however, exceedingly difficult to evaluate the weight of the gland as it continues to grow after birth until puberty and thereafter undergoes progressive atrophy. The hyperplastic gland usually maintains the radiographic characteristics of the normal thymus. Thymic enlargement rarely causes neonatal respiratory distress but should be considered in the differential diagnosis of marked tachypnea in the neonatal period [33].

True thymic hyperplasia is a very rare entity in which the thymus is enlarged without disruption of the normal architecture of the gland or any pattern of abnormal cellular proliferation [34,35]. In such cases the hyperplastic thymus retains most of the radiographic characteristic of the normal thymus [36], but can cause a mass effect on adjacent structures without invasion (Fig. 5).

Thymic hyperplasia may be associated with Graves' disease [37]. Thymic hyperplasia in Graves' disease is more likely to be associated with, rather

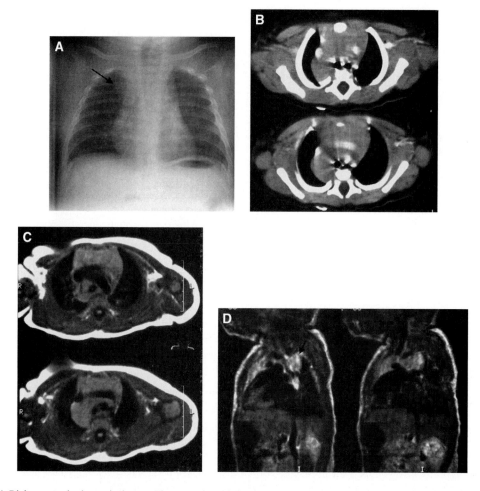

Fig. 4. Right paratracheal ectopic thymus. Three-month-old infant presenting with fever. There is an abnormal contour (*arrow*) along the right upper mediastinal margin on frontal radiograph (*A*). A series of contrast-enhanced axial CT images of the chest (*B*) confirm the posterior location of tissue with attenuation identical to the normally positioned thymus within the anterior mediastinum. Axial (*C*) and sagittal oblique (*D*) contrast-enhanced T1-weighted MR images also demonstrate continuity and identical signal intensity of the ectopic thymus with the anterior thymus (*arrow*).

than the cause of, hyperthyroidism because hyperthyroidism persists after thymectomy [38]. Treatment of the hyperthyroidism in Graves' disease with antithyroid drugs reduces the size of the thymus [39]. Thymic pathology occurs in 80% to 90% of myasthenia gravis patients. Lymphofollicular thymic hyperplasia occurs in 70% of patients with myasthenia gravis, thymoma in 10% to 20%, and thymic atrophy in 10% [40]. Thymic hyperplasia can occur after cytotoxic therapy for various malignancies. The possible cause could be rebound enlargement after initial atrophy caused by these drugs [41]. Thymic hyperplasia may also be associated with thyroid carcinoma and demonstrates increased uptake with

radioiodine scintigraphy even following thyroidectomy [42,43]. Thymic hyperplasia has been associated with anencephaly [44].

Thymomas account for up to 4% of the pediatric mediastinal neoplasms [45,46]. Thymoma has been found to be associated with four organ-specific autoimmune diseases: (1) myasthenia gravis, (2) type 1 diabetes mellitus, (3) autoimmune hepatitis, and (4) Hashimoto's thyroiditis [47]. Thymoma has been associated with pancytopenia [48], myopathy [49], systemic lupus erythematosus [50], aplastic anemia, and hypogammaglobulinemia [51].

The most frequent radiographic appearance of thymoma is a variable-sized, soft tissue mass in the

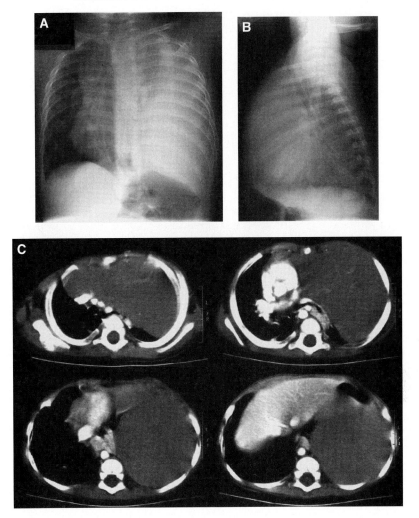

Fig. 5. Thymic hyperplasia. Nine-month-old boy who presented with failure to thrive. Frontal (*A*) and lateral (*B*) radiographs reveal a large, left-sided mass with shift of the mediastinum to the right and loss of volume of the left lung. (*C*) Representative images from an intravenous contrast-enhanced CT examination reveal a large, homogeneous mass in the anterior mediastinum displacing the heart and great vessels posteriorly and to the right. The left lung is severely compressed.

anterior mediastinum (Fig. 6), resulting in smoothly marginated, and often lobulated mass. Possible locations of origin include adjacent to the junction of the great vessels and the pericardium, less commonly the cardiophrenic angle or the adjacent cardiac border, and rarely other mediastinal compartments or the neck. Areas of calcification may be detected on plain radiographs, most commonly linear, thin, and peripheral. Invasive thymomas may demonstrate an irregular interface with the adjacent lung. Rarely, thymoma may manifest as predominantly pleural disease, and may demonstrate nonspecific radiographic patterns, such as pleural

thickening; pleural masses; or diffuse, nodular, circumferential pleural thickening that encases the ipsilateral lung. The latter presentation may mimic the appearance of diffuse malignant mesothelioma or metastatic adenocarcinoma [52,53]. With CT evaluation, thymomas are generally seen as homogeneous, oval, rounded, or lobulated soft tissue masses. In most cases, the contour of the mass is smooth and well defined, and it usually grows asymmetrically to one side of the anterior mediastinum. After intravenous administration of contrast material, the tumor enhances homogeneously. With MR imaging, thymomas are isointense relative to skeletal muscle

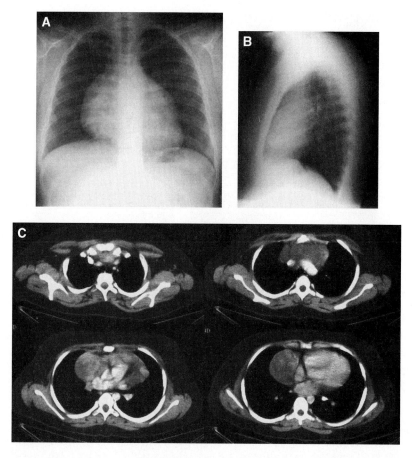

Fig. 6. Thymoma. An otherwise healthy 8-year-old boy presenting with chest pain. Frontal (*A*) and lateral (*B*) chest radiographs demonstrate an anterior mediastinal mass. (*C*) A series of axial intravenous contrast-enhanced images of the chest show a large, lobulated anterior mediastinal mass with irregular enhancement.

on T1-weighted images and have increased, often heterogeneous signal intensity on T2-weighted images [52,54] in addition to irregular margins, mass affect, and size.

Thymic cysts are rare benign lesions that should be considered in the differential diagnosis of cervical and mediastinal masses, especially if cystic, in children [55]. Cysts can be associated with other disorders including HIV infection in children [56], thymoma [57], teratoma [58], and with rhabdomyosarcoma [59].

Lymphoma

Lymphomas are the third most common group of cancers in children and adolescents in the United States, accounting for approximately 13% of newly diagnosed cancers in this age group. Non-Hodgkin's lymphoma represents approximately 60% of these diagnoses, and Hodgkin's disease accounts for the remainder [60–63]. Lymphomas are the most common cause of masses in the pediatric mediastinum. More than 50% of children with lymphoblastic lymphoma present with an anterior mediastinal mass, and more than one third of all patients with non-Hodgkin's lymphoma have their primary sites in the mediastinum. Hodgkin's disease also frequently involves this anatomic compartment with approximately two thirds of all pediatric cases manifesting mediastinal adenopathy [64]. Non-Hodgkin's lymphoma has been associated with Epstein-Barr virus [65].

The disease usually presents as mediastinal mass and adenopathy. The thymus is often infiltrated with the disease and areas of necrosis are present. An enlarged thymic shadow on conventional radiography in a previously normal thymus should alert the physician to the presence of the disease. Mass effects may be present, such as airway compression (Fig. 7), atelectasis, and superior vena cava obstruction and syndrome [66]. Contrast-enhanced CT is more useful based on accurate definition of the location of the lymph node and characterization of the mediastinal mass. Calcifications are rare. MR imaging is a useful imaging tool. [67]Ga scintigraphy is an accurate test for monitoring response to therapy and for early detection of recurrence [67]. Currently, PET (Fig. 8) provides a better assessment of active disease compared with ^{67}Ga scintigraphy [68].

Germ cell tumors

Germ cell tumors are the third most common neoplasm of the mediastinum after lymphoma and neurogenic tumors. Most often they arise within the anterior mediastinum near the thymus gland. A small subset of the germ cell tumors arise from other mediastinal compartments. Germ cell tumors account for 6% to 18% of mediastinal tumors [69]

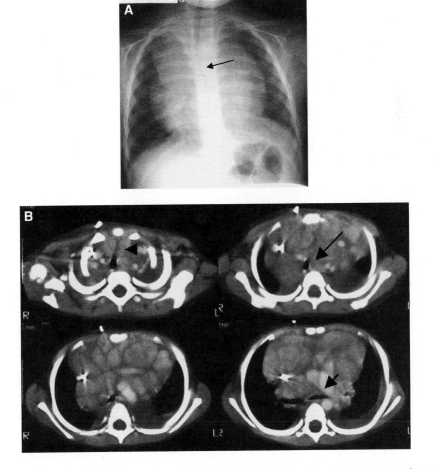

Fig. 7. Lymphoma. A 30-month-old girl presenting with stridor. (*A*) Frontal chest radiograph demonstrates a large mediastinal mass with rightward deviation of the trachea (*arrow*). (*B*) A series of axial intravenous contrast-enhanced CT images of the chest show the anterior and middle mediastinal location of a multilobulated mass with displacement and narrowing of the trachea and the proximal left main stem bronchus (*arrow*). Note also bilateral pleural effusions.

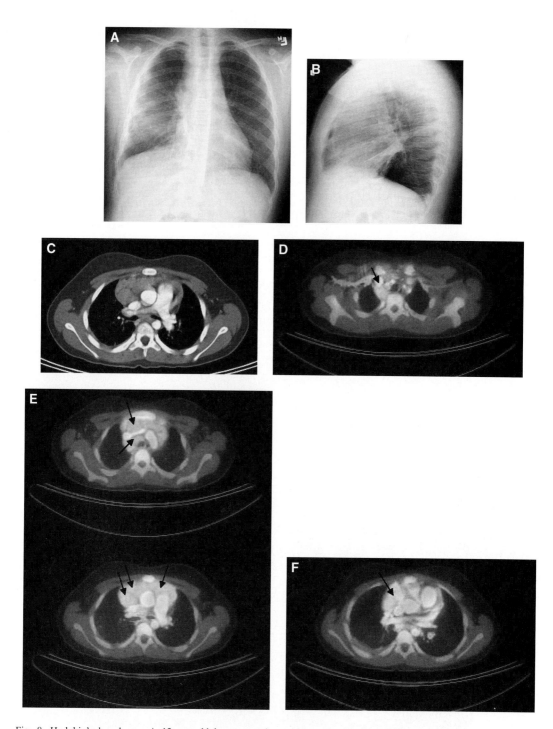

Fig. 8. Hodgkin's lymphoma. A 12-year-old boy presenting with cough. (*A*) Frontal chest radiograph shows a lobular right paratracheal mediastinal silhouette. (*B*) Lateral radiograph demonstrates the anterior location, based on filling in of the clear space with soft tissue. (*C*) Axial contrast-enhanced CT image confirms a right-sided anterior mediastinal lobulated mass. (*D–F*) A series of PET-CT images show intense activity at numerous levels (*arrows*).

and comprise only 1% to 3% of all germ cell tumors [70].

Teratomas (Fig. 9) are the most common mediastinal germ cell tumor, and are divided into mature, immature, and mixed malignant types. Nonteratomatous tumors include seminoma, yolk sac tumor, embryonal carcinoma, choriocarcinoma, and mixed types. Malignant germ cell tumor is a complex tumor of varied histology with frequent coexistence of benign elements (Figs. 10–12). Lesions often have incomplete regression with chemotherapy alone and tumor resection may be undertaken at diag-

nosis or after attempted shrinkage with chemotherapy [71].

The clinical picture is nonspecific. Germ cell tumors are large and produce respiratory distress caused by compression of the tracheobronchial tree. Diminished breath sounds, pain, and cough are usually present. Most children have a subacute course that may span several weeks or longer. Germ cell tumors can be seen in patients with Klinefelter's syndrome and may present with precocious puberty [72].

With chest radiography, teratomas can be rounded or lobulated, and can be large in size. Up to 26%

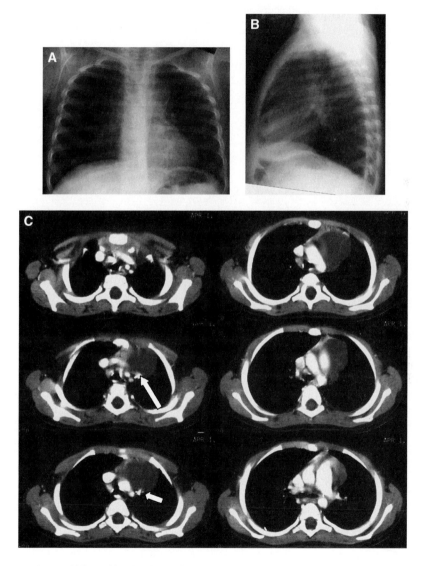

Fig. 9. Teratoma. A 2-year-old boy with wheezing and cough. Frontal (*A*) and lateral (*B*) chest radiographs demonstrate the left anterior mediastinal location of a mass. (*C*) A series of intravenous contrast-enhanced axial CT images illustrates the prominently cystic nature of the mass. Internal calcification is also noted (*arrows*).

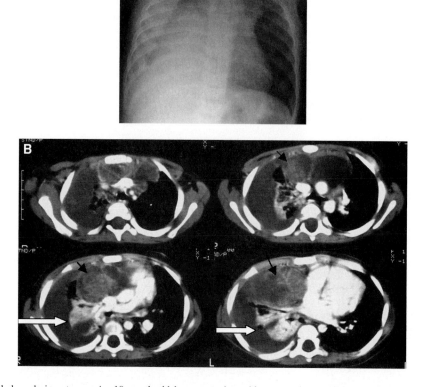

Fig. 10. Endodermal sinus tumor. An 18-month-old boy presenting with progressive respiratory distress. (A) Frontal chest radiograph shows an abnormal contour at the right heart margin, a mass in the region of the aorticopulmonary window, and a large right effusion. (B) A series of axial intravenous contrast-enhanced CT images shows cystic and soft tissue components (*black arrows*) in addition to the large malignant right pleural effusion and enhancing, atelectatic right lung (*white arrows*).

of teratomas exhibit calcification [73]. On CT, teratomas are multilocular cystic tumors with a variable wall thickness [74]. The combination of fluid, soft tissue, calcium, and fat attenuation in the anterior mediastinal mass is highly specific for teratoma [3]. Seminoma manifests as a bulky lobulated mass, which uncommonly invades adjacent structures, but can metastasize to regional lymph nodes and bone [75–77]. Seminoma rarely calcifies [77]. Nonseminomatous malignant germ cell tumors are radiographically large and irregular with extensive heterogeneous areas of low attenuation on CT caused by necrosis, hemorrhage, and cyst formation [76]. Germ cell tumors appear on MR imaging as masses of heterogeneous signal intensity. MR imaging is more sensitive in depicting infiltration of the adjacent structures by fat plane obliteration, and is performed as an ancillary study [78].

Middle mediastinal masses

Duplication cysts

Duplication cysts arise as a result of aberrant fetal development of the primitive foregut, which consists of three distinct cell types. Bronchogenic cysts arise from abnormal budding of the ventral foregut, and enterogenous cysts arise from the dorsal foregut [79]. Congenital duplication cysts are the most common mediastinal cysts, accounting for approximately 20% of mediastinal masses [80]. Bronchogenic cysts represent 50% to 60% of all mediastinal cysts, whereas enterogenous cysts, which include esophageal duplication and neurenteric cysts, constitute 5% to 10% and 2% to 5%, respectively [81]. Bronchogenic cysts are lined by respiratory epithelium and contain cartilaginous plates, bronchial glands, and smooth muscle bundles in the walls [82]. Entero-

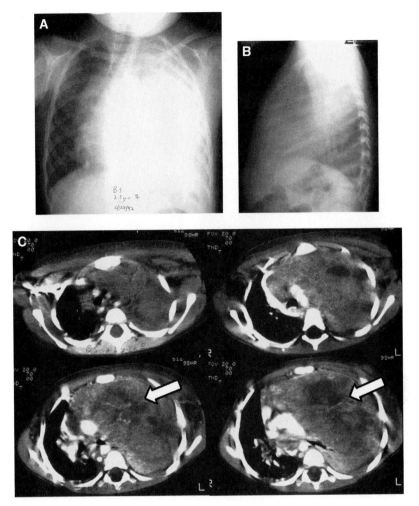

Fig. 11. Mediastinal yolk sac tumor. A 2-year-old girl presenting with progressive dyspnea. Frontal (*A*) and lateral (*B*) chest radiographs demonstrate complete opacification of the right hemithorax with shift of the mediastinum to the right. (*C*) A series of axial intravenous contrast-enhanced CT images demonstrate a large mass with heterogeneous attenuation (*arrows*) arising in the anterior mediastinum and filling much of the left hemithorax. Note the posterior displacement of the great vessels, tracheobronchial tree, and left lung.

genous cysts are usually lined by alimentary epithelium, and 50% to 60% contain gastric mucosa or pancreatic tissue [83,84]. Foregut duplication cysts occur equally in male and female subjects, although a slight male predominance has been reported for neurenteric cysts. Most foregut duplication cysts are located in close relation with the trachea or the esophagus. Rarely, cysts are located in the posterior mediastinum.

Neuroenteric cysts are usually found in the middle mediastinum and have a vertebral body cleft filled with cerebrospinal fluid based on communication with the spinal canal. Most duplication cysts are discovered incidentally, but some manifest in infancy

and childhood. Almost all neuroenteric cysts are discovered in infancy, usually because of signs and symptoms of extrinsic esophageal or tracheobronchial compression [85].

Radiologically, foregut duplication cysts manifest as well-marginated, homogeneous, spherical mediastinal masses ranging in size from 2 to 10 cm (Fig. 13). Cysts typically occur in the paratracheal or subcarinal region but may be found anywhere within the thorax [80,86,87]. With chest CT, cysts are spherical, nonenhancing lesions of variable attenuation (Fig. 14). Enhancement and calcification of the cyst wall may occur [80,86,88–90]. In children, compression of the tracheobronchial tree may produce air trap-

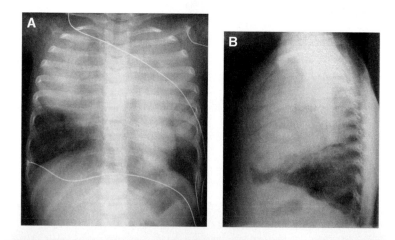

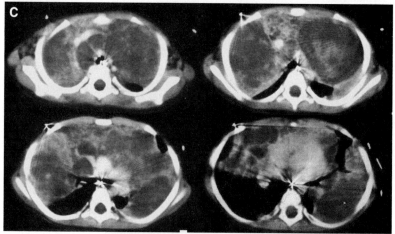

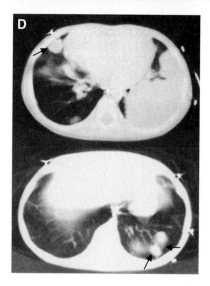

ping, atelectasis, or tracheal deviation [80,91,92]. The cyst may be occult or may be obscured by pulmonary consolidation [92,93]. With MR imaging, cyst contents can exhibit low or high signal intensity on T1-weighted images and high signal intensity on T2-weighted sequences [80].

Vascular anomalies

Both macrocystic (cystic hygromas) and microcystic lymphatic malformations can occur as mediastinal masses. Also known as *lymphangiomas*, lymphatic malformations are rare causes of mediastinal masses [94]. Although these congenital hamartomatous malformations of the lymphatic system are classified as benign, they can be aggressive and, primarily because of mass effect, may be life-threatening [95]. Lymphatic malformations are one of the vascular lesions, a group that also includes venous malformations and hemangiomas. These vascular anomalies together comprise 3% to 6% of mediastinal masses in childhood [94]. With respect to lymphatic malformations, less than 1% localized to the mediastinum [96]. Most mediastinal lymphatic malformations are caused by extension from other sites, such as the neck or axilla [97,98]. The macrocystic lymphatic malformation usually occurs in the neck, axilla, superior mediastinum, or groin.

With chest radiography, lymphatic malformations appear as nonspecific well-defined, round, lobular masses, usually in the anterior or middle mediastinum. A few may occur in the posterior mediastinum. Unilateral or bilateral pleural effusion may be present. In such a situation, the fluid is often chylous. When the chest wall is involved, osseous involvement (eg, displacement, lucent lesions, and abnormalities in thickness) may also be present. Sonographic examination shows a multicystic mass containing internal echoes. CT or MR imaging demonstrates a cystic mass, often multilocular or septated, which envelops or molds to the adjacent mediastinal structures. Intravenous contrast enhancement is usually minimal in lymphatic malformation, and is restricted to the usually thin septae. Areas of fat may also be present. If more than this degree of enhancement is present, it suggests that other tissue, such as a venous malformation or vascular component, is present. This underscores that these vascular malformations may coexist. The more aggressive ones, such as mixed lymphangioma combined with hemangioedothelioma, result in extensive infiltrating soft tissue masses of the mediastinum and pericardium and may cause chylothorax. Parts of the tumor may be insinuated between or adherent to neighboring vital structures, which makes complete excision difficult and hazardous.

Vascular rings are unusual congenital anomalies that occur early in the development of the aortic arch and great vessels. These have been reviewed briefly elsewhere in this issue. The primary symptomatology associated with vascular rings relates to the structures that are encircled by the ring, the trachea and esophagus. Pulmonary sling is created by anomalous origin of the left pulmonary artery from the posterior aspect of the right pulmonary artery. The anomalous left pulmonary artery courses over the right main stem bronchus, posterior to the trachea or carina and anterior to the esophagus, to reach the hilum of the left lung. This compresses the lower trachea and right main stem bronchus, producing upper airway symptoms. Compression caused by the sling can produce obstructive emphysema or atelectasis of the right and left lung.

Other rare vascular masses in the middle mediastinum encountered in the pediatric population include venous and arterial masses. The arterial masses include aortic aneurysms (mycotic or traumatic or syndromic, such as with Marfan syndrome, or other causes of cystic medial necrosis); coronary artery aneurysm (Kawasaki's disease); pulmonary artery aneurysms; and postoperative true aneurysms and pseudoaneurysms almost exclusively seen in the setting of operative intervention for congenital heart disease. The venous masses include dilated azygous vein, dilated superior vena cava, total anomalous pulmonary venous return, arteriovenous malformations, and pulmonary vein varix.

Pericardial cysts

Pericardial cysts are uncommon benign mediastinal lesions and are very rare in children. They are usually unilocular cystic lesions with a thin connective tissue wall and clear fluid contents [99,100].

Fig. 12. Endodermal sinus tumor. A 15-month-old girl with respiratory distress. Frontal (*A*) and lateral (*B*) chest radiographs demonstrate a large mass occupying both sides of the thorax. (*C*) Axial intravenous contrast-enhanced CT images (soft tissue algorithm) demonstrate a large heterogeneous mass within the anterior mediastinum displacing vessels airways and lungs posteriorly. (*D*) Axial CT image (lung algorithm) of the lower chest shows pulmonary metastases (*arrows*).

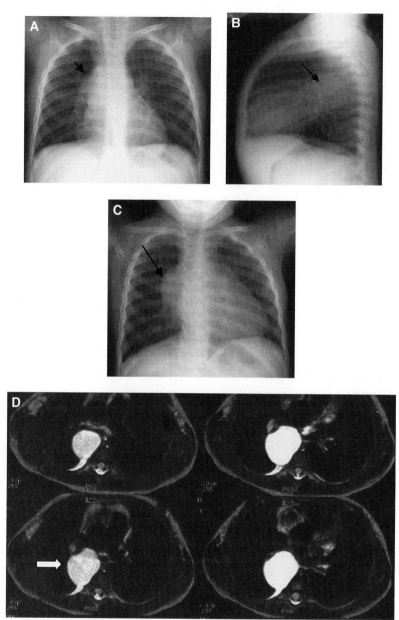

Fig. 13. Bronchogenic cyst. A 2-year-old girl with a history of upper respiratory infections. Frontal (*A*), lateral (*B*), and oblique (*C*) chest radiographs show a rounded middle mediastinal mass (*arrows*). MR images consisting of axial T2-weighted (*D*) and axial (*E*) and coronal (*F*) postcontrast T1-weighted sequences with fat saturation demonstrate the cystic nature of this mass (*arrows*) predominantly in the middle mediastinum.

Pericardial cysts are generally considered developmental abnormalities, although some may be acquired. Complications of pericardial cysts rarely occur [100]. Radiologically, a pericardial cyst manifests as a well-marginated, spherical, or teardrop-shaped mass that characteristically abuts the heart, the anterior chest wall, and the diaphragm [99,101]. Most measure 5 to 8 cm, but some occasionally attain larger sizes. Mural calcification is rare. Approximately 70% were located in the right cardio-

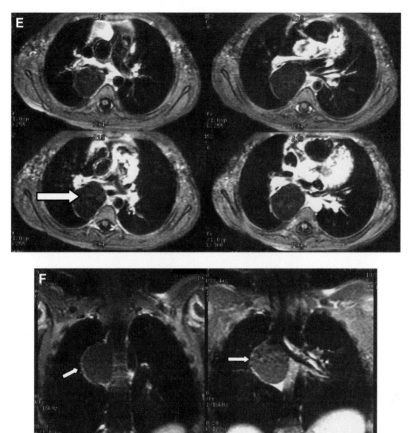

Fig. 13 (*continued*).

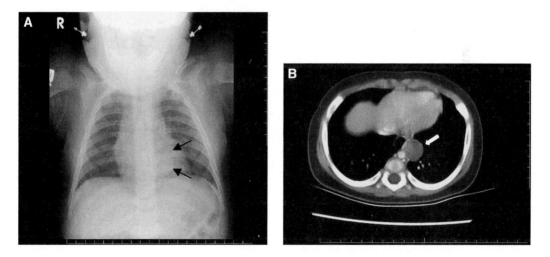

Fig. 14. Esophageal duplication cyst. A 6-year-old girl with a history of chest pain and cough. (*A*) Frontal chest radiograph demonstrates a rounded well-circumscribed opacity (*arrows*). (*B*) Axial intravenous contrast-enhanced CT image at the level of the dome of the liver shows the duplication cyst (*arrow*) located lateral to the esophagus.

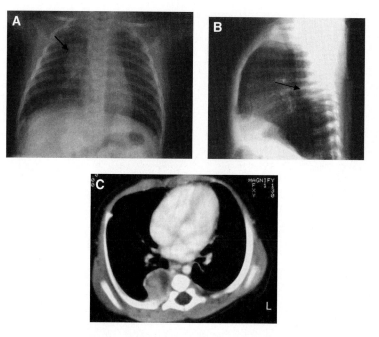

Fig. 15. Neuroblastoma. A 1-month-old girl presenting with one choking episode. Frontal (*A*) and lateral (*B*) chest radiographs show a discrete 2.5 cm right paraspinal rounded soft tissue mass (*arrow*). (*C*) Axial intravenous contrast-enhanced CT image at the mid ventricular level shows the heterogeneous mass without extension into the spinal canal.

phrenic angle, 22% in the left cardiophrenic angle, and the remaining 8% in another paracardiac location [85,99–101]. On CT, pericardial cysts are typically unilocular nonenhancing masses with water attenuation contents and an imperceptible wall. With MR imaging, pericardial cysts have low signal intensity on T1-weighted images and high signal intensity on T2-weighted images [102].

Lymphadenopathy

The lymph node groups that may be visible on chest radiography, when they become enlarged, are in the anterior mediastinal, posterior mediastinal, paratracheal, tracheobronchial, hilar, subcarinal, and paracardiac locations. Because there is little mediastinal fat in children, it is necessary to use intravenous contrast-enhanced CT to visualize the lymph nodes. Unenhanced CT may be necessary before contrast-enhanced CT to detect calcified nodes that suggest granulomatous disease. With T1-weighted MR imaging nodes are similar in signal intensity to muscle. With T2-weighted imaging, nodes are brighter than muscle and become similar in signal intensity to surrounding fat. The signal intensity in MR images

may be similar to the signal intensity of thymus in all sequences [103].

The etiology of lymph node enlargement is extensive. In fact, most middle mediastinal masses are caused by either adenopathy or bronchopulmonary foregut malformations. The most frequent causes of adenopathy are lymphoma; leukemia; tuberculosis; histoplasmosis; sarcoidosis; cystic fibrosis; infectious mononucleosis; Langerhans' cell histiocytosis; Castleman disease; and metastatic neoplasms, such as neuroblastoma in the young child and testicular carcinoma in the teenager that metastasize to mediastinal nodes [103].

Posterior mediastinal masses

Of all pediatric mediastinal masses, 30% to 40% occur in the posterior mediastinum [5]. Most (85%–90%) of these masses are of neurogenic origin [85,104]. Imaging, particularly CT and MR imaging, is used as a guide for determining extent of disease, establishing a differential diagnosis list, and help in judging the efficacy of treatment.

Neurogenic tumors fall into three categories: (1) ganglion cell tumors; (2) nerve sheath and nerve

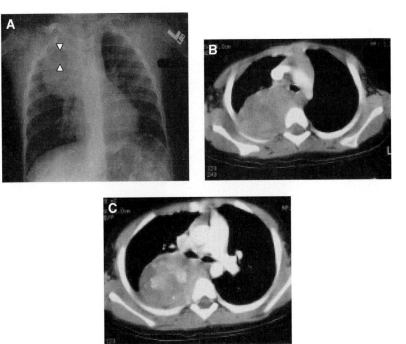

Fig. 16. Neuroblastoma. A 2-year-old girl presenting with cough. (*A*) Frontal chest radiograph shows a large right upper mediastinal soft tissue mass. Note the widening of the third to fourth posterior intercostal space (*arrowheads*). (*B*) Intravenous contrast-enhanced axial CT image at the level of the left pulmonary artery shows a mixed attenuation posterior mediastinal mass with extension into the extradural spinal canal. Note that the mass extends across the midline posterior to the trachea. (*C*) Note calcification within the mass.

tumors; and (3) other nervous tissue tumors, such a paragangliomas. The other, less common posterior mediastinal masses include extramedullary hematopoiesis; lipomatosis; vascular masses, including hemangiomas and vascular malformations; and soft tissue malignancies, such as Ewing's sarcoma, germ cell tumors, and rhabdomyosarcoma.

Ganglion cell tumors

Ganglion cell tumors arise from the sympathetic chain ganglia. These lesions range from malignant masses (neuroblastoma) to benign tumors (ganglioneuroma). Ganglioneuroblastoma has components of both ganglioneuroma and neuroblastoma. All three histologic types are radiographically indistinguishable and the appropriate differential diagnosis is partly determined by the child's age; ganglioneuromas are, in general, seen in an older pediatric population.

Neuroblastoma is the most common extracranial solid tumor in children. Approximately 500 new cases are diagnosed each year in the United States.

It represents 10% of all childhood cancers, and because of its potentially highly aggressive nature, accounts for 15% of cancer deaths [105]. After the abdomen, the thorax is the second most common location of neuroblastoma (15%) followed by the neck (1%–5%) and the pelvis (2%–3%) [106,107].

The child's age is one of the most important criteria when evaluating a patient with a posterior mediastinal mass. Neuroblastoma is a malignancy of young children and is diagnosed at a median age of less than 2 years old and greater than 95% by age 10. In younger patients (less than 5 years old) neuroblastoma is twice as common in boys as girls. As they get older, however, it affects both sexes equally. Fetal or congenital neuroblastoma may even be seen on prenatal ultrasonography. The median age of presentation of ganglioneuroblastoma is 5.5 years of age. Mature ganglioneuroma presents even later in childhood, most often after 10 years of age [105].

Patients with thoracic neuroblastoma can be asymptomatic; masses are found incidentally on chest radiographs. When symptoms do occur, they can be related either to the primary tumor or metastatic

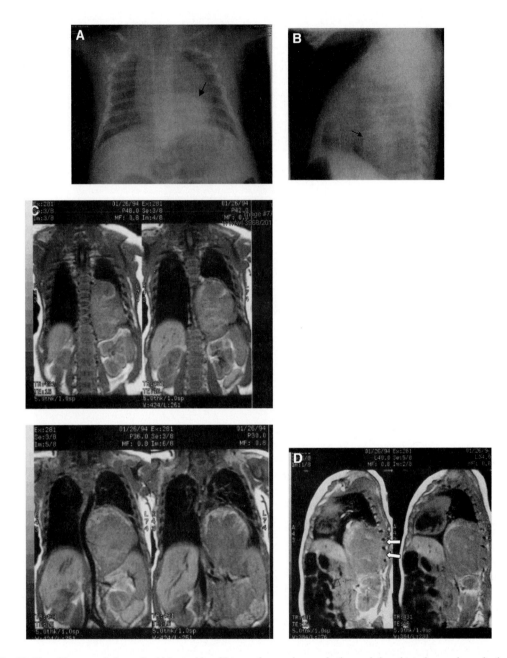

Fig. 17. Neuroblastoma. A 2-month-old boy with a history of meconium aspiration and thought to have a hypoplastic left lung. Frontal (A) and lateral (B) chest radiographs reveal a large dense rounded retrocardiac left posterior mediastinal mass on the left (arrows). (C) Precontrast coronal T1-weighted MR images show a large paraspinal soft tissue mass. (D) Precontrast sagittal T1-weighted MR images show the mass invading the posterior chest wall in the intercostal spaces (arrows). Axial T2-weighted MR images (E) and a coronal contrast-enhanced image (F) demonstrate the intraspinal extension of the tumor through the neural foramina.

disease. Local mass effect or intraspinal extension can lead to symptoms of respiratory distress or cord compression, respectively. Neuroblastoma can secrete catecholamines, such as vanillylmandelic acid and homovanillic acid; however, these catecholamines rarely cause symptoms [104,105]. Finally, patients with widely disseminated disease can present with constitutional symptoms, such as fever, weight loss, and bone pain.

With conventional radiographs of the thorax, ganglion cell tumors appear as paraspinal soft tissue masses that are well-marginated, smooth, and elongated in a superior-to-inferior direction. Calcification can be found in up to 30% of the cases [108]. Chest wall involvement and rib remodeling are common with neuroblastoma. Bony changes associated with intraspinal extension include widening of the intervertebral foramina or pedicle erosion. Because the skeletal system is the most common site of metastasis, an initial skeletal survey with combination of conventional radiographs and bone scintigraphy, including iodine 123 m-iodobenzylguanidine (^{123}I-MIBG), is an essential part of the evaluation for any patient with the diagnosis of neuroblastoma. The role of MR imaging screening has yet to be firmly established for skeletal assessment. Discrete lytic or mixed lytic and sclerotic areas or metaphyseal lucencies are typical of metastatic involvement and aid in determining treatment considerations [106].

CT examination is a commonly used imaging modality for the assessment of thoracic neuroblastoma. CT appearance is that of a soft tissue mass in a paraspinal location (Fig. 15). With contrast enhancement, the mass has attenuation similar to that of muscle and may show low-attenuation areas of necrosis or hemorrhage. With CT, calcification can be seen in up to 80% of patients with neuroblastoma (Fig. 16) [85]. The calcifications can be coarse, mottled, solid, or ring-shaped. CT provides information regarding extent of tumor, regional invasion, metastatic adenopathy, and vascular encasement. The primary tumor can also spread through the neural foramina and extend through it into the spinal canal creating a classic *dumbbell* (Fig. 17). This appearance is seen in up to 28% of patients with thoracic neuroblastoma [105].

The extent of these tumors is best imaged by MR imaging (Fig. 18). The principle advantages of MR imaging are the ability to evaluate the patient in coronal, axial, and sagittal planes together with superior soft tissue (and bone marrow) contrast detail. This provides for accurate evaluation of chest wall involvement and the extent of intraspinal extension. This is critical in assessing response to therapy and for surgical considerations. Bone marrow involvement can also be evaluated by MR imaging and has been shown to correlate well with bone marrow biopsy. On MR imaging, neuroblastoma typically has prolonged T1 and T2 relaxation times with a low signal on T1- and a high signal on T2-weighted sequences. Calcification is not as apparent on MR imaging as CT but the detection of calcification rarely alters the differential considerations. Hemorrhagic and cystic components can be seen on both T1- and T2-weighted sequences with variable signal intensity. Bony marrow metastases appear as areas of low signal intensity on T1-weighted images and areas of high signal intensity on T2-weighted images.

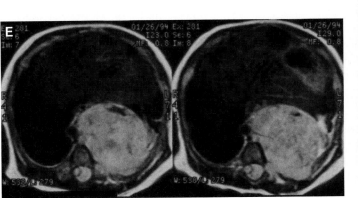
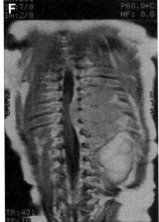

Fig. 17 (*continued*).

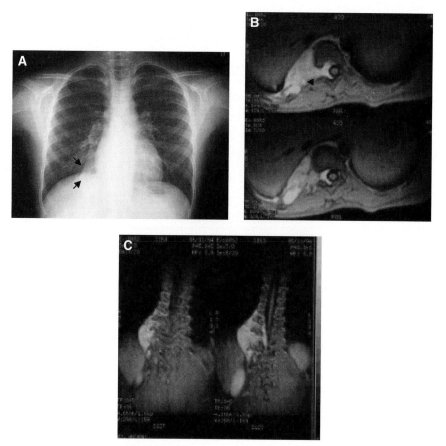

Fig. 18. Neuroblastoma. A 9-year-old boy with a history of trauma 11 months previously. The patient presents now with cough and mild chest pain. Multiple prior chest radiographs (not shown) were interpreted as a right infrahilar pneumonia. (*A*) Frontal chest radiograph reveals a right medial basilar rounded opacity (*arrows*). (*B, C*) T1-weighted intravenous contrast-enhanced MR images show the abnormality is a brightly enhancing right paraspinal posterior mediastinal mass that extends through the neural foramina into the extradural spinal canal.

Nuclear scintigraphy has a role in establishing the staging of neuroblastoma. Technetium 99m (^{99m}Tc) methylene diphosphonate scintigraphy is complementary to skeletal survey with conventional radiography for detecting metastases in the cortical bone [109,110]. Of the nuclear scintigraphic agents available, only ^{99m}Tc methylene diphosphonate can distinguish between involvement of the cortical bone and the bone marrow, which has a prognostic significance [111]. ^{123}I- or ^{131}I-MIBG, an analog to catecholamine precursors, can concentrate in neuroblastic cells. MIBG localizes in primary sites of neuroblastoma and in metastatic sites in 90% to 95% of patients [112–114]. Central nervous system metastatic lesions are rare in neuroblastoma and the ability for detection of central nervous system metastases by MIBG is less certain [115]. MIBG scintigraphy should be performed in all newly diagnosed patients. MIBG findings can result in detection of metastases that are not evident by other imaging studies. Determination of MIBG avidity can influence the choice of follow-up evaluation [111,116].

The role of PET in the management of patients with neuroblastoma has not yet been clearly defined. FDG-PET may offer advantages over MIBG scintigraphy in detecting small lesions or localizing the extent of the disease. In addition, PET can detect lesions in the liver, which are obscured in MIBG scintigraphy by normal MIBG uptake by the liver. PET cannot demonstrate lesions in the cranium because of normal brain avidity [111].

The two most important criteria for establishing prognosis in malignancy is the age of the child and the stage at the time of diagnosis. The staging of neuroblastoma and ganglioneuroblastoma is radiologically or surgically determined by local extent of disease and locating the sites of metastatic involvement [85]. Stage I disease is a well-circumscribed, noninvasive ipsilateral tumor. Complete surgical excision is considered curative in stage I disease and is the treatment of choice. Stage II involves local invasion or ipsilateral nodal invasion. Stage III is the extension of tumor across the midline and lymph node involvement. For stage II and III surgical excision whenever possible plus chemotherapy and radiation are indicated. Stage IV disease is widely metastatic disease and is associated with a dismal outcome. Stage IVS is reserved for children under age 1 year who have metastatic disease limited to liver, skin, or bone marrow but not cortical bone, and has a very good overall prognosis [85]. Children with stages I, II, and IVS tumors have a 3-year event-free survival rate of 75% to 90%. Children less than 1 year with stages of III or IV tumors have a 1-year event-free survival rate of 89% to 90% and 60% to 75%, respectively. Children older than 1 year with stages III and IV tumors have a 3-year event-free survival rate of 50% and 15%, respectively [105]. Furthermore, it is possible for the immature cells found in neuroblastoma and ganglioneuroblastoma to undergo a spontaneous maturation process and follow the benign course of ganglioneuroma. This most often occurs in patients with stage IVS tumors [117].

Nerve sheath and nerve tumors

Nerve sheath tumors are either schwannomas or neurofibromas. Histologically, schwannomas are encapsulated without nerve fibers running through the tissue. Conversely, neurofibromas are unencapsulated with nerve fibers running though the tissue. These nerve sheath tumors are most commonly benign and asymptomatic and are rarely seen in less than 20 years of age [118]. They often arise from intercostals or sympathetic nerves and are more common in patients with neurofibromatosis type II. Schwannomas constitute 75% of nerve sheath tumors.

Radiologically, schwannomas and neurofibromas are indistinguishable and are usually sharply marginated, spherical, and lobulated paraspinal masses [119]. Bony abnormalities, such as rib erosion and splaying of the ribs, are more common to nerve sheath tumors than ganglion cell tumors and can be seen up to 50% of the time. Ten percent of peripheral nerve sheath tumors have been shown to have intraspinal extension. On MR imaging and T1-weighted sequences, neurofibromas and schwannomas typically appear homogenous in signal. On T2-weighted sequences, they exhibit a target appearance with a high signal intensity in the periphery and intermediate signal intensity in the central zone [107]. Malignant degeneration of these neurofibromas and schwannomas is rare in the pediatric population and involves less than 5% of nerve sheath tumors. Benign lesions can either be observed or resected; however, malignant lesions require complete surgical resection for cure. For malignant tumors, adjuvant chemotherapy and radiation do not seem to improve survival. Local recurrence is common and the prognosis is poor [119].

Plexiform neurofibroma is a well-defined nonencapsulated tumor that can occur at any location, and a single one is pathognomic for neurofibroma type I [85]. These masses are multifocal myxoid lesions and have the appearance of a *bag of worms* on cross-sectional imaging consisting of peripheral regions of high-signal myxoid material with central low-signal fibrous material seen with T2-weighted sequences.

Paragangliomas

Although most pediatric posterior mediastinal masses are of ganglion cell or nerve sheath or nerve origin, other nervous tissue tumors must be considered when formulating a complete differential diagnosis. Paragangliomas or extra-adrenal pheochromocytomas are rare tumors of chromaffin cells of the sympathetic nervous tissue that can be seen in the posterior mediastinum within the paravertebral sulcus. Patients with these lesions often present with signs of catecholamine excess [120]. Less than 2% of these tumors are malignant [121]. Treatment consists of surgical resection; however, recurrence can occur and close follow-up after excision is recommended.

On cross-sectional imaging, either CT or MR imaging show a paraspinal soft tissue mass that can be larger than 3 cm with extension into the spinal canal. On CT, the attenuation of the tumor is similar to that of liver but may appear inhomogeneous secondary to necrosis or hemorrhage. Calcification is rare. On MR imaging, the mass is hypointense to isointense to the liver on T1-weighted sequences and highly intense on T2-weighted sequences. The mass also diffusely enhances with gadolinium contrast.

Nonneurogenic posterior mediastinal masses

Extramedullary hematopoiesis is often clinically asymptomatic; however, it may present as signs of spinal cord compression. Extramedullary hematopoiesis is seen in hematologic disorders, most commonly

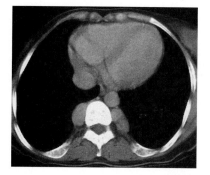

Fig. 19. Extramedullary hematopoiesis. A preteenage boy with thalassemia who has bilateral soft tissue masses. The posterior ribs are broadened and there is left gynecomastia. The latter is a rare site of extramedullary hematopoeisis. (Courtesy of Lynne Hurwitz-Koweek, MD, Durham, North Carolina.)

thalassemia (Fig. 19). The actual pathogenesis of this disorder, however, is unknown. Bilateral paraspinal masses with smooth margins are the classic presentation on chest radiographs. The soft tissue mass may contain fat and is almost always seen within the lower thorax. These masses are either observed if clinically silent or may be surgically resected.

Lipomatosis is a deposit of mature fat in the extrapleural and mediastinal spaces, commonly associated with long-term steroid administration [122]. On CT or MR imaging, the appearance is that of the normal subcutaneous fat.

Vascular masses, including hemangiomas (true neoplasms) and vascular malformations, can occur in the posterior mediastinum, although they rarely isolate to the posterior mediastinum. The CT or MR imaging appearance depends on the type of vascular malformation (cystic spaces, large blood vessels, fatty components) or stage of hemangioma. Hemangiomas densely enhance in the proliferative stage (Fig. 20), with eventual fibrofatty replacement during involution.

The differential diagnosis of nonneurogenic posterior mediastinal masses also includes primary soft tissue malignancies, such as Ewing's sarcoma (Fig. 21), germ cell tumor, and rhabdomyosarcoma. All of these malignancies can arise in the paraspinal area and can dumbbell into the spinal canal [123,124]. Adenopathy, both infectious and meta-

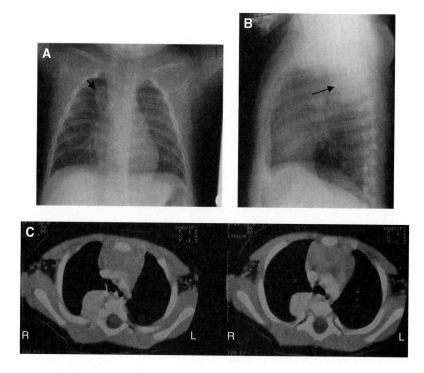

Fig. 20. Hemangioma. A 5-month-old girl with recurrent upper respiratory infections. Frontal (A) and lateral (B) radiographs show a medial right upper mediastinal rounded opacity (arrows). (C) Intravenous contrast-enhanced CT images at the upper portion of the aortic arch demonstrate a brightly enhancing right posterior mediastinal mass with a small amount of right extradural intraspinal extension.

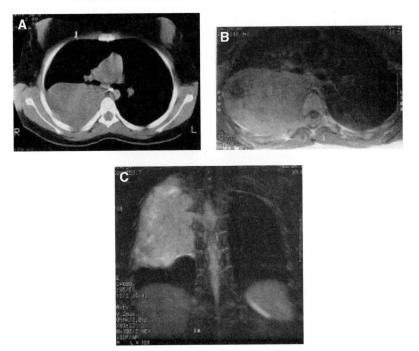

Fig. 21. Soft tissue Ewing's sarcoma. A 14-year-old girl with a past history of medulloblastoma at 3 years of age and meningioma at age 11 years now presented with chest pain. (*A*) Axial unenhanced chest CT demonstrates a large posterior mediastinal soft tissue mass with likely intraspinal extension. Axial MR postcontrast T1-weighted image (*B*) and coronal fat-suppressed T2-weighted MR image (*C*) show the mass with obvious intraspinal extension of the tumor.

static, is also a consideration. Other potential masses are included in Box 3.

Summary

Mediastinal masses consist of a variety of tumors that are classified according to their anatomic location and their histologic characteristics. Occasionally, the mass can arise in a different compartment. It may be difficult to localize an extensive mass to its anatomic compartment. A thorough knowledge of the radiologic characteristics of each mass and the anatomic compartment of origin can help the radiologist to construct and refine an appropriate differential diagnosis of the mass, instrumental for clinical management.

References

[1] Wychulis AR, Payne WS, Clagett OT, et al. Surgical treatment of mediastinal tumors. J Thorac Cardiovasc Surg 1971;62:379–92.

[2] Fraser RS, Pare JAP, Fraser RG. The normal chest. In: Fraser RS, Pare JAP, Fraser RG, editors. Synopsis of diseases of the chest. 2nd edition. Philadelphia: WB Saunders; 1994. p. 1–116.

[3] Strollo DC, Rosado de Christenson ML, Jett JR. Primary mediastinal tumors. Part 1: tumors of the anterior mediastinum. Chest 1997;112:511–22.

[4] Freud E, Ben-Ari J, Schonfeld T, et al. Mediastinal tumors in children: a single institution experience. Clin Pediatr 2002;41:219–23.

[5] Meza MP, Benson M, Slovis TL. Imaging of mediastinal masses in children. Radiol Clin North Am 1993;31:583–604.

[6] Hasselbalch H, Jeppesen DL, Ersboll AK, et al. Thymus size evaluated by sonography: a longitudinal study on infants during the first year of life. Acta Radiol 1997;38:222–7.

[7] Hasselbalch H, Jeppesen DL, Ersboll AK, et al. Sonographic measurement of thymic size in healthy neonates: relation to clinical variables. Acta Radiol 1997; 38:95–8.

[8] Adam EJ, Ignotus PI. Sonography of the thymus in healthy children: frequency of visualization, size, and appearance. AJR Am J Roentgenol 1993;161: 153–5.

[9] Lemaitre L, Marconi V, Avni F, et al. The sonographic evaluation of normal thymus in infants and children. Eur J Radiol 1987;7:130–6.

[10] Han BK, Babcock DS, Oestreich AE. Normal thymus in infancy: sonographic characteristics. Radiology 1989;170:471–4.

[11] Ben-Ami TE, O'Donovan JC, Yousefzadeh DK. Sonography of the chest in children. Radiol Clin North Am 1993;31:517–31.

[12] Sklair-Levy M, Agid R, Sella T, et al. Age-related changes in CT attenuation of the thymus in children. Pediatr Radiol 2000;30:566–9.

[13] Takahashi K, Inaoka T, Murakami N, et al. Characterization of the normal and hyperplastic thymus on chemical-shift MR imaging. AJR Am J Roentgenol 2003;180:1265–9.

[14] Hibi S, Todo S, Imashuku S. Thymic localization of gallium-67 in pediatric patients with lymphoid and nonlymphoid tumors. J Nucl Med 1987; 28:293–7.

[15] Handmaker H, O'Mara RE. Gallium imaging in pediatrics. J Nucl Med 1977;18:1057.

[16] Johnson PM, Berdon WE, Baker DH, et al. Thymic uptake of gallium-67 citrate in a healthy 4 year old boy. Pediatr Radiol 1978;7:243–4.

[17] Michigishi T, Mizukami Y, Shuke N, et al. Visualization of the thymus with therapeutic doses of radioiodine in patients with thyroid cancer. Eur J Nucl Med 1993;20:75–9.

[18] Fletcher BD. Thymic concentration of radiolabeled octreotide. J Nucl Med 1999;40:1967.

[19] Connolly LP, Connolly SA. Thymic uptake of radiopharmaceuticals. Clin Nucl Med 2003;28:648–51.

[20] Patel PM, Alibazoglu H, Ali A, et al. Normal thymic uptake of FDG on PET imaging. Clin Nucl Med 1996;21:772–5.

[21] Nakahara T, Fujii H, Ide M, et al. FDG uptake in the morphologically normal thymus: comparison of FDG positron emission tomography and CT. Br J Radiol 2001;74:821–4.

[22] Alibazoglu H, Alibazoglu B, Hollinger EF, et al. Normal thymic uptake of 2-deoxy-2[F-18]fluoro-D-glucose. Clin Nucl Med 1999;24:597–600.

[23] Saggese D, Compadretti GC, Cartaroni C. Cervical ectopic thymus: a case report and review of the literature. Int J Pediatr Otorhinolaryngol 2002;66: 77–80.

[24] Malone PS, Fitzgerald RJ. Aberrant thymus: a misleading mediastinal mass. J Pediatr Surg 1987;22:130.

[25] Saade M, Whitten DM, Necheles TF, et al. Posterior mediastinal accessory thymus. J Pediatr 1976; 88:71–2.

[26] Baysal T, Kutlu R, Kutlu O, et al. Ectopic thymic tissue: a cause of emphysema in infants. Clin Imaging 1999;23:19–21.

[27] Bach AM, Hilfer CL, Holgersen LO. Left-sided posterior mediastinal thymus: MR imaging findings. Pediatr Radiol 1991;21:440–1.

[28] Bar-Ziv J, Barki Y, Itzchak Y, et al. Posterior mediastinal accessory thymus. Pediatr Radiol 1984;14: 165–7.

[29] Cohen MD, Weber TR, Sequeira FW, et al. The diagnostic dilemma of the posterior mediastinal thymus: CT manifestations. Radiology 1983;146:691–2.

[30] Rollins NK, Currarino G. Case report: MR imaging of posterior mediastinal thymus. J Comput Assist Tomogr 1988;12:518–20.

[31] Slovis TL, Meza MP, Kuhn JP. Aberrant thymus: MR assessment. Pediatr Radiol 1992;22:490–2.

[32] Kuhn JP. Pediatric thorax. In: Nadich DP, Zerhouni EA, Siegelman SS, editors. Computed tomography and magnetic resonance of the thorax. New York: Raven Press; 1998. p. 505.

[33] Dimitriou G, Greenough A, Rafferty G, et al. Respiratory distress in a neonate with an enlarged thymus. Eur J Pediatr 2000;159:237–8.

[34] Rice HE, Flake AW, Hori T, et al. Massive thymic hyperplasia: characterization of a rare mediastinal mass. J Pediatr Surg 1994;29:1561–4.

[35] Judd RL. Massive thymic hyperplasia with myoid cell differentiation. Hum Pathol 1987;18:1180–3.

[36] Parker LA, Gaisie G, Scatliff JH. Computerized tomography and ultrasonographic findings in massive thymic hyperplasia: case discussion and review of current concepts. Clin Pediatr 1985;24: 90–4.

[37] Budavari AI, Whitaker MD, Helmers RA. Thymic hyperplasia presenting as anterior mediastinal mass in 2 patients with Graves disease. Mayo Clin Proc 2002;77:495–9.

[38] Van Herle AJ, Chopra IJ. Thymic hyperplasia in Graves' disease. J Clin Endocrinol Metab 1971;32: 140–6.

[39] Murakami M, Hosoi Y, Negishi T, et al. Thymic hyperplasia in patients with Graves' disease: identification of thyrotropin receptors in human thymus. J Clin Invest 1996;98:2228–34.

[40] Marx A, Muller-Hermelink HK, Strobel P. The role of thymomas in the development of myasthenia gravis. Ann N Y Acad Sci 2003;998:223–36.

[41] Mishra SK, Melinkeri SR, Dabadghao S. Benign thymic hyperplasia after chemotherapy for acute myeloid leukemia. Eur J Haematol 2001;67:252–4.

[42] Lin EC. Iodine-131 uptake in thymic hyperplasia with atypical computed tomographic features. Clin Nucl Med 2000;25:375.

[43] Veronikis IE, Simkin P, Braverman LE. Thymic uptake of iodine-131 in the anterior mediastinum. J Nucl Med 1996;7:991–2.

[44] Shin YK, Lee GK, Kook MC, et al. Reduced expression of CD99 and functional disturbance in anencephalic cortical thymocytes. Virchows Arch 1999; 434:443–9.

[45] Kuleva SA, Kolygin BA. Malignant mediastinal neoplasms in children. Vestn Khir Im I I Grek 2003;162: 46–8.

[46] Takeda S, Miyoshi S, Akashi A, et al. Clinical spectrum of primary mediastinal tumors: a comparison of adult and pediatric populations at a single Japanese institution. J Surg Oncol 2003;83:24–30.

[47] Asakawa H, Kashihara T, Fukuda H, et al. A pa-

tient with thymoma and four different organ-specific autoimmune diseases. Neth J Med 2002;60: 292–5.

[48] Spedini P, D'Adda M, Blanzuoli L. Thymoma and pancytopenia: a very rare association. Haematologica 2002;87:EIM18.

[49] Herrmann DN, Blaivas M, Wald JJ, et al. Granulomatous myositis, primary biliary cirrhosis, pancytopenia, and thymoma. Muscle Nerve 2000;23: 1133–6.

[50] Bozzolo E, Bellone M, Quaroni N, et al. Thymoma associated with systemic lupus erythematosus and immunologic abnormalities. Lupus 2000;9:151–4.

[51] Montresor E, Falezza G, Vassia S, et al. Thymoma, aplastic anemia, hypogammaglobulinemia and malignant pulmonary neoplasm: a case report. G Chir 1998;19:92–5.

[52] Rosado-de-Christenson ML, Galobardes J, Morán CA. Thymoma: radiologic- pathologic correlation. Radiographics 1992;12:151–68.

[53] Thomas CR, Wright CD, Loeherer PJ. Thymoma: state of the art. J Clin Oncol 1999;17:2280–9.

[54] Santana L, Givica A, Camacho C. Best cases from the AFIP: thymoma. Radiographics 2002;22:95–102.

[55] Hendrickson M, Azarow K, Ein S, et al. Congenital thymic cysts in children: mostly misdiagnosed. J Pediatr Surg 1998;33:821–5.

[56] Kontny HU, Sleasman JW, Kingma DW, et al. Multilocular thymic cysts in children with human immunodeficiency virus infection: clinical and pathologic aspects. J Pediatr 1997;131:264–70.

[57] Liang SB, Ohtsuki Y, Sonobe H, et al. Multilocular thymic cysts associated with thymoma: a case report. Pathol Res Pract 1996;192:1283–7.

[58] Rakheja D, Weinberg AG. Multilocular thymic cyst associated with mature mediastinal teratoma: a report of 2 cases. Arch Pathol Lab Med 2004;128:227–8.

[59] Chetty R, Reddi A. Rhabdomyomatous multilocular thymic cyst. Am J Clin Pathol 2003;119:816–21.

[60] Sandlund JT, Downing JR, Crist WM. Medical progress: non-Hodgkin's lymphoma in childhood. N Engl J Med 1996;334:1238–48.

[61] Robison LL. General principles of the epidemiology of childhood cancer. In: Pizzo PA, Poplack DG, editors. Principles and practice of pediatric oncology. 2nd edition. Philadelphia: JB Lippincott; 1993. p. 3–10.

[62] Magrath IT. Malignant non-Hodgkin's lymphomas in children. In: Pizzo PA, Poplack DG, editors. Principles and practice of pediatric oncology. 2nd edition. Philadelphia: JB Lippincott; 1993. p. 537–75.

[63] Young Jr JL, Ries LG, Silverberg E, et al. Cancer incidence, survival, and mortality for children younger than age 15 years. Cancer 1986;58:598–602.

[64] Glick RD, La Quaglia MP. Lymphomas of the anterior mediastinum. Semin Pediatr Surg 1999;8:69–77.

[65] Sandlund JT, Gorban ZI, Berard CW, et al. Large proportion of Epstein-Barr virus-associated small noncleaved cell lymphomas among children with non-Hodgkin's lymphoma at a single institution in Moscow, Russia. Am J Clin Oncol 1999;22:523–5.

[66] Arya LS, Narain S, Tomar S, et al. Superior vena cava syndrome. Indian J Pediatr 2002;69:293–7.

[67] Front D, Bar-Shalom R, Epelbaum R, et al. Early detection of lymphoma recurrence with gallium-67 scintigraphy. J Nucl Med 1993;34:2101–4.

[68] Bar-Shalom R, Yefremov N, Haim N, et al. Camera-based FDG PET and ^{67}Ga SPECT in evaluation of lymphoma: comparative study. Radiology 2003; 227:353–60.

[69] Billmire DF. Germ cell, mesenchymal, and thymic tumors of the mediastinum. Semin Pediatr Surg 1999; 8:85–91.

[70] Nichols CR. Mediastinal germ cell tumors: clinical features and biologic correlates. Chest 1991;99: 472–9.

[71] Billmire D, Vincour C, Rescorla F, et al. Malignant mediastinal germ cell tumors: an intergroup study. J Pediatr Surg 2001;36:18–24.

[72] Bebb GG, Grannis Jr FW, Paz IB, et al. Mediastinal germ cell tumor in a child with precocious puberty and Klinefelter syndrome. Ann Thorac Surg 1998; 66:547–8.

[73] Lewis BD, Hurt RD, Payne WS, et al. Benign teratoma of the mediastinum. J Thorac Cardiovasc Surg 1983;86:727–31.

[74] Brown LR, Muhm JR, Aughenbaugh GL, et al. Computed tomography of benign mature teratomas of the mediastinum. J Thorac Imaging 1987;2:66–71.

[75] Aygun C, Slawson RG, Bajaj K, et al. Primary mediastinal seminoma. Urology 1984;23:109–17.

[76] Lee KS, Im JG, Han CH, et al. Malignant primary germ cell tumors of the mediastinum: CT features. AJR Am J Roentgenol 1989;153:947–51.

[77] Shin MS, Ho KJ. Computed tomography of primary mediastinal seminomas. J Comput Assist Tomogr 1983;7:990–4.

[78] Drevelegas A, Palladas P, Scordalaki A. Mediastinal germ cell tumors: a radiologic-pathologic review. Eur Radiol 2001;11:1925–32.

[79] Kirwan WO, Walbaum PR, McCormack RJM. Cystic intrathoracic derivatives of the foregut and their complications. Thorax 1973;28:424–8.

[80] Snyder ME, Luck SR, Hernandez R, et al. Diagnostic dilemmas of mediastinal cysts. J Pediatr Surg 1985;20:810–5.

[81] Sirivella S, Ford WB, Zikria EA, et al. Foregut cysts of the mediastinum. J Thorac Cardiovasc Surg 1985; 90:776–82.

[82] Abell MR. Mediastinal cysts. Arch Pathol Lab Med 1956;61:360–79.

[83] Reed JC, Sobonya RE. Morphologic analysis of foregut cysts in the thorax. AJR Am J Roentgenol 1974; 120:851–60.

[84] Kuhlman JE, Fishman EK, Wang KP, et al. Esophageal duplication cyst: CT and transesophageal needle aspiration. AJR Am J Roentgenol 1985;145: 531–2.

[85] Strollo DC, Rosado-de-Christenson ML, Jett JR. Primary mediastinal tumors. Part II: tumors of the middle and posterior mediastinum. Chest 1997;112: 1344–57.

[86] Salyer DC, Salyer WR, Eggleston JC. Benign developmental cysts of the mediastinum. Arch Pathol Lab Med 1977;101:136–9.

[87] Reed JC, Sobonya RE. Morphologic analysis of foregut cysts in the thorax. AJR Am J Roentgenol 1974;120:851–60.

[88] Nakata H, Nakayama C, Kimoto T, et al. Computed tomography of mediastinal bronchogenic cysts. J Comput Assist Tomogr 1982;6:733–8.

[89] Mendelson DS, Rose JS, Efremidis SC, et al. Bronchogenic cysts with high CT numbers. AJR Am J Roentgenol 1983;140:463–5.

[90] Bergstrom JF, Yost RV, Ford KT, et al. Unusual roentgen manifestations of bronchogenic cysts. Radiology 1973;107:49–54.

[91] Tobert DG, Midthun DE. Bronchogenic cyst. J Bronch 1996;3:295–9.

[92] Eraklis AJ, Griscom NT, McGovern JB. Bronchogenic cysts of the mediastinum in infancy. N Engl J Med 1969;281:1150–4.

[93] Estrera AS, Landay MJ, Pass LJ. Mediastinal carinal bronchogenic cyst: is its mere presence an indication for surgical excision? South Med J 1987;80: 1523–6.

[94] Fishman SJ. Vascular anomalies of the mediastinum. Semin Pediatr Surg 1999;8:92–8.

[95] Kataria R, Bhatnagar V, Gupta SD, et al. Mediastinal lymphangiomyoma in a child: report of a case. Surg Today 1998;28:1084–6.

[96] Adil A, Ksiyer M. Unusual mediastinal cystic lymphangioma: apropos of a case and review of the literature. Ann Radiol 1996;39:249–52.

[97] Sumner TE, Volberg FM, Kiser PE, et al. Mediastinal cystic hygroma in children. Pediatr Radiol 1981; 11:160–2.

[98] Antuaco EJ, Jimenez JF, Burrow P, et al. Lymphatic-venous malformation (lymphohemangioma) of mediastinum. J Comput Assist Tomogr 1983;7:895–7.

[99] Feigin D, Fenoglio JJ, McAllister HA, et al. Pericardial cysts: a radiologic-pathologic correlation and review. Radiology 1977;125:15–20.

[100] Prader E, Kirschner PA. Pericardial diverticulum. Dis Chest 1969;55:344–6.

[101] Abell MR. Mediastinal cysts. Arch Pathol Lab Med 1956;61:360–79.

[102] Murayama S, Murakami J, Watanabe H, et al. Signal intensity characteristics of mediastinal cystic masses on T sub 1-weighted MR imaging. J Comput Assist Tomogr 1995;19:188–91.

[103] Kuhn JP. Middle mediastinal masses. In: Kuhn JP, Slovis TL, Haller JO, editors. Caffey's pediatric diagnostic imaging. St. Louis: Mosby; 2004. p. 1160–240.

[104] Frush DP. Pediatric mediastinal masses. Ann Acad Med Singapore 2003;32:525–35.

[105] Lonergan GJ, Schwab CM, Suarez ES, et al. Neuroblastoma, ganglioneuroblastoma, and ganglioneuroma: radiologic-pathologic correlation. Radiographics 2002;22:911–34.

[106] Hiorns MP, Owens CM. Radiology of neuroblastoma in children. Eur Radiol 2001;11:2071–81.

[107] Daldrup HE, Link TM, Wortler K, et al. MR imaging of thoracic tumors in pediatric patients. AJR Am J Roentgenol 1998;170:1639–44.

[108] Sofka CM, Semelka RC, Kelekis NL, et al. Magnetic resonance imaging of neuroblastoma using current techniques. Magn Reson Imaging 1999;17: 193–8.

[109] Howman-Giles RB, Golday DL, Ash JM. Radionuclide skeletal survey in neuroblastoma. Radiology 1997;131:497–502.

[110] Heisel MA, Miller JH, Reid BS, et al. Radionuclide bone scan in neuroblastoma. Pediatrics 1983; 71:206–9.

[111] Kushner BH. Neuroblastoma: a disease requiring a multitude of imaging studies. J Nucl Med 2004; 45:1172–88.

[112] Montalldo PG, Lanciotti M, Casalaro A, et al. Accumulation of m-iodobenzylguanidine by neuroblastoma cells results from independent uptake and storage mechanism. Cancer Res 1991;51:4342–6.

[113] Iavarone A, Lasorella A, Servidei T, et al. Uptake and storage of m-iodobenzylguanidine are frequent neuronal functions of human neuroblastoma cell line. Cancer Res 1993;53:304–9.

[114] Biasotti S, Garavanta A, Villavecchia GP, et al. False-negative metaiodobenzylguanidine scintigraphy at diagnosis of neuroblastoma. Med Pediatr Oncol 2000;35:153–5.

[115] Mathay KK, Brisse H, Couanet D, et al. Central nervous system metastases in neuroblastoma: radiologic, clinical, and biologic features in 23 patients. Cancer 2003;98:155–65.

[116] Suc A, Lumbroso J, Rubie H, et al. Metastatic neuroblastoma in children older than one year: prognostic significance of the initial metaiodobenzylguanidine scan and proposal for a scoring system. Cancer 1996;77:805–11.

[117] Perel Y, Conway J, Kletzel M, et al. Clinical impact and prognostic value of metaiodobenzylguanidine imaging in children with metastatic neuroblastoma. Pediatr Hematol Oncol 1999;21:13–8.

[118] Laurent F, Latrabe V, Lecesne R, et al. Mediastinal masses: diagnostic approach. Eur Radiol 1998;8: 1149–59.

[119] Inci I, Turgut M. Neurogenic tumors of the mediastinum in children. Childs Nerv Syst 1999;15:372–6.

[120] Spector J, Willis D, Ginsburg H. Paraganglioma (pheochromocytoma) of the posterior mediastinum: a case report and review of the literature. J Pediatr Surg 2003;38:1114–6.

[121] Hutchins K, Dickson D, Hameed M, et al. Sudden death in a child due to an intrathoracic paraganglioma. Am J Forensic Med Pathol 1999;20: 338–42.

[122] Pungavkar S, Shah J, Patkar D, et al. Isolated symmetrical mediastinal lipomatosis. J Assoc Physicians India 2001;49:1026–8.

[123] Siebenrock K, Nascimento A, Rock M. Comparison of soft tissue Ewing's sarcoma and peripheral neuroectodermal tumor. Clin Orthop 1996;329: 288–99.

[124] Cohen M. Tumors involving multiple tissues or organs. In: Imaging of children with cancer. St. Louis: Mosby; 1992. p. 342–58.

ELSEVIER
SAUNDERS

Radiol Clin N Am 43 (2005) 355 – 370

RADIOLOGIC
CLINICS
of North America

Imaging Evaluation of Chest Wall Disorders in Children

Nancy R. Fefferman, MD*, Lynne P. Pinkney, MD

Division of Pediatric Radiology, Department of Radiology, New York University School of Medicine, 560 First Avenue,
RIRM 234, New York, NY 10016, USA

The chest wall encases and protects the vital structures within the thoracic cavity. The chest wall comprises multiple layers, including skin, subcutaneous fat, muscle, bone, cartilage, and pleura. Chest wall disorders may be congenital, developmental, or acquired and typically involve one or more of these layers. Acquired pathologic processes may be infectious, neoplastic, or traumatic. Imaging often plays an integral role in the evaluation of symptomatic and asymptomatic chest wall abnormalities. Symptomatic chest wall pathology usually requires imaging evaluation to assist in localization and characterization of lesions. Although asymptomatic palpable chest wall lesions tend to be benign or reflect normal developmental variations, imaging is still often requested [1,2].

Imaging modalities and techniques

Radiography

Conventional radiography of the chest or osseous structures is often the primary screening modality for palpable, symptomatic, or asymptomatic chest wall disorders as well as for symptomatic nonpalpable processes. Palpable but otherwise asymptomatic osseous abnormalities, including congenital and developmental variants involving the ribs and sternum, can sometimes be recognized on chest radiographs or on dedicated radiographs, avoiding further imaging evaluation. Chest or rib radiographs may be the only imaging study necessary for definitive diagnosis of benign osseous lesions. Additionally, chest radiography can be useful in the preliminary assessment of suspected malignant osseous lesions and can help direct the imaging work-up.

Cross-sectional imaging

CT

CT has a pivotal role in the evaluation of chest wall pathology. Recent technological advances in CT allowing improved spatial resolution, multiplanar capabilities, and faster examination times minimizing respiratory artifact have increased the appeal of this imaging modality in children. Additionally, the rapid scan time with multidetector helical CT (MDCT) has helped to overcome the need for sedation in younger children [3]. Concerns regarding the radiation dose associated with CT in children and the potential carcinogenic effects [4,5] remain important considerations when using CT. CT may be indicated for further evaluation when plain radiographs are normal or inconclusive. In particular, CT is excellent for defining lesion extent, including involvement of adjacent structures, for providing information that can be important for determining the nature of the disorder, or for narrowing the range of differential considerations.

Examinations for chest wall pathology can be performed using single-detector or multidetector CT. The smallest possible field of view should be used to maximize spatial resolution. When diagnostic

* Corresponding author.
E-mail address: nancy.fefferman@nyumc.org
(N.R. Fefferman).

considerations include infectious and neoplastic processes, non-ionic intravenous contrast material is used. A suggested dose is 2.0 mL/kg, with an injection rate 1 to 1.5 mL/s, and a scan delay from the start of the injection of 35 seconds for single-detector CT and 50 seconds for MDCT. Single-detector CT images are acquired with a slice collimation of 5 to 7 mm, depending on patient size, pitch of 1.5, peak kilovoltage (kVp) of 120, and milliampere-seconds (mAs) determined by patient weight [6]. The images are reconstructed in both standard and edge-enhanced algorithms. MDCT protocols vary depending on the vendor. At The New York University School of Medicine, when CT is indicated, the authors currently use a 16-slice MDCT scanner (Siemens Sensation, Siemens Medical Systems, Erlangen, Germany) for evaluation of pediatric chest wall abnormalities. The images are acquired with 1.5-mm acquisition collimation, feed/rotation of 24 mm, kVp 120, and mAs determined by Siemens weight-based criteria. The images are reconstructed at 4-mm intervals using both soft tissue and bone algorithms.

MR imaging

MR imaging is an excellent cross-sectional imaging modality that offers superior contrast and excellent spatial resolution without the use of ionizing radiation or iodinated contrast. Its application in smaller children is more limited, however, because of the relatively long duration of examination, often requiring sedation, and the inherent respiratory artifact from non–breath-holding. For these reasons, successful MR imaging in children can be challenging, and at the New York University School of Medicine it is often reserved for problem solving in specific cases and for the evaluation of vascular anomalies that can affect the chest wall.

The authors use a 1.5-T system (Vision, Symphony, or Avanto; Siemens Medical Systems, Erlangen, Germany) together with a head coil for infants and toddlers and a phased-array surface coil for older children or larger areas of coverage. The MR imaging approach for achieving optimal spatial and temporal resolution in children includes using the smallest field of view possible and minimizing patient motion and scan time. Intravenous contrast is used in most cases. The specific MR imaging protocol for chest wall lesions is determined by the suspected location of chest wall involvement; protocols for visualizing osseous pathology and soft tissue pathology can differ.

MR imaging of chest wall soft tissue pathology typically includes multiplanar T1-weighted turbo spin echo (TSE) and a fat-suppression sequence such as an inversion-recovery (STIR) or T2-weighted TSE with fat suppression (in two planes that will best demonstrate the abnormality). Three-dimensional gradient echo T1-weighted imaging with fat suppression, both before and after administration of contrast (gadopentate dimeglumine, Magnevist; Berlex, Wayne, New Jersey) at a dose of 0.1 mmol/kg body weight by rapid bolus, is often employed for evaluation of lesions suspected to be neoplastic, infectious, or vascular in origin.

Examinations are tailored further to the specific clinical indication using additional sequences. They may include time-resolved MR angiography for dynamic characterization of vascular anomalies. Time-resolved MR angiography is performed using a fat-suppressed T1-weighted volumetric spoiled gradient echo sequence for rapid acquisition of repeated serial images through a region of interest after contrast administration. This technique offers excellent temporal resolution at the expense of decreased spatial resolution.

At the New York University School of Medicine, postprocessing techniques, including subtraction, multiplanar reconstruction and maximal-intensity projections (MIPs), are routinely performed. These techniques often help further define and characterize chest wall pathology.

Routine MR imaging of the chest wall for evaluation of bone abnormalities includes multiplanar spin echo T1- and T2-weighted sequences for assessment of marrow signal. Additional sequences with fat saturation may be helpful for delineating changes in the adjacent soft tissues.

Ultrasonography

Ultrasound is being used with increasing frequency in the evaluation of palpable, superficial chest wall pathology [7]. The relatively risk-free, non-invasive nature and the fast examination time of this imaging modality make ultrasound a useful screening tool, especially for children. Using a high-frequency linear transducer, ultrasound can aid in determining whether a lesion is present and potentially can characterize a palpable lesion as cystic or solid. Additionally, color Doppler ultrasound and spectral tracings can provide important information regarding vascular flow, particularly in the evaluation of vascular masses such as malformations and hemangiomas [8]. The inability to see deeper structures (such as the spinal foramina or mediastinum) and to penetrate or evaluate bone limits usefulness in sufficiently assessing lesions that are other than superficial and soft tissue in nature.

Soft tissue abnormalities

Congenital abnormalities

Poland syndrome

Poland syndrome is a rare congenital malformation of the chest wall consisting of hypoplasia or aplasia of the pectoralis major muscle and adjacent cartilaginous, osseous, and soft tissue structures. Poland syndrome is hypothesized to occur as a result of ipsilateral subclavian artery disruption. Brachysyndactly also occurs as an associated abnormality of the upper extremity. Although the degree of involvement varies, this condition is nearly always unilateral. Males are affected more frequently than females (2–3:1), and the right side is involved in approximately 60% to 75% of cases [9,10].

Asymmetry of the chest wall is apparent clinically. Radiographically, hypoplasia of the chest wall soft tissues results in a relative hyperlucency of the affected hemithorax. The differential diagnosis includes pulmonary entities that cause air trapping. such as congenital lobar emphysema, obstruction from a foreign body, or Swyer-James syndrome. Because the extent of chest wall deformity is difficult to determine by physical examination and chest radiography, multiplanar cross-sectional imaging with MR imaging or CT scanning using three-dimensional reformatting can be helpful in presurgical planning [11].

Vascular malformations

Lymphatic malformation

Lymphatic malformations, formerly known as lymphangiomas, are part of the spectrum of congenital abnormalities of the lymphatic system. Histologically, lymphatic malformations are composed of an increased number of dilated lymphatic channels lined by endothelium. They have been classified as microcystic, macrocystic, or combined. Lymphatic malformations can occur anywhere but are most commonly located in the axilla, chest, and cervicofacial region. In the chest, lymphatic malformations can be focal or diffuse masses confined to the subcutaneous tissues or can involve the spine or mediastinum [12,13].

Superficial lesions can be imaged easily with ultrasound. Because it can be difficult to determine the true extent of vascular malformations with sonography, cross-sectional imaging (preferably MR imaging) is usually indicated. Sonographically, macrocystic lymphatic malformations are predominantly anechoic masses that may contain septations of variable thickness. Color Doppler interrogation may demonstrate arterial or venous flow within the septations [14]. Microcystic lesions tend to be more echogenic.

When the lesion clearly is not confined to the subcutaneous layer, MR imaging can best assess the extent of the abnormality. Macrocystic lymphatic malformations are composed of discrete cystic structures with intervening septations. The cysts have homogenously high signal intensity on T2-weighted sequences and low signal intensity on T1-weighted sequences. Blood or protein products within the cysts can result in fluid–fluid levels. The septations are low signal on both T1- and T2-weighted sequences and may demonstrate contrast enhancement (Fig. 1). Because the cysts in microcystic lymphatic malformations are often too small to resolve, these lesions tend to have diffuse low signal intensity on T1-weighted images and high signal intensity on T2-weighted images. After administration of intravenous contrast the microcystic lymphatic malformations may demonstrate mild diffuse enhancement resulting from enhancement of the closely packed contiguous cyst walls, mimicking solid soft tissue masses [15].

Venous malformation

Venous malformations represent a spectrum of congenital abnormalities of the deep or superficial venous system. These malformations manifest as isolated or multiple dilated, tortuous venous structures that, histologically, are composed of dilated, thin-walled channels. Although they are usually present at birth, they may not become symptomatic until later in life. Like lymphatic malformations, venous malformations can range from focal abnormalities within the subcutaneous soft tissues to more diffuse involvement of the deeper soft tissues and bone as well as extensive infiltration of the body wall, extremities, and organs. Venous malformations affect the chest wall less commonly than lymphatic malformations [13].

On ultrasound, venous malformations may be hypoechoic, isoechoic, or hyperechoic to subcutaneous soft tissues. Internal, shadowing, echogenic foci representing phleboliths may also be identified. Color Doppler spectral tracings demonstrate either low-flow venous patterns or no flow [8,14].

In the management of venous malformations, MR imaging is the imaging modality of choice with respect to extent of involvement and characterization of flow. These lesions are typically multiloculated structures with a lobulated contour. They have high signal intensity on T2-weighted sequences and low

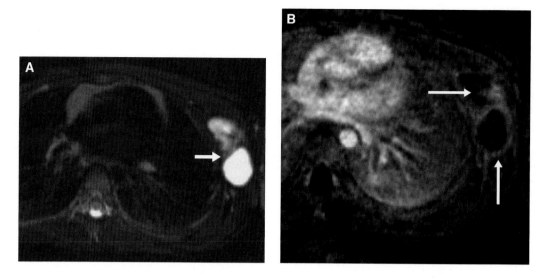

Fig. 1. A 2-year-old boy who has left lateral chest wall lymphatic malformation. (*A*) Axial T2-weighted MR image of the chest demonstrates a multiloculated high-signal-intensity left lateral chest wall mass with internal septations (*arrow*). (*B*) Axial fat-saturated, T1-weighted postcontrast MR image demonstrates low signal intensity of the cystic component and enhancement of the walls and septations (*arrows*).

signal intensity on corresponding T1-weighted sequences. Focal round signal voids, consistent with the presence of phleboliths, are often present on T1- and T2-weighted sequences. Venous malformations enhance diffusely during the venous phase after intravenous contrast administration, best demonstrated with time-resolved MR angiography (Fig. 2) [15].

Benign soft tissue masses

Hemangioma

Hemangiomas, the most common soft tissue tumors of infancy and childhood, are benign soft tissue neoplasms composed of abnormally proliferating

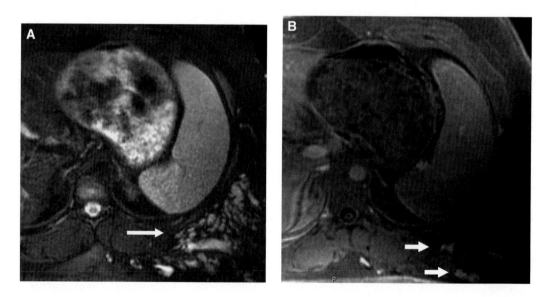

Fig. 2. A 10-year-old boy who has left posterolateral chest wall venous malformation. (*A*) Axial MR STIR image demonstrates a cluster of serpiginous high-signal structures within the posterolateral left chest wall (*arrow*). (*B*) Axial postcontrast T1-weighted MR image shows late venous-phase enhancement of abnormal vascular structures in the posterolateral left chest wall (*arrows*).

endothelial cells. These soft tissue masses are typically located within the subcutaneous soft tissues, most commonly in the head and neck, chest wall, and extremities. Hemangiomas may be present at birth or appear in the first few weeks or months of life. These lesions typically undergo an early proliferative phase, followed by a plateau and subsequent involutional phase during which about 70% to 90% of hemangiomas spontaneously regress almost completely [16]. Small, superficial hemangiomas are most often clinically insignificant, but larger, more extensive hemangiomas can be disfiguring or compromise the function of adjacent structures such as the airway.

Superficial subcutaneous hemangiomas can usually be diagnosed clinically by their characteristic cutaneous appearance. Imaging may be indicated for deeper or larger lesions. Ultrasound is often the initial imaging modality used to evaluate these palpable soft tissue masses. Subcutaneous lesions typically are well-defined hypoechoic or, less commonly, hyperechoic masses. Larger hemangiomas may have a complex echotexture containing dilated vascular channels during the proliferative and plateau phases. These lesions are hypervascular with color Doppler sonography demonstrating high-velocity arterial and venous flow (Fig. 3) [8,17,18]. Although ultrasound

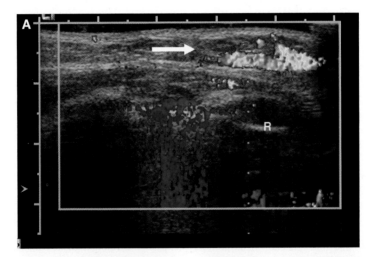

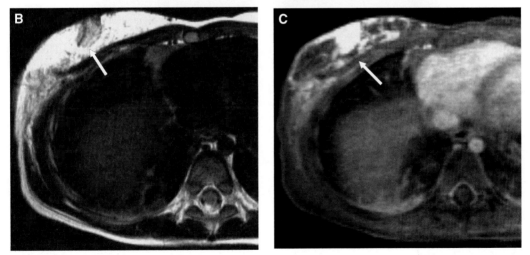

Fig. 3. An 8-month-old girl who has right anterior chest wall hemangioma. (*A*) Transverse sonographic image of the right anterior chest wall with color Doppler shows a hypervascular hypoechoic mass in the subcutaneous soft tissues. R, rib. (*B*) Axial T2-weighted MR image demonstrates diffuse abnormal high signal in the subcutaneous soft tissues of the right anterior chest wall (*arrow*). (*C*) Axial postcontrast T1-weighted MR image shows focal regions of enhancement. The areas of decreased signal within the mass (*arrow*) represent fibrofatty replacement that occurs during the involutional phase.

can be diagnostic in the evaluation of hemangiomas, MR imaging is useful in assessing the extent of involvement and the anatomic relationship to adjacent structures before surgical intervention. With MR imaging, hemangiomas in the proliferative or plateau phase are well-circumscribed, lobulated soft tissue masses isointense to muscle on T1-weighted images and hyperintense on T2-weighted images. On T1- and T2-weighted sequences they often contain tubular signal voids reflecting the high-flow vessels. Hemangiomas demonstrate profound diffuse enhancement after administration of intravenous gadolinium. During the involutional phase, the fibrofatty replacement that occurs results in increasing T1 signal intensity, decreased T2 signal intensity, and decreased contrast enhancement (Fig. 3) [15].

Other benign soft tissue masses

Other, more rare benign soft tissue masses that can affect the chest wall include lipoblastoma, fibrous tumors of childhood such as fibroma, fibromatosis, fibrous hamartoma of infancy [19], and infantile myofibromatosis [20]. Neurogenic tumors such as schwannomas and neurofibromas arising from the intercostal nerves or sympathetic ganglia can result in secondary erosive or destructive changes to the adjacent rib. Children with underlying neurofibromatosis type I are susceptible to extensive involvement of the chest wall with plexiform neurofibromas. Primary osseous abnormalities related to neurofibromatosis, including the ribbon appearance of the ribs, kyphoscoliosis, and dorsal scalloping of the vertebral bodies, are often present in these cases.

Lipoblastoma is a rare benign but locally aggressive mesenchymal tumor of embryonal fat that occurs in infants and children. Whereas lipoblastoma may demonstrate the typical findings associated with fat-containing lesions, such as increased echogenicity on ultrasound and increased signal intensity on T1-weighted sequences, imaging is often nonspecific with respect to definitive diagnosis within the spectrum of fibrous tumors of childhood [21]. Because local excision is the usual treatment, cross-sectional imaging can aid in the evaluation of the extent of the lesion and the relationship to adjacent structures [22].

Osseous abnormalities

Congenital/Developmental abnormalities

Congenital and developmental variations in the chest wall typically involve the sternum, ribs, and costal cartilage. Many of the asymptomatic palpable chest wall masses in children are developmentally normal anatomic osseous and cartilaginous variants Cross-sectional imaging may confirm the benign nature of these chest wall variants but is often not necessary [1]. In the absence of clinical signs suggesting an aggressive lesion such as pain, interval increase in size, or constitutional symptoms, chest radiography is usually adequate for excluding the possibility of an aggressive condition when evaluating focal, palpable chest wall masses.

Anatomic variations affecting the sternum that can manifest as a physical chest wall abnormality include tilting of the sternum, pectus excavatum, and pectus carinatum. Sternal tilting refers to deviation of the typical horizontal positioning of the sternum in the transverse axis of the body. Although sternal tilting is usually not apparent on conventional radiographs, the secondary lateral displacement of the medial ends of the adjacent clavicles may be helpful. Sternal tilting can also be associated with anterior subluxation of the adjacent clavicular head or abnormal convexity of the adjacent rib resulting in a palpable chest wall bump [1,2].

Pectus excavatum is a deformity of the chest wall in which the inferior aspect of the sternum is depressed posteriorly, resulting in a relative concavity that can vary from mild to severe. In addition to the cosmetic issues, severe pectus excavatum has been associated with mitral valve prolapse and compromise of cardiopulmonary function. On the frontal chest radiograph the soft tissue depression results in silhouetting of the right heart border simulating a right middle lobe consolidation. CT is an excellent imaging modality to assess the anatomic severity of the pectus excavatum defect (Fig. 4). The ratio of the transverse diameter of the chest to the anteroposterior diameter of the chest at its narrowest dimension on CT, known as the pectus or Haller index, can be used to characterize the degree of chest wall deformity. Haller et al [23] found that children requiring surgical correction for pectus excavatum on the subjective basis of abnormal chest wall dynamics or general distortion of the chest wall configuration had a pectus index greater than 3.25, compared with less than 3.25 in normal controls. Pectus carinatum is a less common chest wall deformity characterized by convexity of the chest wall resulting from anterior protrusion of the superior aspect of the sternum. Although pectus excavatum and pectus carinatum can be isolated abnormalities, they may be associated with Marfan syndrome, congenital heart disease, and scoliosis [24].

Congenital sternal-fusion abnormalities are rare and include a broad spectrum of deformities includ-

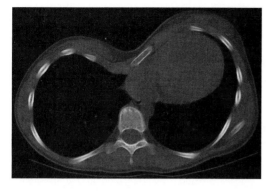

Fig. 4. A 12-year-old girl who has pectus excavatum. Axial noncontrast CT image of the chest demonstrates marked depression of the sternum.

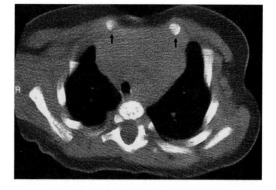

Fig. 6. A 1-month-old boy who has bifid sternum. Axial noncontrast CT image shows marked separation of the clavicular heads (*arrows*) and depression of the intervening soft tissues in the expected location of the absent upper sternum.

ing bifid or cleft sternum and complete absence of sternal fusion (Fig. 5). The bifid sternum may be an isolated abnormality requiring surgical correction to prevent cardiopulmonary compromise (Fig. 6) [25]. At the severe end of sternal-fusion abnormalities, there is often associated congenital heart disease such as ectopia cordis (extrathoracic heart) and pentalogy of Cantrell [26,27], a combination of severe defects of the middle of the chest including the sternum, diaphragm, heart, and abdominal wall.

Common congenital anomalies affecting the ribs include agenesis, hypoplasia, and a bifid configuration. Developmental anatomic variations of the ribs and costal cartilage can present as asymptomatic palpable chest wall masses. These variations include prominent convexity of an anterior rib or costal carti-

lage, prominence of the costochondral junction, and small parachondral nodules of unknown origin [2].

The scapula is also subject to a spectrum of congenital anomalies. The most notable of these affecting the chest wall is failure of descent of the scapula known as Sprengel's deformity. Although Sprengel's deformity may be an isolated abnormality, it has been associated with Klippel-Feil syndrome. In some patients with Sprengel's deformity, the scapula is tethered to the spine by an osteocartilaginous connection referred to as the omohyoid bone.

Benign osseous lesions

Osteochondroma and enchondroma

The osseous structures of the chest wall can be affected by benign neoplastic lesions. The most common benign neoplasm involving the osseous components of the chest wall is an osteochondroma or exostosis. Osteochondromas are osseous excrescences composed of cortical and medullary bone with a hyaline cartilaginous cap that arise from the surface of the bone. These bony outgrowths most commonly involve the metaphysis of tubular bones, but they can also affect the ribs, vertebra, clavicle, scapula, and sternum [20,28]. Osteochondromas may be solitary or multiple. The majority of solitary osteochondromas occur in children and adolescents. Multiple bilateral osteochondromas occur with the autosomal dominant disorder, multiple hereditary exostosis. Although osteochondromas typically present as nontender chest wall masses, they can cause symptoms related to compression of adjacent structures such as nerves or vessels. Malignant transformation is a rare complication that has been reported to occur with an incidence

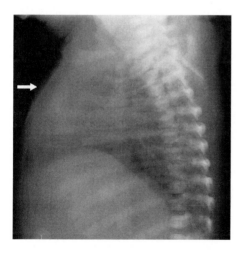

Fig. 5. A 9-month-old girl who has an absent sternum. Lateral radiograph of the chest demonstrates complete absence of the sternum and sternal ossification centers (*arrow*).

less than 1% in solitary osteochondromas and up to 25% for multiple osteochondromas. Over 90% of the malignant transformations result in chondrosarcoma [29]. Clinical signs of malignant transformation include new onset of pain and continued growth after skeletal maturity.

Osteochondromas are characterized radiographically by an osseous protrusion from a bone composed of both spongiosa and cortex that is continuous with the adjacent bone. These exophytic excrescences may be pedunculated or sessile and can result in secondary deformity of the bone (Fig. 7). Osteochondromas usually stop growing at the time of growth plate fusion. Cross-sectional imaging usually is reserved for surgical planning in cases of larger, more complicated, or symptomatic lesions and for evaluation for possible malignant degeneration. CT is helpful in characterizing internal matrix. Asymptomatic rib or scapular lesions may be detected as incidental findings on CT performed for other indication. With CT, osteochondromas appear as a contour irregularity of the bone that is contiguous with the cortex of the adjacent donor bone. Although the cartilaginous cap in superficial lesions can be visualized with ultrasound [30], MR imaging is more widely used for evaluation of the cartilaginous cap, which should not be greater than 2 cm in thickness [29]. The benign cartilaginous cap appears as a thin, uniform layer of high signal on T2-weighted gradient echo sequences. Thickening and irregularity of the cartilaginous cap is suspicious for malignant transformation. Differen-

tiation of early chondrosarcoma from osteochondroma can be difficult with MR imaging, because both entities have demonstrated septal enhancement after contrast administration [31]. These entities can be differentiated better by dynamic contrast-enhanced MR imaging [32].

Enchondromas are less common in children and typically occur in the third and fourth decades of life. The rib is the most commonly affected osseous structure of the chest wall [33]. The solitary enchondroma is a benign neoplasm composed of hyaline cartilage that originates in the medullary cavity. Radiographically, enchondromas are characterized by a well-defined medullary lesion with a lobulated contour and endosteal scalloping. The lesions may be expansile and may contain chondroid matrix [34]. Multiple enchondromas occur in Ollier's syndrome and are associated with multiple vascular masses, including hemangiomas, in Mafucci's syndrome (Fig. 8).

Fibrous dysplasia

Fibrous dysplasia is a developmental anomaly of bone-forming mesenchyme in which the osteoblasts fail to undergo normal morphologic differentiation Fibrous dysplasia has been reported to represent up to 20% to 30% of chest wall masses [33], with the ribs most commonly affected. Radiographically, a wide spectrum of rib changes is associated with fibrous dysplasia. Involvement can be characterized by a focal, expansile, multiloculated lucent lesion or fusiform enlargement with a ground-glass or sclerotic appearance. Adjacent extraosseous dysplastic soft tissue has also been described [35]. Although cross-sectional imaging is not typically required, fibrous dysplasia may be an incidental finding on CT (Fig. 9).

Rib changes similar to those seen with fibrous dysplasia have also been described in patients with tuberous sclerosis [36,37]. Radiographic findings include subperiosteal thickening, sclerosis, and cystic changes.

Infection

Chest wall infections are relatively rare in children. Infection occurs by hematogenous spread or direct extension and can involve the soft tissues, cartilage, and osseous structures. Both bacterial and fungal infections of the chest wall have been described in children [38–43]. Organisms include *Staphylococcus aureus*, *Mycobacterium tuberculosis*, *Actinomyces*, *Nocardia*, *Aspergillus*, and *Candida* [44,45]. Fungal infections more commonly affect immunocompromised patients. Empyema necessitatis

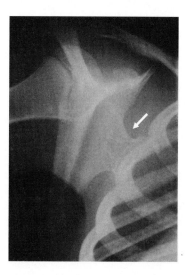

Fig. 7. A 6-year-old girl who has right scapular osteochondroma. Oblique radiograph of the right scapula demonstrates an osseous excrescence (*arrow*) projecting from the ventral aspect with contiguity of the cortical and medullary bone.

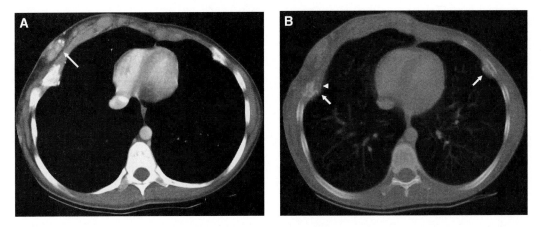

Fig. 8. An 8-year-old girl who has Mafucci syndrome. (*A*) Intravenous contrast–enhanced axial CT image of the chest shows a heterogeneously enhancing subcutaneous soft tissue mass in the right anterior chest wall representing a hemangioma (*arrow*). (*B*) Bone windows at the same level demonstrate lucent lesions involving anterolateral ribs on the right and left (*arrows*) in this patient with multiple enchondromatosis. Cartilaginous matrix is present in the right rib lesion (*arrowhead*).

is a rare complication of empyema characterized by extension from the pleural space into the chest wall [39]. Infection usually presents with clinical symptoms of pain and fever. Signs of local infection including erythema and swelling may be apparent.

Ultrasound can be helpful to localize a focal abscess and direct drainage for superficial lesions. On ultrasound, a chest wall abscess has the typical appearance of an encapsulated, predominantly anechoic mass with posterior acoustic enhancement and substantial peripheral flow demonstrated with color Doppler interrogation. Cross-sectional imaging better delineates the extent of more complex and deeper infectious processes (Fig. 10). Chest wall abscesses are peripherally enhancing, low-attenuation lesions with surrounding inflammation on contrast-enhanced CT examination. Chest wall infections may also appear as complex inflammatory masses without focal abscess formation. Adjacent rib destruction is easily detected on CT. MR imaging

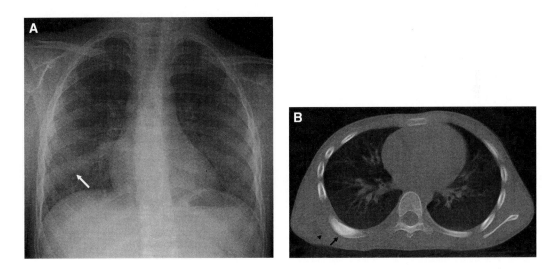

Fig. 9. A 5-year-old boy who has tuberous sclerosis and isolated rib fibrous dysplasia. (*A*) Frontal radiograph of the chest shows subtle, diffuse expansion and increased density of the right eighth posterior rib with a ground-glass appearance (*arrow*). (*B*) Axial CT image of the chest confirms a diffuse, expansile lesion of the rib (*arrow*) with abnormal adjacent soft tissue (*arrowhead*).

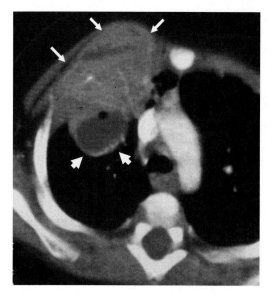

Fig. 10. A 6-month-old boy who has autosomal recessive severe combined immunodeficiency of unknown molecular cause and Candida organism chest wall infection. Axial contrast-enhanced CT scan of upper chest shows a mixed-attenuation mass consisting of abscess containing air and fluid in lung (*large arrows*) with invasion of anterior chest wall (*small arrows*). (*From* Yin EZ. Primary immunodeficiency disorders in pediatric patients: clinical features and imaging findings. AJR Am J Roentgenol 2001;176:1541–52; with permission.)

findings include abnormal increased signal on T2-weighted sequences. MR imaging is more sensitive for marrow edema without frank osseous destruction in early osteomyelitis.

Langerhans' cell histiocytosis

Langerhans' cell histiocytosis (LCH) can arise in the osseous structures of the chest wall including the ribs, clavicles, scapula, and vertebral bodies. The classic change associated with vertebral body involvement is vertebral body flattening known as vertebra plana. LCH affecting the ribs, clavicles, and scapula has a variable appearance ranging from poorly defined, expansile, lytic lesions to sharply marginated, sclerotic lesions [46]. Additionally, an adjacent soft tissue mass may be present [47]. The appearance is nonspecific and includes infection and neoplasm in the differential diagnosis. The margins may be ill defined or sharply marginated with or without surrounding sclerosis (Fig. 11) [48].

Benign masses

Mesenchymal hamartoma

Mesenchymal hamartoma of the chest wall is a rare, benign soft tissue mass originating from the rib that occurs most commonly in infancy. Histopathologically, this lesion is composed of both cystic and solid components. The solid component comprises normal maturing mesenchymal tissues including bone, cartilage, fat, and fibroblasts. The cystic component reflects the presence of hemorrhagic cavities related to the associated secondary aneurysmal bone formation [49–51].

Clinically, this lesion typically presents as a palpable, hard chest wall mass that, depending on size, may deform the chest wall or cause respiratory symptoms such as dyspnea. On chest radiography, mesenchymal hamartoma is a destructive, expansile lytic lesion involving one or more ribs with a large extrapleural soft tissue mass that may be partially calcified. Osteoid or chondroid matrix may be seen as well. Both CT and MR imaging demonstrate a large extrapleural soft tissue mass with associated expansion and destruction of contiguous ribs (Fig. 12). The heterogeneous nature of the lesion is well depicted with CT, which shows the low-attenuating cystic components, matrix mineralization, and heterogeneous, diffuse contrast enhancement. The mass demonstrates intermediate signal intensity relative to adjacent muscle on T1-weighted sequences with foci of high signal reflecting hemorrhage. T2-weighted sequences also show predominantly intermediate signal intensity with areas of high signal intensity and fluid levels in the regions of hemorrhagic cystic cavities. The solid components of the mass generally show diffuse enhancement after administration of gadolinium contrast [49].

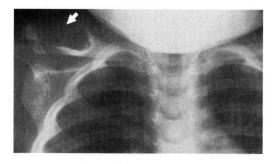

Fig. 11. A 1-year-old boy who has right-clavicular Langerhans' cell histiocytosis. Frontal radiograph of the upper chest demonstrates a sharply marginated, expansile, lytic lesion involving the mid and distal right clavicle (*arrow*).

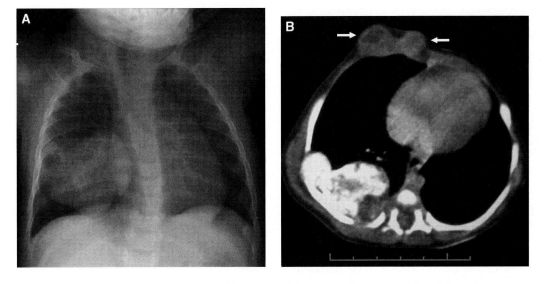

Fig. 12. A 3-month-old boy who has mesenchymal hamartoma of the chest wall. (*A*) Frontal chest radiograph demonstrates a well-defined mass in the right lower thorax. (*B*) Axial contrast-enhanced CT image demonstrates enhancement of the mass. Two other nodules (*arrows*) seen anteriorly also are believed to be mesenchymal hamartomas. (*From* Donnelly LF. Pediatric multidetector body CT. Radiol Clin North Am 2003;41:637–55.)

Although mesenchymal hamartomas are rare, it is important to consider this entity in the differential diagnosis of a complex cystic and solid chest wall mass containing mineralized elements that presents in early infancy or childhood. Surgical excision is curative, and there is no malignant potential.

Malignant soft tissue masses

Malignant soft tissue masses of the chest wall include primary soft tissue neoplasms in addition to soft tissue extension of a primary osseous neoplasm or a primary mediastinal neoplasm infiltrating the chest wall. Chest wall malignancies often involve many layers of the chest wall because of their aggressive nature.

Primitive neuroectodermal tumor (Askin's tumor) and Ewing's sarcoma

The Ewing's sarcoma family of tumors (ESFT), including primitive neuroectodermal tumor of the chest wall (also known as Askin's tumor [52]), Ewing's sarcoma of bone, and extraosseous Ewing's sarcoma, are the most common malignancy to affect the chest wall in children. These tumors can be difficult to differentiate both macroscopically and microscopically, requiring electron microscopic identification of neurosecretory granules and immunohis-

tochemical analysis for neuron-specific enolase to make the diagnosis [53]. ESFT share similar histology, consisting of small, round, blue-staining cells. They contain the same balanced translocation between chromosome 11 and 22 [54–56] and express the protein product of the *MIC2* gene on their surface [57,58].

The clinical presentation of these tumors includes a painful, palpable chest wall mass, cough, and dyspnea. Chest radiography often shows a thoracic soft tissue opacity with associated erosion or destruction of the adjacent rib. CT demonstrates a large, heterogeneously enhancing extrapleural mass with adjacent rib destruction (Fig. 13). Pleural effusions have also been described [59]. MR imaging shows a large soft tissue mass with abnormal heterogeneous high signal intensity on T2-weighted images and postcontrast T1-weighted images. Although the CT and MR imaging features of these tumors are nonspecific, these imaging modalities are essential in the assessment of local extension of the tumor, which helps direct treatment options. CT is better at detecting lung metastases, which are also common at presentation [34]. MR imaging can be superior to CT for defining tumor extension within the chest wall.

These tumors have a poor prognosis and a high recurrence rate. The best chance of cure is complete tumor resection. Extensive lesions may require chemotherapy or radiation to reduce the size of the mass before surgery. Cross-sectional imaging is important

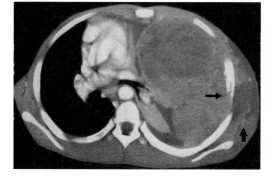

Fig. 13. A 10-year-old boy who has a left chest wall Askin tumor. Intravenous contrast–enhanced axial CT image of the chest demonstrates a large, heterogeneous soft tissue mass in the left chest displacing the mediastinal structures to the right. The mass is contiguous with the left chest wall, demonstrates rib destruction (*thin arrow*), and extends into the left lateral chest wall (*thick arrow*).

in assessing tumor response to chemotherapy and in the postoperative setting to ensure complete resection. Necrosis and cystic transformation of the tumor after chemotherapy have been described [60]. Surveillance imaging is also critical to detect early recurrence. Pleural and interlobar fissure nodules and subpleural plaques at the resection site have been described in cases of local recurrence [60].

Rhabdomyosarcoma

Rhabdomyosarcoma is the most common soft tissue sarcoma in children and is the second most common malignancy of the pediatric chest wall [61].

These tumors can arise in any site; approximately 7% affect the chest wall [62]. Prognosis has been related to multiple variables including the site of origin and histologic subtype (embryonal, alveolar, pleomorphic). Those arising in the genitourinary tract and orbit and the embryonal subtype tend to have the better prognosis; those originating in the chest wall have a poorer prognosis [62]. The most common histologic subtype of rhabdomyosarcoma affecting the chest wall is the embryonal form [61].

Chest radiography demonstrates nonspecific soft tissue opacity over the thorax with variable adjacent rib changes. Although CT and MR imaging are important to assess disease extension, the cross-sectional imaging characteristics are nonspecific (Fig. 14). CT demonstrates a large, heterogeneously enhancing soft tissue mass of the chest wall with adjacent rib destruction and possible pleural effusion. The mass demonstrates heterogeneous increased signal intensity on both T1- and T2-weighted MR imaging and heterogeneous contrast enhancement on T1-weighted, fat suppressed sequences, probably reflecting tumor necrosis [63].

Lymphoma

Although thoracic lymphoma is most commonly associated with mediastinal masses, both Hodgkin's and non-Hodgkin's lymphoma can involve the chest wall by direct mediastinal or parenchymal extension or as an isolated soft tissue mass. Chest wall involvement occurs with both primary lymphoma and recurrent disease. Because staging and therapeutic options are determined by disease extent, cross-

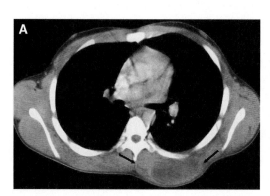

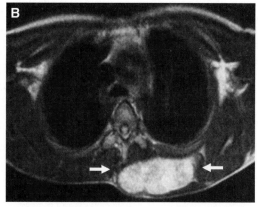

Fig. 14. A 12-year-old boy who has left posterior chest wall rhabdomyosarcoma (*A*) Intravenous contrast–enhanced axial image of the chest shows a heterogeneously low-attenuation mass (*arrows*) in the left posterior chest wall with subtle adjacent rib destruction. (*B*) Corresponding axial T2-weighted MR image demonstrates a well-circumscribed, homogenous high-signal-intensity soft tissue mass (*arrows*).

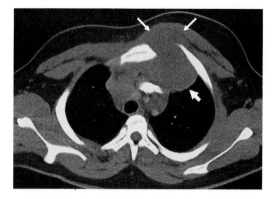

Fig. 15. An 8-year-old boy who has Hodgkin's lymphoma. Intravenous contrast–enhanced axial CT image of the chest shows a large anterior and middle mediastinal mass (*thick arrow*) with extension into the anteromedial left chest wall (*thin arrows*).

sectional imaging has become instrumental in the management of lymphoma. Demonstration of chest wall involvement may alter the radiation portals and administration of chemotherapy [64].

On CT, lymphomatous extension of a large mediastinal mass often occurs in the parasternal region and appears as a fairly homogeneous soft tissue mass displacing normal structures of the chest wall and obliterating normal fat planes (Fig. 15). There may be lytic destruction of adjacent osseous structures such as ribs or sternum. Isolated chest wall involvement appears as homogeneous soft tissue masses deep to or within the pectoralis major and minor muscles [62].

Although CT has been the imaging modality most commonly used in the evaluation and staging of lymphoma, MR imaging has also been shown to be sensitive to chest wall involvement. MR imaging demonstrates abnormal increased signal intensity on T2-weighted sequences in the region of the chest wall abnormality [65,66].

Other malignant soft tissue masses

Other less common malignant soft tissue masses involving the chest wall in children include congenital fibrosarcoma, malignant peripheral nerve sheath tumors, mesenchymal chondrosarcoma, neuroblastoma, and osteosarcoma.

Neuroblastoma can invade the chest wall by direct extension, usually from the posterior mediastinum [67]. MR imaging is the best imaging modality to assess tumor extent and involvement of the neural foramina. These tumors demonstrate abnormal high signal intensity on T2-weighted sequences and show

heterogeneous enhancement after administration of gadolinium [44].

Congenital fibrosarcoma, also referred to as fibrosarcoma of infancy, is a rare neoplasm that typically occurs in the axilla and thigh as well as other regions of the upper and lower extremities. These masses often are misdiagnosed as hemangiomas or vascular malformations. Although these lesions are histologically similar to adult fibrosarcomas, congenital fibrosarcomas reportedly have a more favorable prognosis than fibrosarcomas occurring in adults [61,68–70]. On MR imaging, these tumors are described as isointense to muscle on T1-weighted sequences, hyperintense on T2-weighted sequences, and demonstrate heterogeneous gadolinium contrast enhancement [20].

Although chondrosarcoma of the chest wall is rare, the ribs and mandible are the bones most frequently involved with mesenchymal chondrosarcoma. [38] These lesions are usually large soft tissue masses arising from bone with low signal intensity on T1-weighted MR images and high signal intensity on T2-weighted images. Cross-sectional imaging of chondrosarcoma with CT may demonstrate central, poorly defined calcifications reflecting the cartilaginous matrix [71].

Primary osteosarcoma of the ribs and other osseous structures of the chest wall account for about 3% to 10% of all osteosarcomas [71] and are extremely rare in children. Radiographs demonstrate a destructive bone lesion with an associated soft tissue mass and presence of osteoid matrix. Cross-sectional imaging typically shows a large, heteroge-

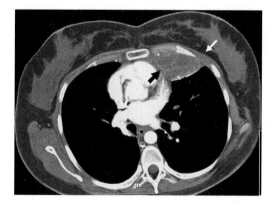

Fig. 16. An 18-year-old woman who has recurrent metastatic osteogenic sarcoma involving the left anterior chest wall. Intravenous contrast–enhanced CT of the chest demonstrates a pleural based heterogeneous soft tissue mass (*black arrow*) in the anteromedial aspect of the left chest with extension into the chest wall (*white arrow*).

neously enhancing soft tissue mass arising from bone
with destruction of the adjacent bone. Secondary
chest wall osteosarcoma in patients with metastatic
osteosarcoma from a remote primary site may also
occur by direct extension from a subpleural pulmonary metastasis (Fig. 16).

An excellent recent review of the general category
of pediatric soft tissue masses has been published
recently [72].

Summary

Although plain radiography still has an essential
role in the initial evaluation of chest wall pathology
in children, the recent technological advances in
cross-sectional imaging have expanded the capabilities
for lesion characterization, localization, and extension.
The role of the radiologist is central and pivotal.
Understanding the spectrum of pediatric chest wall
variations as well as pathology and the associated
imaging findings can enable the radiologist to limit
the differential considerations, make a specific diagnosis, or suggest potential management options.

References

[1] Donnelly LF, Taylor CNR, Emery KH, et al. Asymp-
    tomatic chest wall lesions in children: is cross sectional
    imaging necessary? Radiology 1997;202:829–31.
[2] Donnelly LF, Frush DP, Foss JN, et al. Anterior chest
    wall: frequency of anatomic variations in children.
    Radiology 1999;212:837–40.
[3] Pappas JN, Donnelly LF, Frush DP. Reduced fre-
    quency of sedation of young children with multisec-
    tion helical CT. Radiology 2000;215:897–9.
[4] Brenner DJ, Elliston CD, Hall EJ, et al. Estimated risks
    of radiation induced fatal cancer from pediatric CT.
    AJR Am J Roentgenol 2001;176:289–96.
[5] Hall EJ. Lessons we have learned from our children:
    cancer risks from diagnostic radiology. Pediatr Radiol
    2002;32:700–6.
[6] Donnelly LF, Emery KH, Brody AS, et al. Minimizing
    radiation dose for pediatric body applications of single-
    detector helical CT: strategies at a large children's
    hospital. AJR Am J Roentgenol 2001;176:303–6.
[7] Kim OH, Kim WS, Kim MJ, et al. US in the diagnosis
    of pediatric chest diseases. Radiographics 2000;20:
    653–71.
[8] Paltiel HJ, Burrows PE, Kozakewich HPW, et al. Soft
    tissue vascular anomalies: utility of US for diagno-
    sis. Radiology 2000;214:747–54.
[9] Fokin AA, Robicsek F. Poland's syndrome revisited.
    Ann Thorac Surg 2002;74:2218–25.
[10] Mentzel HJ, Seidel J, Sauner D, et al. Radiologic

[11] Hurwitz DJ, Stofman G, Curtin H. Three-dimensional
    imaging of Poland's syndrome. Plast Reconstr Surg
    1994;94:719–23.
[12] Faul JL, Berry GJ, Colby TV, et al. Thoracic
    lymphangiomas, lymphangiectasis, lymphangiomato-
    sis, and lymphatidic dysplasia syndrome. Am J Respir
    Crit Care Med 2000;161:1037–46.
[13] Mulliken JB, Fishman SJ, Burrows PE. Vascular
    anomalies. Curr Prob Surg 2000;37:517–84.
[14] Siegel M. Face and neck. In: Siegel M, editor. Pediatric
    sonography. 3rd edition. New York: Lippincott Wil-
    liams & Wilkins; 2002. p. 123–66.
[15] Konez O, Burrows PE. Magnetic resonance of vascular
    anomalies. Magn Reson Imaging Clin N Am 2002;10:
    363–88.
[16] Low DW. Hemangiomas and vascular malformations.
    Semin Pediatr Surg 1994;3:40–61.
[17] Siegel M. Chest. In: Siegel M, editor. Pediatric
    sonography. 3rd edition. New York: Lippincott Wil-
    liams & Wilkins; 2002. p. 167–211.
[18] Boon LM, Enjolras O, Mulliken JB. Congenital
    hemangiomas: evidence of accelerated involution.
    J Pediatr 1996;128:329–35.
[19] Lee GT, Girvan DP, Armstrong RF. Fibrous hamar-
    toma of infancy. J Pediatr Surg 1988;23:759–61.
[20] Eich GF, Hoeffel JC, Tshappeler H, et al. Fibrous
    tumors in children: imaging features of a heteroge-
    neous group of disorders. Pediatr Radiol 1998;28:
    500–9.
[21] Leonhardt J, Schirg E, Schmidt H, et al. Imaging
    characteristics of childhood lipoblastoma [abstract in
    English]. Rofo Fortschr Geb Rontgenstr Neuen
    Bildgeb Verfahr 2004;176:972–5 [in German].
[22] Chun YS, Kim WK, Park KW, et al. Lipoblastoma.
    J Pediatr Surg 2001;36:905–7.
[23] Haller JA, Kramer SS, Lietman SA. Use of CT scans in
    selection of patients for pectus excavatum surgery:
    a preliminary report. J Pediatr Surg 1987;10:904–6.
[24] Shamberger RC, Welch KJ, Castaneda AR. Anterior
    chest wall deformities and congenital heart disease.
    J Thorac Cardiovasc Surg 1988;96:427–32.
[25] Domini M, Cupaioli M, Rossi F, et al. Bifid sternum:
    neonatal surgical treatment. Ann Thorac Surg 2000;
    69:267–9.
[26] Morales JM, Patel SG, Duff JA, et al. Ectopia cordis
    and other midline defects. Ann Thorac Surg
    2000;70:111–4.
[27] Martin RA, Cunniff C, Erickson L, et al. Pentalogy of
    Cantrell and ectopia cordis, a familial developmental
    field complex. Am J Med Genet 1992;42:839–41.
[28] Franken Jr EA, Smith JA, Smith WL. Tumors of the
    chest wall in infants and children. Pediatr Radiol 1977;
    6:13–8.
[29] Lee KC, Davies AM, Cassar-Pullicino VN. Imaging
    the complications of osteochondromas. Clin Radiol
    2002;57:18–28.

[30] Malghem J, Berg BV, Noel H, et al. Benign osteo-chondromas and exostotic chondrosarcomas: evaluation of cartilage cap thickness by ultrasound. Skel Radiol 1992;21:33–7.

[31] Beukeleer LHL, Schepper AMA, Ramon F, et al. Magnetic resonance imaging of cartilaginous tumours: a retrospective study of 79 patients. Eur J Radiol 1995; 21:34–40.

[32] Geirnaerdt MJA, Hogendoorn PCW, Bloem JL, et al. Cartilaginous tumors: fast contrast-enhanced MR imaging. Radiology 2000;214:539–46.

[33] Stelzer P, Gay WA. Tumors of the chest wall. Surg Clin North Am 1980;60:779–91.

[34] Karmazyn B, Davis MM, Davey MS, et al. Imaging evaluation of chest wall tumors in children. Acad Radiol 1998;5:642–54.

[35] Feldman F. Tuberous sclerosis, neurofibromatosis, and fibrous dysplasia. In: Resnick D, editor. Bone and joint imaging. Philadelphia: W.B. Saunders; 1989. p. 1218–32.

[36] Dutton RV, Singleton EB. Tuberous sclerosis: a case report with aortic aneurysm and unusual rib changes. Pediat Radiol 1975;3:184–6.

[37] Ng Sh, Ng KK, Pai SC, et al. Tuberous sclerosis with aortic aneurysm and rib changes: CT demonstration. J Comput Assist Tomogr 1988;12:666–8.

[38] Faro SH, Mahboubi S, Ortega W. CT diagnosis of rib anomalies, tumors and infection in children. Clin Imaging 1993;17:1–7.

[39] Hachitanda Y, Nakagawara A, Ikeda K. An unusual anterior chest wall tumor due to actinomycosis in a child. Pediatr Radiol 1989;20:96.

[40] Freeman AF, Ben Ami T, Shulman ST. Streptococcus pneumoniae empyema necessitates. Pediatr Infect Dis J 2004;23:177–9.

[41] Goussard PM, Gie R, Kling S, et al. Thoracic actinomycosis mimicking primary tuberculosis. Pediatr Infect Dis J 1999;18:473–5.

[42] Hsieh MJ, Liu HP, Chang JP, et al. Thoracic actinomycosis. Chest 1993;104:366–70.

[43] Thomas KE, Owens CM, Veys PA, et al. The radiological spectrum of invasive aspergillosis in children: a 10 year review. Pediatr Radiol 2003;33:453–60.

[44] Watt AJB. Chest wall lesions. Pediatr Respir Rev 2002;3:328–38.

[45] Wong K, Hung IJ, Wang CR, et al. Thoracic wall lesions in children. Pediatr Pulmonol 2004;37:257–64.

[46] Guttentag AR, Salwen JK. Keep your eyes on the ribs: the spectrum of normal variants and diseases that involve the ribs. Radiographics 1999;19:1125–42.

[47] Resnick D. Lipoidoses, histiocytoses and hypoproteinemias. In: Resnick D, editor. Diagnosis of bone and joint disorders. 3rd edition. Philadelphia: W.B. Saunders; 1995. p. 2215–7.

[48] Glass RB, Norton KI, Mitre SA, et al. Pediatric ribs: a spectrum of abnormalities. Radiographics 2002;22: 87–104.

[49] Groom KR, Murphey MD, Howard LM, et al. Mesenchymal hamartoma of the chest wall: radiologic manifestations with emphasis on cross-sectional imaging and histopathologic comparison. Radiology 2002; 222:205–11.

[50] Kabra NS, Bowen JR, Christie J, et al. Mesenchymal hamartoma of chest wall in a newborn. Indian Pediatr 2000;37:1010–3.

[51] Gwyther SJ, Hall CM. Mesenchymal hamartoma of the chest wall in infancy. Clin Radiol 1991;43:24–5.

[52] Askin FB, Rosai J, Sibley RK, et al. Malignant small cell tumour of the thoracopulmonary region in childhood. A distinctive clinicopathological entity of uncertain histiogenesis. Cancer 1979;43:2438–51.

[53] Schulman H, Newman-Heinman N, Kurtzbart E, et al. Thoracoabdominal peripheral primitive neuroectodermal tumors in childhood: radiologic features. Eur Radiol 2000;10:1649–52.

[54] Burchill SA. Ewing's sarcoma: diagnostic, prognostic and therapeutic implications of molecular abnormalities. J Clin Pathol 2003;56:96–102.

[55] Aurias A, Rimbaut C, Buffe D, et al. Translocation involving chromosome 22 in Ewings sarcoma. A cytogenetic study of four fresh tumors. Cancer Genet Cytogenet 1984;12:21–5.

[56] Turc-Carel C, Philip I, Berger MP, et al. Chromosome study of Ewings sarcoma (ES) cell lines consistency of reciprocal translocation +(11;22)(q24;q12). Cancer Genet Cytogenet 1984;12:1–19.

[57] Ambros IM, Ambros PF, Strehl S, et al. MIC 2 is a specific marker for Ewings sarcoma and primitive neuroectodermal tumors: evidence for a common histiogenesis of Ewing sarcoma and peripheral primitive neuroectodermal tumors for n MIC 2 expression and specific chromosome aberration. Cancer 1991;67: 1886–93.

[58] Shamberger RC, Tarbell NJ, Perez-Atayde AR, et al. Malignant small round cell tumor (Ewing's PNET) of the chest wall in children. J Pediatr Surg 1994;29: 179–85.

[59] Saiffuddin A, Robertson RJH, Smith SEW. The radiology of Askin tumours. Clin Radiol 1991;43:19–23.

[60] Sallustio G, Pirronti T, Lasorella A, et al. Diagnostic imaging of primitive neuroectodermal tumour of the chest wall (Askin tumour). Pediatr Radiol 1998;28: 697–702.

[61] Shamberger RC, Grier HE. Chest wall tumors in infants and children. Semin Pediatr Surg 1994;3:267–76.

[62] Saenz NC, Ghavimi F, Gerald W, et al. Chest wall rhabdomyosarcoma. Cancer 1997;80:1513–7.

[63] Kim EE, Valenzuela RF, Kumar AJ, et al. Imaging and clinical spectrum of rhabdomyosarcoma in children. Clin Imaging 2000;24:257–62.

[64] Press GA, Glazer HS, Wasserman TH, et al. Thoracic wall involvement by Hodgkin disease and non-Hodgkin lymphoma: CT evaluation. Radiology 1985; 157:195–8.

[65] Carlsen SE, Bergin CJ, Hoppe RT. MR imaging to detect chest wall and pleural involvement in patients with lymphoma: effect on radiation therapy planning. AJR 1993;160:1191–5.

[66] Bergin CJ, Healy MV, Zincone GE, et al. MR evaluation of chest wall involvement in malignant lymphoma. J Comput Assist Tomogr 1990;14:928–32.

[67] Wyttenbach R, Vock P, Tschappeler H. Cross sectional imaging with CT and/or MRI of pediatric chest tumors. Eur Radiol 1998;8:1040–9.

[68] Pousti TJ, Upton J, Loh M, et al. Congenital fibrosarcoma of the upper extremity. Plast Reconstr Surg 1998;102:1158–62.

[69] Stout AP. Fibrosarcoma in infants and children. Cancer 1962;15:1028–40.

[70] Coffin CM, Jaszcz W, O'Shea PA, et al. So-called congenital infantile fibrosarcoma: does it exist and what is it? Pediatr Pathol 1994;14:133–50.

[71] Jeung MY, Gangi A, Gasser B, et al. Imaging of chest wall disorders. Radiographics 1999;19:617–37.

[72] Laor T. MR imaging of soft tissue tumors and tumor-like lesions. Pediatr Radiol 2004;34:24–37.

ELSEVIER
SAUNDERS

Radiol Clin N Am 43 (2005) 371–389

RADIOLOGIC
CLINICS
of North America

Imaging Evolution of Airway Disorders in Children

Frederick R. Long, MD[a,b,*]

[a]Body CT/MR Imaging, Department of Radiology, Columbus Children's Hospital, 700 Children's Drive, A-1010,
Columbus, OH 43205, USA
[b]Department of Radiology, College of Medicine and Public Health, Ohio State University, Columbus, OH, USA

The radiographic evaluation of the airways in infants and young children is demanding because of the inherent technical challenges of imaging young children. Not only are the airways of young children small, but typically young children cannot cooperate with breathholding maneuvers and are breathing rapidly during the examination. Respiratory motion, alone or in combination with the relatively low lung volumes that occur during tidal breathing, may obscure abnormal findings or create artifacts resulting in a false-positive finding [1]. These problems are noticeable on CT studies, especially when attempting high-resolution CT (HRCT) with thin slices.

The inability to acquire motionless images of the lungs in infants and young children at end-inspiratory and end-expiratory lung volumes, which is routine for studies done in adults, limits the information obtainable from CT. Depending on the clinical indication, these limitations may be minor and do not affect diagnostic accuracy, or they may be severe, rendering the study nondiagnostic. Examples of conditions that can usually be accurately diagnosed with CT in young children while breathing include tracheal stenosis and vascular rings. Examples of studies that are severely limited include HRCT of the lungs to assess airway changes in cystic fibrosis (CF) and HRCT applied to differentiate patterns of diffuse

lung disease. If clinical circumstances dictate that a high-quality examination of the lungs is needed, then the usual approach is to use general anesthesia along with endotracheal intubation to control respiratory motion and lung volumes during imaging. Although effective, this method is invasive, expensive, and not without significant risk. Consequently, HRCT has been underused in infants and young children. In a recent review of the work-up of diffuse interstitial lung disease in infants and small children, HRCT was not even mentioned [2].

If HRCT is to be a practical clinical imaging tool in the evaluation and treatment of respiratory disease in the lungs of infants and young children, an alternative method to general anesthesia for HRCT imaging is desirable and necessary. To this goal, a technique was developed at the author's institution called controlled ventilation CT (CVCT), which allows one to control respiration during imaging without intubation and general anesthesia [3]. CVCT uses positive pressure facemask ventilation to hyperventilate a sedated child, who is otherwise breathing on his or her own, and images are acquired during the hyperventilation-induced transient respiratory pause [3]. CVCT has proved to be a safe and reliable means for acquiring motionless CT images in infants and young children at full inflation and expiratory lung volumes. The first case was done in 1997, and over 400 CVCT examinations have been successfully performed since January of 2001 (70% for respiratory conditions and 30% for problems arising from congenital heart disease).

Coinciding with the development of CVCT, there has been increasing interest in using HRCT to evaluate and manage children for both medically

This work was supported by a grant from the Radiological Society of North America Research and Education Foundation.

* Department of Radiology, Columbus Children's Hospital, 700 Children's Drive, A-1010, Columbus, OH 43205.
  E-mail address: flong@chi.osu.edu

and surgically treatable respiratory conditions [4–6]. The areas of greatest current interest are in children with CF, interstitial lung disease, asthma, bronchopulmonary dysplasia, stridor, and congenital heart disease. This article discusses and illustrates the new information and insights gained from imaging the lungs of infants and young children using controlled ventilation techniques in health and disease.

Controlled-ventilation technique

Controlled ventilation does not require endotracheal intubation or specialized equipment but does require deep conscious sedation (also known as "moderate sedation") and positive pressure facemask ventilation to hyperventilate the child and induce a transient respiratory pause. The study is facilitated at the author's institution by having dedicated nurses who specialize in sedating children for imaging studies, and respiratory therapists who are trained in controlled ventilation technique. Sedation is accomplished using the same conscious sedation protocol for other imaging studies done in the radiology department (75–100 mg/kg of oral chloral hydrate or 2–6 mg/kg of intravenous pentobarbital).

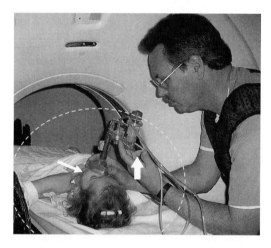

Fig. 1. Patient supine head first on CT gantry with neck extended. One operator applies positive pressure augmented breaths by facemask held over nose and mouth. Pressure is generated after occluding manually the expiratory port (*thick arrow*). A second operator applies gentle cricoid pressure (*thin arrow*) to prevent air from entering the esophagus during inflations.

The EKG and pulse oximeter are continuously monitored while the children are sedated.

After sedation is achieved, the child is positioned while asleep feet first on the CT scan table. A facemask attached to a source of flowing room air is placed over the nose and mouth (Fig. 1). The child can breathe at any time while the mask is held in place. With the facemask and airflow system, the child is given a few (approximately 3–10) deep breaths at 25 cm H_2O pressure timed to coincide with normal tidal breathing. The induced hypocarbia removes the need for the child to take another breath for a short period (5–20 seconds) similar to a diver who hyperventilates to swim longer underwater. During the pause, the CT images are acquired. By applying or removing pressure at the facemask, the lungs can be imaged at correspondingly different lung volumes. Typically, positive pressure is applied at 25 cm H_2O pressure to image the lungs at end inspiration or full inflation. For expiratory imaging, no mask pressure is applied and the lungs assume their resting state near functional residual capacity. The number of consecutive augmented breaths required to induce transient apnea sufficient for imaging varies depending on the age of the child and the child's level of respiratory distress. Younger children generate carbon dioxide faster than older children and require a greater degree of augmented ventilation to produce the desired state of hypocarbia. This also means that respiratory pause lengths are shorter in younger children. As a rule of thumb, children less than 3 years of age require approximately five to six consecutive augmented breaths and older children may need only two to three augmented breaths [4].

Because CVCT requires deep conscious sedation and hyperventilation and is used to evaluate children with respiratory problems who may have critical airways, it is important to evaluate children for potential contraindications or who are at risk for sedation before scheduling. This is accomplished in part by a screening sheet filled in by the requesting physician in which the indications for the examination are reviewed and the absence of potential contraindications are documented, which includes a history of apnea, enlarged tonsils, previous problems with sedation, and seizure disorder. After scheduling but before the study, sedation nurses also interview the parents by telephone regarding any potential sedation issues. To date, even though indications have been expanded to include children with central airway problems (with ear-nose-throat consultation and following bronchoscopy) and children with complex congenital heart disease (after cardiology consultation), no complications have been experienced at the authors' institution, including prolonged apnea, seizure, or pneumothorax.

Quantitative assessment: lung density and spatial resolution

At birth, the human lung contains only one third to one half of the number of alveoli that eventually develop [7]. Hence, the lungs as measured by CT are denser than those of adults. The period of rapid alveolar growth occurs between 0 and 2 years of age (Fig. 2), with continued growth at a much slower rate to about 8 years of age. One would hypothesize that as the lung grows exponentially by adding alveoli, the gas volume per gram of lung increases at the same rate. By measuring lung volume and density using CT in children ranging in age from 15 days to 17 years, however, de Jong et al [8] estimated lung weight and thereby degree of lung expansion (mL gas/g tissue) occurring at various ages [2]. They found a paradoxical decrease in lung expansion from birth to 2 years. This was hypothesized to be caused by the septation of the growing alveoli. The relationship between lung density and volume seems to be more complex than one would predict just on the basis of an increase in number of alveoli, at least during the period of rapid growth in the first 2 years.

By imaging the lungs at full inflation with no respiratory motion using a small field of view (13–15 cm) and thin 1-mm sections, one can resolve pixels that are 0.25 mm in diameter. This degree of resolution is sufficient to resolve the walls of the segmental and subsegmental airways in infants and young children, which have lumen diameters that range between 0.5 and 1.5 mm [9]. This degree of resolution conflicts with statements in the literature that airways located in the periphery of the lung, which are less than 2 mm in diameter, are not commonly seen [10]. This may be true of less than 2 mm airways in adults that have already undergone multiple branchings and have thin, noncartilaginous walls. In young children, the same-sized airways represent the segmental and subsegmental airways, which are still cartilaginous and presumably easier to resolve.

The increased resolution afforded by controlled ventilation gives the pediatric radiologist the opportunity to apply quantitative HRCT measures to pediatric lung disease. This is an important new direction to take full advantage of the potential of HRCT imaging as a clinical and research tool. Central to this goal is the development of specialized computer programs that can objectively measure airway wall thickness, airway lumen diameters, and cross-sectional lumen and wall areas [11]. Ideally, such a program would be able to take into account the fact that the airways for the most part course obliquely to the orthogonal axial imaging plane. For these programs to be effective and for measured values to be meaningful, a reproducible high-quality imaging dataset is essential. This is especially true in young children because quantitative accuracy declines exponentially as the structure measured approaches the limits of spatial resolution.

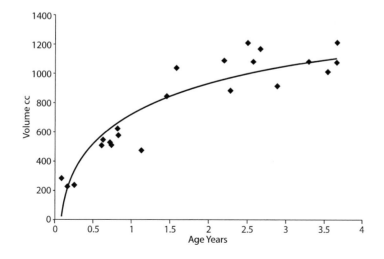

Fig. 2. Scatter plot shows the increase in total lung capacity (in mL) from birth to 4 years measured by CVCT at 25 cm H_2O pressure or total lung capacity in a group of children who had chest CT for reasons other than respiratory disease.

Quantitative assessment: airway-vessel measurements

With regards to airway pathology, bronchiectasis is an important finding, associated with considerable morbidity, and is a cardinal sign of chronic, progressive lung disease [12]. The radiographic diagnosis of bronchiectasis is made on the basis of the relationship of the cross-sectional diameters of a bronchus and its accompanying artery. Normally, the outer diameter of a bronchus and its accompanying artery should be approximately equal in both children and adults [13]. Bronchiectasis is diagnosed in routine radiographic practice, however, when the bronchial lumen or inner diameter exceeds the adjacent pulmonary artery diameter [14]. This working radiographic definition of bronchiectasis is not precise because the bronchial lumen or inner diameter is normally smaller than the accompanying artery diameter, but as a matter of practice, a lumen diameter greater than vessel diameter is easy to recognize and implies that the airway in question is irreversibly damaged. Such damaged airways have lost their structural integrity and normal compliance and remain dilated irrespective of the phase of respiration, whether at full inflation or at end exhalation. Typically, such airways clear secretions poorly, are thick walled, and chronically inflamed. The result is a vicious circle of poor clearance of airway secretions, infection, and progressive lung damage.

In assessing bronchiectasis on CT, the radiologist should consider potential confounding variables. (1) A bronchus may appear larger than the adjacent artery if the scan plane traverses a bronchus-vessel pair near a branch point, when the bronchus has not yet divided but the accompanying artery has. In this situation, two artery branches are seen to lie adjacent to a "dilated" bronchus; (2) In studies with normal controls in adults, bronchi with a lumen diameter larger than the artery diameter [15] can be found and are of unclear significance; (3) hypoxia is a known cause of both vasoconstriction and bronchial dilatation and may be a confounding factor in children with respiratory disease [16] or in comparing the lungs from patients living at different altitudes [17]; and (4) It is not known if the measured bronchoarterial ratio changes with lung volume.

In children with chronic inflammatory airways disease, such as CF, the etiology of bronchial dilatation leading to bronchiectasis is believed to be secondary to increased levels of free elastase that seem to act on elastin in airway walls, weakening the airway wall, decreasing elastic recoil, and potentially making the airways more compliant. Levels of free elastase in bronchoalveolar lavage fluid have been found to be markedly elevated in infants with CF [18,19].

The normal airway lumen diameter to vessel diameter ratio, or bronchoarterial ratio, is reported to be 0.62 ± 0.02 when measured in adult lungs fixed and inflated at 25 cm H_2O pressure [13]. This ratio was found to be independent of position in the lungs [13,20]. In infants and small children, the measured bronchoarterial ratio is slightly smaller, averaging 0.58 ± 0.10 when measured at 25 cm H_2O pressure using CVCT (Fig. 3). The bronchoarterial ratio

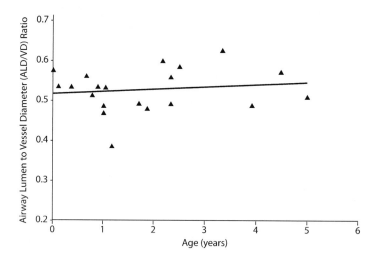

Fig. 3. Scatter plot of mean airway lumen to accompanying vessel diameter ratio (bronchoarterial ratio) for normal control subjects versus age with linear regression. (*Modified from* Long FR, Williams RS, Castile RG. Structural airway abnormalities in infants and young children with cystic fibrosis. J Pediatr 2004;144:154–61; with permission.)

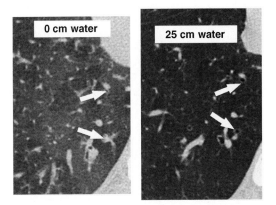

Fig. 4. Controlled ventilation high-resolution CT (CV-HRCT) images of the right lower lobe obtained in a 3-year-old child with cystic fibrosis. There is mild bronchial dilatation (*arrows*) at 25 cm H_2O pressure not appreciable at the same level (*arrows*) at 0 cm H_2O pressure.

gradually increases with age, approaching 0.79 in older adults [20].

Airways that are mildly dilated, with an airway lumen diameter to vessel diameter ratio greater than 0.6 but less than 1, are difficult to discern visually but are detectable using quantitative methods [9]. This early bronchial dilation may not be detectable on expiratory images but only revealed with full lung inflation that unmasks the abnormal compliance or distensibility of the weakened airway wall (Fig. 4). The significance of these mildly dilated bronchi that do not meet the common criteria for the diagnosis of frank bronchiectasis (airway lumen diameter to vessel diameter greater than 1) is yet to be elucidated but likely important in children with chronic respiratory disease, such as CF [9]. One could hypothesize that in children with a chronic inflammatory process that affects the whole lung [21], in which bronchiectasis is a common final pathway, airways would be found at various stages of damage, some frankly bronchiectatic and others in a precursor stage, signified by mild dilatation, but not yet irreversibly damaged. The hope is that early identification of these airways and the institution of appropriate therapy delays or stops the progression of disease (Fig. 5). Support for such a hypothesis was suggested in a recent study of infants with CF [9]. In this study, the measured bronchoarterial ratios in CF infants were found to be greater than in normal control infants and progressively worsened with age (Fig. 6) [9].

Bronchial wall thickening is another important sign of airways disease, reflecting inflammation and airway wall edema or thick viscid mucus that is associated with airway obstruction. The reliability of the visual assessment of bronchial wall thickening at HRCT in infants has not been reported, in part because no clear definition of wall thickening in infants exists and applying such a definition is difficult

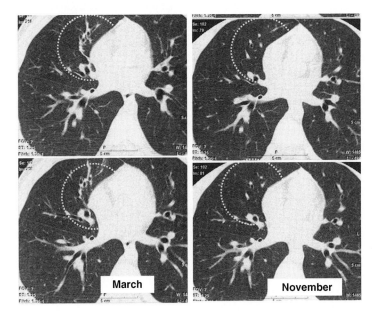

Fig. 5. Three-year-old child with cystic fibrosis. Series of 1.25-mm inspiratory CV-HRCT images of the right middle lobe done 8 months apart. Dashed circle indicates bronchiectatic airways in March study that resolved at follow-up in November study after intravenous antibiotics.

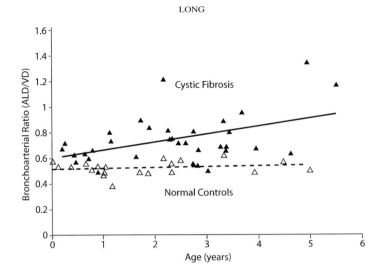

Fig. 6. Scatter plot of mean bronchoarterial ratios for young children with cystic fibrosis and age-matched normal control subjects versus age with linear regression. (*Modified from* Long FR, Williams RS, Castile RG. Structural airway abnormalities in infants and young children with cystic fibrosis. J Pediatr 2004;144:154–61; with permission.)

because of the small diameters of the airway walls in small children. In general, the thickness of the wall of a bronchus or bronchiole less than 5 mm in diameter should measure from one sixth to one tenth of its diameter [22]; in young children this translates to a normal wall thickness of 0.1 to 0.5 mm for the visible airways, which is at the limit of CT spatial resolution. Consequently, measurements of wall thickness in children have an inherent increased variability compared with adults. The variability of measurement for a 1-mm airway at HRCT is about 10% and increases exponentially for structures less than 1 mm in diameter [23].

In the assessment of airway wall thickness, one must also consider how or if it changes with bronchial diameter. The reported wall thickness of conducting bronchi and bronchioles is approximately proportional to their diameter, at least at the subsegmental level [13,22]. The bronchial lumen ratio, defined as the inner diameter of the bronchus divided by its outer diameter, is expected to be uniform throughout the lungs. In a study of the subsegmental bronchi by Kim et al [24] in adults, the average bronchial lumen ratio was 0.66 ± 0.06 and no significant difference was found in bronchial lumen ratio between segments, lobes, and lungs. A related ratio is the wall thickness to bronchial diameter ratio, which seems to be relatively independent of age [20]. The average wall thickness to bronchial diameter ratio in adults was 0.20 ± 0.01 [20]. How wall thickness to bronchial diameter changes with different lung volumes is unknown but has important implications for visually interpreting airway wall

thickening in children who are quietly breathing, near functional residual capacity, versus children whose lungs are at total lung capacity (Fig. 7).

The effect respiratory motion and lung volumes have on the ability visually to identify and quantify

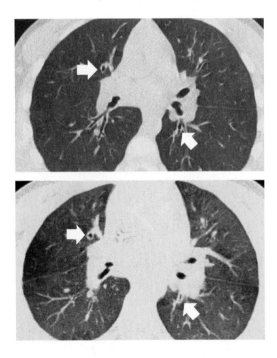

Fig. 7. Three-year-old child with cystic fibrosis. (*Top*) Inspiratory CV-HRCT image shows probable airway wall thickening (*arrows*). (*Bottom*) Matched expiratory CV-HRCT image. The airways appear in general thicker (*arrows*).

airway abnormalities and air trapping at HRCT has not been systematically studied. The same can be said for the interplay between these factors and the radiation dose used to acquire the study. An understanding of these effects, however, is particularly important in young children to understand and design the optimal imaging protocol for a given indication at the lowest acceptable radiation dose. It has been demonstrated that the presence of respiratory motion limits the degree to which one can decrease the radiation dose before sacrificing necessary diagnostic information. In a study by Lucaya et al [25], it was demonstrated that the image quality of thin-section CT deteriorates below an exposure of 40 mA in quietly breathing young children, whereas lower doses were acceptable in children who could cooperate with breathholding [25].

The effect that the degree of lung expansion has on resolution and the ability to lower radiation dose while maintaining diagnostic quality is unknown. The effect could be significant because the degree of lung expansion approximately doubles from tidal volumes to total lung capacity. The criteria used for diagnosis, whether qualitative or quantitative, may also change depending on degree of lung expansion. As even faster scan speeds become possible with increasing numbers of detector arrays with multislice CT scanners, providing snapshots of the lungs, problems resulting from respiratory motion will diminish but limitations related to the degree of lung expansion at the time of imaging will persist. These limitations include but are not limited to the following: airway resolution, ability to lower radiation dose, ability to apply quantitative measures to airway analysis, and ability to diagnose early bronchiectasis.

Pulmonary function tests

Both CVCT and raised volume infant pulmonary function tests (PFTs) [26] use a similar technique for inducing a respiratory pause. Instead of imaging during the pause, flow volume curves are generated using a rapid chest compression method [26]. Values for the forced vital capacity, the forced expiratory volume at 0.5 seconds, and the forced expiratory flows between 25% and 75% of expired vital capacity have been generated and normalized to the child's height and weight. By performing controlled ventilation maneuvers in an enclosed container, otherwise known as "whole-body plethysmography," fractional lung volumes, including residual volume, functional residual capacity, and total lung capacity, can be obtained.

The same sedation used to prepare a child for CVCT or infant PFTs is of sufficient duration that in over 90% of cases both studies can be done consecutively the same day. The child needs only to undergo sedation once. In children referred for respiratory conditions, the ability to obtain a full set of PFTs along with HRCT is a major additional advantage of CVCT. The combination of structural

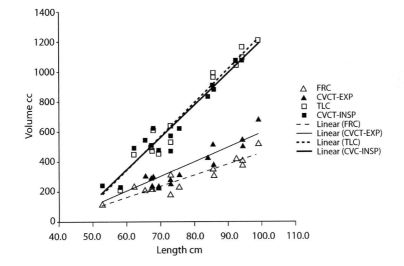

Fig. 8. Scatter plot of estimated lung volumes at total lung capacity and functional residual capacity with linear regression in children with cystic fibrosis who were considered clinically well at the time of the studies as measured by CVCT and by infant pulmonary function tests. CVCT-EXP, controlled ventilation expiratory; CVCT-INSP, controlled ventilation inspiratory; FRC, functional residual capacity; TLC, total lung capacity.

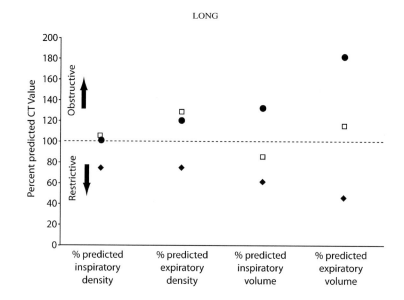

Fig. 9. Scatter plot of percent predicted mean inspiratory and expiratory lung density and lung volume measured using CVCT in three infants. Two children had obstructive physiology (biopsy-proved neuroendocrine cell hyperplasia of infancy ●; bronchiolitis obliterans □). One child had restrictive disease (nonspecific diffuse interstitial disease ◆).

and functional information enhances the ability to differentiate various types of respiratory disease and provide more powerful predictive outcome measures [27]. Because both CVCT and raised volume infant PFTs are done using similar techniques, the data are complementary and reproducible. Lung volumes, for example, determined by CVCT using simple thresholding techniques that isolate lung from surrounding soft tissues are highly correlated with PFT measures of total lung capacity and functional residual capacity using whole-body plethysmography (Fig. 8) [28]. Small differences in the actual values obtained are systematic and predictable. Consequently, the combination of inspiratory and expiratory CVCT can provide information on lung volumes similar to PFTs. If percent predicted values for CT lung density and lung volumes at mask pressures of 25 cm and 0 cm H_2O were determined, inferences about the obstructive and restrictive nature of airway pathology that is done using PFTs could be accomplished using CVCT (Fig. 9).

Quantitative assessment: air trapping

A good example of the potential of CT to provide quantitative functional correlates to PFTs is in the evaluation of air trapping. Air trapping on expiratory HRCT is a frequently associated finding in patients with obstructive airways disease, and may be particu-

larly severe in infants, who may trap gas more readily because of their smaller airways and relatively poorer collateral airway conductance in comparison with adults [29]. Air trapping is commonly identified on expiratory CT images as areas of the lung that are of abnormally low attenuation [30]. Normally, as air is exhaled, the lung increases in density, with the greatest increase in density being in the dependent portions of the lung because of the gravity gradient in a supine patient [31]. The low attenuation seen in the region of lung involved with air trapping results from a lack of an appropriate increase in density with exhalation, which is often clearly demarcated by surrounding normal and denser lung on expiratory HRCT images.

Air trapping may be identified on expiratory HRCT before structural airway abnormalities are visible if the involved airways are small, below the limits of resolution. This has been termed "small airways disease" [32]. The identification of this air trapping may be important because it represents the earliest sign of airways disease on CT. In some cases, however, it may not be possible to distinguish early pathologic air trapping from that which can occur in normal lungs. There have been several reports of air trapping found on expiratory HRCT in asymptomatic adults who have normal PFTs [33]. In infants, modest amounts of gas trapping have been found in the lungs of normal controls as measured using nitrogen washout [34]. The finding of air trapping on expiratory HRCT in normal infants and young children

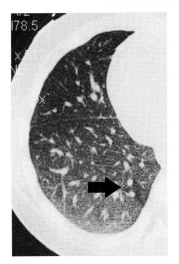

Fig. 10. One-year-old child with Wilms' tumor. CT study done for staging. Expiratory CV-HRCT image shows subsegmental air trapping (*arrow*) in the medial aspect of the right lower lobe.

has not been reported in the literature but has been observed (Fig. 10).

The severity of air trapping is typically assessed by visually estimating the percent of lung that is of abnormal low attenuation on expiratory images. A limitation of the visual approach is that some regions of lung that are of abnormally low attenuation may have more trapped gas than others, even though they may be equal in area.

Most quantitative approaches to estimating air trapping reported in the literature do not attempt to account for both the area of lung involved and the density differences between inspiration and expiration for each lung region. Instead, simpler methods have been used that include differences in whole mean expiratory lung density, differences in whole mean inspiratory minus mean expiratory density, and the percentage of lung below a density threshold believed to be in the air trapping density range, the pixel index [35–37]. Of these quantitative methods for estimating air trapping, the most promising method is probably the pixel index [36]. In adults, a pixel index of −900 HU, a density value at approximately 2 standard deviations below the mean, has been used. If the pixel index is applied to the whole lung density histogram, there is the same limitation arising from the fact that different thresholds exist for different lung regions on the bases of the supine density gradient. The pixel index could conceivably be adjusted for location if normative

data for different levels in the lung were available, but in children adjustments also have to be made for age. Nevertheless, the pixel index can be quickly measured and likely is more robust than measuring shifts in the mean whole lung expiratory density.

The difficulty in quantifying air trapping and developing percent predicted CT values for air trapping is compounded by the fact that the normal expiratory lung density for any given individual is variable caused by hereditary differences in number of alveoli [7]. This variability is probably more apparent in children than in adults because density differences are accentuated at smaller lung volumes.

One potential approach to quantifying air trapping that addresses the additional problem of individual variability is to use each individual as their own control. This was done by Goris et al [38] by adjusting the expiratory pixel index thresholds used relative to the inspiratory histogram. The rational for this is that the whole lung inspiratory histogram does not change much in the presence of air trapping, particularly the mild amounts of air trapping encountered in young children. Using this method with an automated approach, Goris et al [38] was able to discriminate normal school-aged children from children with mild CF disease. Such a method required anatomically matched inspiratory and expiratory HRCT images. This was achieved by spirometrically triggered HRCT data acquisition in older children who could cooperate with breathholding maneuvers [39]. The six inspiratory-expiratory histograms obtained using this method was compared at different anatomic levels and there was some adjustment on the basis of lung location. Bonnel et al [40] expanded the work to include the effects of two different expiratory lung volumes, functional residual capacity and residual volume, on the percentage of visual air trapping and expiratory lung density in CF subjects. Lung density measurements and percentage of air trapping better discriminated differences between CF and normal groups than PFTs [40]. Measurements made on expiratory scans near functional residual capacity showed significantly higher values for air trapping than those made near residual volume. In young children, controlled ventilation rather than spirometric triggering could be used to obtain the necessary matched inspiratory and expiratory images to use this method.

There have been a number of proposed methods for how to obtain adequate diagnostic images to evaluate air trapping in young children who cannot cooperate with breathholding. These include lateral decubitus positioning to obtain an expiratory image [41], cine CT to plot density changes in the lung in a fixed region of interest during several respiratory cycles [42], electron beam CT to assess density changes during quiet breathing at multiple levels [43], general anesthesia and endotracheal intubation, or controlled ventilation technique. Using controlled ventilation, one can compare inspiratory and expiratory information in matched lung regions. This allows for an accurate and simple method for quantification of air trapping.

Clinical examples

An important development in the ability to diagnose and better characterize airway abnormalities in both adults and children has been the development of multidetector array CT, also referred to as "multislice CT," with multiplanar reformats and multislice three-dimensional volumetric rendering techniques [44]. When combined with controlled ventilation, the resultant image quality is so impressive that in many instances invasive procedures, such as endoscopy, that would have previously been done routinely, can be avoided (Fig. 11). This is true not only for airway abnormalities but also in the assessment of extra-

cardiac vascular anatomy in children with congenital heart disease.

To study the airways and lungs of infants and small children, the authors use a multislice helical technique ideal for three-dimensional imaging and decrease the radiation exposure to settings below the usual low-dose settings described in the literature, largely because they are using controlled ventilation technique [45]. The customary 120 kilovolt (peak) (kV[p]) is decreased to 100 kV(p) and the mA are decreased to 20 for full inspiration and 10 mA for expiration. These ultra low-dose settings combined with the speed of a multislice scanner result in a low-dose exposure to the patient (Fig. 12). The estimated effective dose of a controlled ventilation helical chest CT in a 10-kg child using an eight-slice scanner [General Electric Healthcare, Milwaukee, Wisconsin; 8 × 1.25 mm, 13.5 mm/rotation, 0.5 rotation speed, 100 kV(p), 40 mA] is between 25 and 50 mrem (0.25–0.5 mSv) or 0.25 and 0.50 mGy [46].

The standard approach to diagnosis of various airway abnormalities in infants and young children is shown in Table 1, in which the uses of various imaging modalities are compared. The text discussion follows the outline in Table 1. Examples of the use of

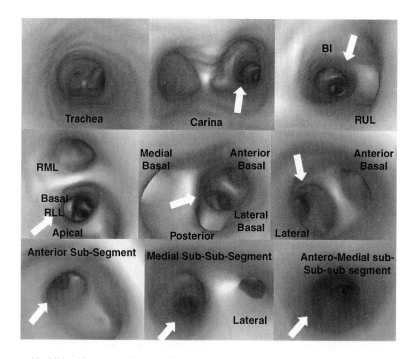

Fig. 11. Two-year-old child with suspected cystic fibrosis, later ruled out. Virtual bronchoscopic images acquired using CVCT at resting end exhalation. Arrows indicate path of the virtual bronchoscope.

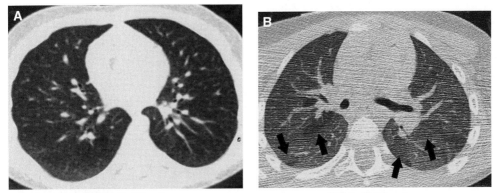

100 kvP, 20 mAs   100 kvP, 10 mAs

Fig. 12. Twelve-month-old girl with cystic fibrosis. (*A*) 1.25-mm CVCT image at full inflation at 100 kilovolt (peak) and 20 mA using 0.5 rotation speed. (*B*) 1.25-mm CVCT image at resting end exhalation at 120 kilovolt (peak) and 10 mA using 0.5 rotation speed. Note air trapping (*arrows*).

controlled ventilation for the diagnosis of various pathologies are highlighted.

Congenital anomalies: bronchopulmonary foregut malformations

Congenital anomalies of the airways are important causes for respiratory distress in the newborn. Some are incompatible with life, such as tracheal agenesis, whereas others may be found incidentally in adulthood, such as bronchogenic cysts. These abnormalities are called bronchopulmonary foregut malformations on the basis of their embryologic origins. A failure of separation of the alimentary and respiratory tracts results in a tracheoesophageal fistula, one of the most common congenital anomalies. This is easily diagnosed clinically in combination with conventional radiographs. During development, disruption of the pulmonary arterial supply may be the cause of lung agenesis, whereas a local interruption of blood supply with continued development of lung distally, supplied by a persistent primitive systemic capillary supply, could result in tracheal or bronchial stenosis, bronchogenic cyst, cystic congenital adenomatoid malformation (CCAM), and bronchopulmonary sequestration [47].

Table 1
Airway abnormalities

Diagnosis	CXR	Fluoro	CT
Congenital anomalies:			
Tracheal agenesis, fistula/stenosis, tracheal bronchus	● +		● ++
Lung agenesis and hypoplasia: Scimitar syndrome; esophageal and horseshoe lung	● +		● ++
Bronchial stenosis/atresia	● +		● ++
Bronchogenic cyst	● +		● ++
CCAM, CLE, sequestration	● +		● ++
Extrinsic compression			
Vascular rings: double arch,right arch/aberrant left subclavian artery innominate artery syndrome, pulmonary sling	●	● +	● ++
Tracheobronchomalacia	●	● +	● ++
Bronchial carcinoid tumor	●		● ++
Inflammatory/small airways disease: cystic fibrosis, bronchiolitis, bronchiolitis obliterans, asthma, aspiration	●		● ++
Lung disease of prematurity	● +		● ++

Abbreviations: CXR, chest radiograph; Fluro, fluoroscopy; ●, useful in detection; +, narrows differential diagnosis; ++, diagnostic.

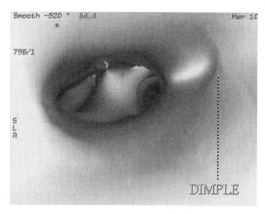

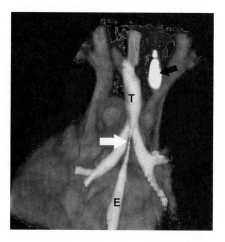

Fig. 13. Seven-week-old child with hypoplastic left lung. Virtual bronchoscopic image obtained from a helical full inflation CVCT demonstrates a dimple at the expected take-off of the lingula confirming lingular atresia.

Fig. 14. Newborn with esophageal atresia and tracheo-esophageal fistula (*white arrow*) arising from distal trachea. Coronal volume-rendered image from a helical CVCT at full inflation was performed without using Sellick maneuver to allow air to outline the fistula. The distance from the end of the proximal pouch as demarcated by the Replogle tube (*black arrow*) from the origin of the fistula (*white arrow*) was clearly depicted. T, trachea; E, esophagus.

Pulmonary hypoplasia may result from inadequate space for lung growth or inadequate vascular supply. Inadequate space for lung growth can occur in congenital diaphragmatic hernia, extralobar sequestration, Jeune's syndrome, or oligohydramnios. In children with pulmonary hypoplasia, there may be various stages of incomplete development of the lungs; the affected segments and subsegments can be defined using CVCT (Fig. 13). Other entities associated with lung hypoplasia include scimitar syndrome, also called venolobar syndrome, which is a rare anomaly characterized by hypoplasia of the right lung with anomalous systemic arterial supply and systemic pulmonary venous drainage to the inferior vena cava, resulting in right-to-left shunt. The diagnosis is made usually by chest radiograph in adult-age patients [47]. Horseshoe lung and esophageal lung are also rare congenital anomalies that can be characterized with CVCT. For example, after the prerequisite number of augmented breaths needed to induce transient apnea, cricoid pressure can be released during the scan, thereby allowing air to distend the esophagus with the application of positive pressure used to inflate the lungs. Air can then delineate the esophageal bronchus or potentially a tracheoesophageal fistula (Fig. 14).

Bronchopulmonary foregut malformations may be diagnosed on chest radiographs but usually require other imaging modalities for full characterization. The trachea on chest radiographs may be difficult to see, particularly in young children, and a high index of suspicion must be maintained not to miss a tracheal abnormality as the cause of respiratory distress in infants. In such cases, airway fluoroscopy may be

used to screen for a mass compressing the airway and to assess noninvasively the severity of the lesion before endoscopy and surgery. Endoscopy may not be necessary if a helical multislice CT study using low-dose technique and intravenous contrast can be accomplished with or without controlled ventilation.

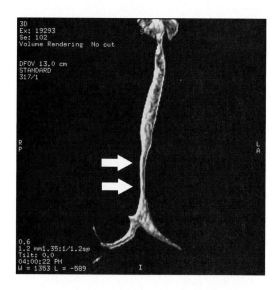

Fig. 15. Two-month-old child with focal congenital tracheal stenosis. Three-dimensional coronal volume-rendered image from a helical full inflation CVCT shows the nature and extent of the stenosis (*arrows*).

A CVCT could potentially follow an endoscopic procedure if endoscopy results indicated that sedation can be safely used. One of the advantages of CVCT is that all important findings potentially contributing to the clinical presentation, including tracheal or bronchial stenosis, tracheobronchomalacia, vascular rings, extrinsic masses, and underlying lung disease, can be assessed and quantified. Another advantage is that CVCT is much less operator dependent than endoscopy.

Congenital tracheal stenosis is rare and presents with biphasic stridor usually in the first year of life. The classic lesion is the long funnel-shaped stenosis seen with complete cartilaginous rings, but tracheal stenosis, when present, is most frequently focal (Fig. 15). Like tracheal stenosis, bronchial stenosis and atresia are rare. The bronchi distal to the stenosis or atresia may become filled with mucus forming a bronchocele. Another possible presentation is focal air trapping. A tracheal bronchus, or pig bronchus, is relatively more common, often asymptomatic, and may be difficult to see when it is a supernumerary bronchus that ends blindly (Fig. 16). The tracheal bronchus usually supplies a small segment of the right upper lobe but can involve the left lung [48]. It should be mentioned that tracheal and bronchial anomalies are often associated with congenital heart disease. Many of the tracheal abnormalities reported are minor, such as bilateral trifurcate bronchi or right upper lobe tracheal bronchus, but more serious anomalies, such as tracheal stenosis, have also been reported [49].

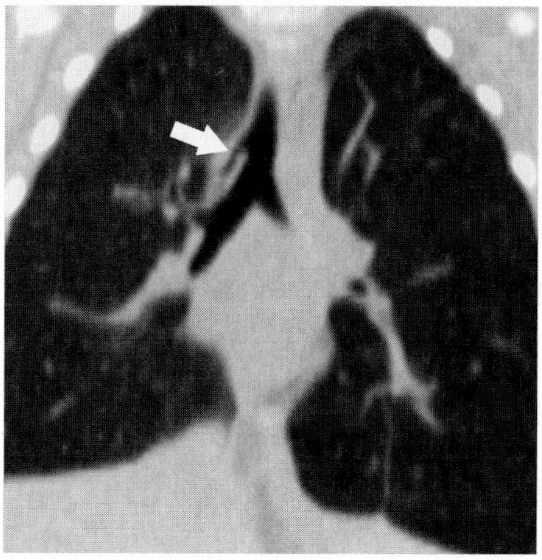

Fig. 16. Three-year-old girl with recurrent pneumonias. Coronal reconstructed reformatted image from a CVCT examination at full inflation shows a right-sided tracheal bronchus (*arrow*).

The other bronchopulmonary foregut malformations, which include bronchogenic cyst, congenital lobar emphysema (CLE), sequestration, and CCAM, are much more common. These lesions may present at any time in life, but large lesions, typically CCAM and CLE, are more likely to present shortly after birth with respiratory distress, whereas sequestration and bronchogenic cyst tend to present later in life with infection. CCAM and CLE are often identified on chest radiographs at presentation but require CT for a more definitive diagnosis and for therapeutic planning. CCAM lesions may be difficult to differentiate by CT from pneumatoceles or lung abscesses. CLE is typified by a hyperinflated lobe secondary to bronchial obstruction, either primary in origin or secondary to an extrinsic compression. CVCT may delineate the nature of the obstruction and establish accurately the lobes involved. Sequestrations are diagnosed by identifying a systemic arterial supply to the lesion. The two types of sequestration, intralobar and extralobar, are differentiated on the basis of whether the lesion is contained within the normal visceral pleura and has normal pulmonary venous drainage. Typically, sequestrations can be diagnosed using a number of modalities, including ultrasound, CT, and MR imaging [47].

Tracheomalacia

Although not considered typically a bronchopulmonary foregut malformation, tracheomalacia is an important cause of respiratory distress in the infant and small child and is the most frequent cause of stridor [50]. Tracheomalacia is responsible for considerable difficulties and occasionally mortality in the operating room and intensive care unit [51]. It is characterized by a floppy, hypercompliant airway secondary to deficiency of the supporting cartilage. The abnormal floppiness or compliance results in airway collapse or obstruction during breathing, characteristically during exhalation, in which there is a drop in intraluminal pressure secondary to increased airflow and a concomitant increase in extraluminal or intrapleural pressure. Tracheomalacia may be primary or secondary in origin. Secondary causes are more common and result from extrinsic compression that interferes with cartilage development. Examples of structures causing extrinsic compression on the trachea associated with tracheomalacia include the dilated proximal esophageal pouch in a child with esophageal atresia and distal tracheal esophageal fistula, and vascular rings. Vascular compression arising from the innominate artery as it crosses anterior to the trachea may also result in tracheomalacia [52].

Although secondary causes are more common, diffuse primary tracheomalacia that also involves the mainstem bronchi is an important cause for morbidity and mortality in the intensive care unit [53]. In a study of children diagnosed following bronchography with tracheomalacia or stenosis of the airways in an intensive care unit setting, at least half of the children with tracheomalacia also had bronchomalacia, 62% affecting the left main bronchus and 51% affecting the right side. Children in this study with severe tracheobronchomalacia had a very poor prognosis [53]. This study was unique in that it used cinetracheobronchography. In those children who underwent both bronchoscopy and cinetracheobronchography, bronchoscopy was found to be much less sensitive in detecting bronchomalacia, which is likely related to stenting and distortion of the airway secondary to the presence of the endotracheal tube.

There are a number of pitfalls in the diagnosis of tracheomalacia and bronchomalacia that should be discussed. Because tracheomalacia presents in infants who have small airways and are breathing fast, the diagnosis is not easy. The lateral chest radiograph may be misleading because the trachea can collapse or appear narrowed depending on whether the child was forcibly exhaling (eg, crying) at the moment the film was taken. Airway fluoroscopy has similar problems because of the inability to be able to control and monitor the dynamic pressure changes acting on the tracheal wall and compare those changes with tracheal lumen area or diameter. The same factors limit the endoscopic evaluation, which is additionally hampered by the presence of the endotracheal tube, which may alter the flow dynamics in the airway.

CVCT is an ideal method for tracheomalacia evaluation, whether performed under deep conscious sedation or in the intubated and ventilated child who has a critical airway. By using controlled ventilation technique, the dynamic pressures acting on the airway wall are controlled and these pressure changes can be correlated with precise measurements of changes in lumen area or diameter. The CVCT assessment of tracheomalacia does not depend on a subjective assessment of the degree of collapsibility during exhalation, but rather is based on the degree of distensibility of the trachea as a result of increased intraluminal pressure applied by the facemask in a controlled and reproducible manner (Fig. 17). Malacic airways, because of their loss of supportive cartilage, are more distensible than normal airways when positive intraluminal pressure is applied and also assume a more round shape.

Additional advantages of controlled ventilation for assessment of tracheomalacia include the ability to make a distensibility map of the entire trachea including the bronchi (Fig. 18). Because controlled ventilation can be combined with infant PFTs, functional correlation with the anatomic changes can also be made. It is hoped that an objective assessment of tracheomalacia will yield insights into the natural history of this abnormality and aide in management decisions.

Because of the small size and oblique course of the bronchi, assessment of bronchomalacia by CVCT is more difficult and the findings less certain. An example of bronchomalacia identified by CVCT involving the left mainstem bronchus is shown in (Fig. 19). In children with bronchopulmonary dysplasia or cardiomegaly and refractory respiratory distress, the issue of whether bronchomalacia is a cause is important but difficult to answer even with CVCT. For example, it is unclear whether bronchomalacia or extrinsic compression is the reason a bronchus that was visible at full inflation disappears at end exhalation. It is also unclear how diffuse

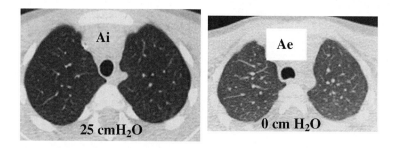

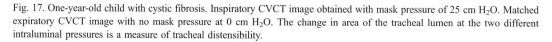

Fig. 17. One-year-old child with cystic fibrosis. Inspiratory CVCT image obtained with mask pressure of 25 cm H_2O. Matched expiratory CVCT image with no mask pressure at 0 cm H_2O. The change in area of the tracheal lumen at the two different intraluminal pressures is a measure of tracheal distensibility.

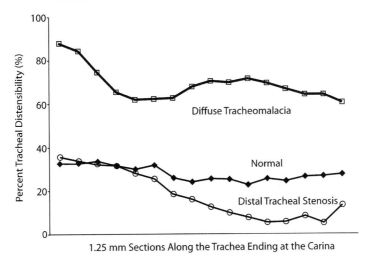

Fig. 18. Line graphs depicting the distensibility measurements at 1.25-mm intervals along the trachea from the thoracic inlet to carina: 8-month-old child with diffuse tracheomalacia, asymptomatic infant with cystic fibrosis (normal), and a 2-year-old child with distal congenital tracheal stenosis.

fibrosis or air trapping may alter the distensibility measurements of the trachea and bronchi in response to intraluminal pressure changes. Not enough information is available to evaluate and compare CVCT with cinebronchography in the diagnosis of tracheobronchomalacia in small infants.

Bronchial lesions and inflammation

In the differential diagnosis of respiratory distress, one must include intraluminal foreign bodies and masses. Intraluminal masses are rare, particularly in infants and small children. The most common intraluminal mass is the carcinoid tumor, which may present in young adulthood and is associated with abnormal neuroendocrine secretion [54]. Foreign bodies may be difficult to differentiate from carcinoid tumor; however, usually the clinical history, such as witnessed choking episode, narrows the differential. It is important to realize that inspiratory and expiratory chest radiographs may be normal in the setting of an aspirated foreign body, particularly in the acute stage [55]. When an acute or possibly a chronic foreign body aspiration is suspected, and chest radiographs are unremarkable, helical CT with or without controlled ventilation may prove useful in excluding a foreign body, saving the child a bronchoscopic examination.

Inflammation of the bronchi and bronchioles is common in children and the chest radiograph findings of hyperinflation with increased perihilar markings are well known. In children with diffuse lung disease and chronic respiratory symptoms, a similar nonspecific chest radiograph pattern may be seen, but the underlying pathology may be quite different, including both predominately interstitial and airway disease processes [56]. The HRCT findings in pediatric diffuse lung disease have not been well defined because there are only few reports in small numbers of children [6,56,57]. One reason for the

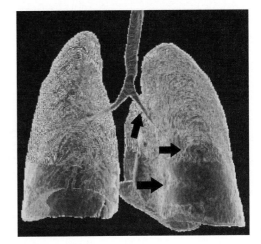

Fig. 19. Coronal three-dimensional volume-rendered image of the lungs in a 3-year-old child with left mainstem bronchomalacia (*upper arrow*) from a volumetric expiratory CVCT study. Note resultant area of air trapping (*lower arrows*) involving the left lower lobe.

paucity of literature is that HRCT has not typically been used in the evaluation of children with diffuse lung disease because of poor image quality.

One of the most common diffuse airway disease processes presenting with chronic respiratory symptoms is constrictive bronchiolitis or bronchiolitis obliterans. Although it may present as a unilateral hyperlucent lung, the Swyer-James syndrome, it more commonly presents with bilateral disease characterized by a prominent mosaic attenuation pattern with bronchial abnormalities, including bronchiectasis, and air trapping on expiratory images [58,59]. The pattern can be identical to that seen in CF or severe asthma. There are many causes of bronchiolitis obliterans including infection (viral or mycoplasma); toxic and fume exposure; collagen vascular disease, such as

rheumatoid arthritis; and as a complication of bone marrow transplant and heart lung transplant [32].

Bronchiectasis is another common cause of chronic respiratory symptoms in children and usually manifests as recurrent pneumonias [55]. Bronchiectasis is caused primarily by chronic inflammation, which damages the supporting structure of the airway resulting in dilatation (the hallmark) and often wall thickening and mucus plugging secondary to poor clearance. The abnormal mucus produced in children with CF or the poor clearance of mucus in children with primary ciliary dyskinesia or bronchial obstruction secondary to adenopathy leads to progressive bronchiectasis. Similarly, chronic inflammation secondary to immunodeficiency states may lead to bronchiectasis. Aspiration with or without

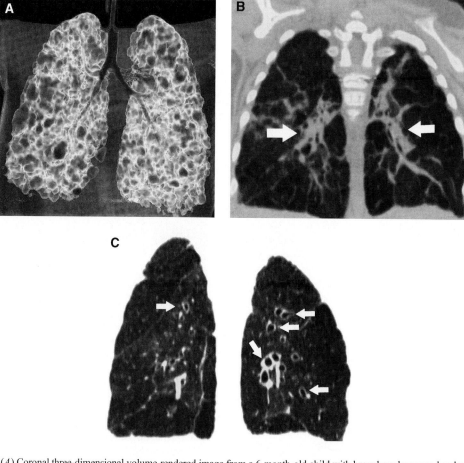

Fig. 20. (*A*) Coronal three-dimensional volume-rendered image from a 6-month-old child with bronchopulmonary dysplasia who has diffuse replacement of normal lung by air-filled cystic cavities. (*B*) Reformatted coronal image obtained 6 months later from a repeat examination shows more normal hyperinflated lung parenchyma with scarring along the bronchovascular bundles (*arrows*). (*C*) Reformatted coronal image obtained at 2 years of age shows more normal hyperinflated lung parenchyma with diffuse cylindrical bronchiectasis (*arrows*).

gastroesophageal reflux is commonly implicated in respiratory disease in infants and young children. The HRCT appearance of the lungs in the setting of chronic aspiration has not been described but bronchiectasis secondary to chronic inflammation has been postulated. As in other airway diseases, bronchiectasis is commonly not appreciable on chest radiograph in children or is underestimated. HRCT at end inspiration is the diagnostic technique of choice.

Other causes of small airways disease include extrinsic allergic alveolitis or hypersensitivity pneumonitis, which results in a cellular bronchiolitis, characterized by diffuse small ill-defined centrilobular nodules acutely and in the subacute or chronic stage by a mosaic attenuation pattern at inspiration with expiratory air trapping caused by partial bronchial obstruction [32]. Diffuse pan-bronchiolitis, an exudative bronchiolitis characterized by a diffuse tree in bud pattern, is an important cause of progressive obstructive lung disease in Asia. It is characterized by the presence of small centrilobular nodular and linear opacities diffusely distributed in both lungs. Follicular bronchiolitis, defined as lung hyperplasia of the bronchus associated lymphoid tissue, is another cause of chronic respiratory symptoms characterized by obstructive lung disease [60] that in addition to expiratory air trapping consists of areas of ground glass capacity presumably secondary to peribronchial nodules. A unique form of airway disease occurs in the lungs of premature infants with bronchopulmonary dysplasia, in which destructive diffuse lung disease is occurring in the setting of rapid alveolar growth. The potential role of HRCT in management of this condition is as yet relatively unexplored (Fig. 20). Currently, HRCT is helpful to the extent that it excludes other causes for refractory respiratory distress, such as central airway lesions.

Summary

Many new avenues of investigation and new insights into pediatric respiratory disease should result from the application of a noninvasive and reproducible method for obtaining motionless HRCT images of the airways and lungs at end-inspiratory and end-expiratory lung volumes in infants and young children who cannot cooperate with breathholding.

Acknowledgments

This work would not have been possible without the support of the RSNA Research and Education Foundation; the encouragement of William E. Shiels, DO; the guidance and mentoring of Robert G. Castile, MD; the assistance of my colleagues; and the dedication of the CT radiology technologists, sedation nurses, and respiratory therapists at Columbus Children's Hospital who perform the controlled ventilation studies.

References

[1] Long FR. High-resolution CT of the lungs in infants and young children. J Thorac Imaging 2001;16:251–8.

[2] Fan LL, Langston C. Chronic interstitial lung disease in children. Pediatr Pulmonol 1993;16:184–96.

[3] Long FR, Castile RG, Brody AS, et al. Lungs in infants and children: improved thin-section CT with a non-invasive controlled-ventilation technique-initial experience. Radiology 1999;212:588–93.

[4] Long FR, Castile RG. Technique and clinical applications of full-inflation and end-exhalation controlled-ventilation chest CT in infants and young children. Pediatr Radiol 2001;31:413–22.

[5] Sibtain NA, Padley SP. HRCT in small and large airways diseases. Eur Radiol 2004;14:L31–43.

[6] Owens C. Radiology of diffuse interstitial pulmonary disease in children. Eur Radiol 2004;14:L2–12.

[7] Thurlbeck WM. Postnatal growth and development of the lung. Am Rev Respir Dis 1975;111:803–44.

[8] de Jong PA, Nakano Y, Lequin MH, et al. Estimation of lung growth using computed tomography. Eur Respir J 2003;22:235–8.

[9] Long FR, Williams RS, Castile RG. Structural airway abnormalities in infants and young children with cystic fibrosis. J Pediatr 2004;144:154–61.

[10] King GG, Muller NL, Pare PD. Evaluation of airways in obstructive pulmonary disease using high-resolution computed tomography. Am J Respir Crit Care Med 1999;159:992–1004.

[11] Nakano Y, Whittall KP, Kalloger SE, et al. Development and validation of human airway analysis algorithm using multidetector row CT. Medical Imaging 2002; 460–9.

[12] Coleman LT, Kramer SS, Markowitz RI, et al. Bronchiectasis in children. J Thorac Imaging 1995; 10:268–79.

[13] Berend N, Woolcock AJ, Marlin GE. Relationship between bronchial and arterial diameters in normal human lungs. Thorax 1979;34:354–8.

[14] Kim JS, Muller NL, Park CS, et al. Cylindrical bronchiectasis: diagnostic findings on thin-section CT. AJR Am J Roentgenol 1997;168:751–4.

[15] Lynch DA, Newell JD, Tschomper BA, et al. Uncomplicated asthma in adults: comparison of CT appearance of the lungs in asthmatic and healthy subjects. Radiology 1993;188:829–33.

[16] Wetzel RC, Herold CJ, Zerhouni EA, et al. Hypoxic bronchodilation. J Appl Physiol 1992;73:1202–6.

[17] Kim JS, Muller NL, Park CS, et al. Bronchoarterial ratio on thin section CT: comparison between high altitude and sea level. J Comput Tomogr 1997;21: 306–11.

[18] Armstrong DS, Grimwood K, Carzino R, et al. Lower respiratory infection and inflammation in infants with newly diagnosed cystic fibrosis. BMJ 1995;310: 1571–2.

[19] Khan TZ, Wagener JS, Bost T, et al. Early pulmonary inflammation in infants with cystic fibrosis. Am J Respir Crit Care Med 1995;151:1075–82.

[20] Matsuoka S, Uchiyama K, Shima H, et al. Broncho-arterial ratio and bronchial wall thickness on high-resolution CT in asymptomatic subjects: correlation with age and smoking. AJR Am J Roentgenol 2003;180:513–8.

[21] Brody AS, Klein JS, Molina PL, et al. High-resolution computed tomography in young patients with cystic fibrosis: distribution of abnormalities and correlation with pulmonary function tests. J Pediatr 2004; 145:32–8.

[22] Webb WR, Muller NL. HRCT of the lung. Philadelphia: Lippincott Williams and Wilkins; 2001.

[23] McNamara AE, Muller NL, Okazawa M, et al. Airway narrowing in excised canine lungs measured by high-resolution computed tomography. J Appl Physiol 1992;73:307–16.

[24] Kim SJ, Im JG, Kim IO, et al. Normal bronchial and pulmonary arterial diameters measured by thin section CT. J Comput Tomogr 1995;19:365–9.

[25] Lucaya J, Piqueras J, Garcia-Pena P, et al. Low-dose high-resolution CT of the chest in children and young adults: dose, cooperation, artifact incidence, and image quality. AJR Am J Roentgenol 2000;175: 985–92.

[26] Castile R, Filbrun D, Flucke R, et al. Adult-type pulmonary function in infants without respiratory disease. Pediatr Pulmonol 2000;30:215–27.

[27] Robinson TE, Leung AN, Northway WH, et al. Composite spirometric-computed tomography outcome measure in early cystic fibrosis lung disease. Am J Respir Crit Care Med 2003;168:588–93.

[28] Kauczor HU, Heussel CP, Fischer B, et al. Assessment of lung volumes using helical CT at inspiration and expiration: comparison with pulmonary function tests. AJR Am J Roentgenol 1998;171:1091–5.

[29] Griscom NT. Diseases of the trachea, bronchi, and smaller airways. Radiol Clin North Am 1993;31: 605–15.

[30] Arakawa H, Webb WR. Expiratory high-resolution CT scan. Radiol Clin North Am 1998;36:189–209.

[31] Verschakelen JA, Van Fraeyenhoven L, Laureys G, et al. Differences in CT density between dependent and nondependent portions of the lung: influence of lung volume. AJR Am J Roentgenol 1993;161:713–7.

[32] Hansell DM. Small airways diseases: detection and insights with computed tomography. Eur Respir J 2001;17:1294–313.

[33] Lee KW, Chung SY, Yang I, et al. Correlation of aging and smoking with air trapping at thin-section CT of the lung in asymptomatic subjects. Radiology 2000; 214:831–6.

[34] Castile RG, Iram D, McCoy K. Gas trapping in normal infants and infants with cystic fibrosis. Pediatr Pulmonol 2004;37:461–9.

[35] Chen D, Webb WR, Storto ML, et al. Assessment of air trapping using postexpiratory high-resolution computed tomography. J Thorac Imaging 1998;13: 135–43.

[36] Newman KB, Lynch DA, Newman LS, et al. Quantitative computed tomography detects air trapping due to asthma. Chest 1994;106:105–9.

[37] Tanaka N, Matsumoto T, Suda H, et al. Paired inspiratory-expiratory thin-section CT findings in patients with small airway disease. Eur Radiol 2001; 11:393–401.

[38] Goris ML, Zhu HJ, Blankenberg F, et al. An automated approach to quantitative air trapping measurements in mild cystic fibrosis. Chest 2003;123: 1655–63.

[39] Robinson TE, Leung AN, Moss RB, et al. Standardized high-resolution CT of the lung using a spirometer-triggered electron beam CT scanner. AJR Am J Roentgenol 1999;172:1636–8.

[40] Bonnel AS, Song SM, Kesavarju K, et al. Quantitative air-trapping analysis in children with mild cystic fibrosis lung disease. Pediatr Pulmonol 2004; 38:396–405.

[41] Choi SJ, Choi BK, Kim HJ, et al. Lateral decubitus HRCT: a simple technique to replace expiratory CT in children with air trapping. Pediatr Radiol 2002;32: 179–82.

[42] Johnson JL, Kramer SS, Mahboubi S. Air trapping in children: evaluation with dynamic lung densitometry with spiral CT. Radiology 1998;206:95–101.

[43] Webb W, Stern E, Kanth N, et al. Dynamic pulmonary CT: findings in healthy adult men. Radiology 1993; 186:117–24.

[44] Remy J, Remy-Jardin M, Artaud D, et al. Multiplanar and three-dimensional reconstruction techniques in CT: impact on chest diseases. Eur Radiol 1998;8: 335–51.

[45] Jung KJ, Lee KS, Kim SY, et al. Low-dose, volumetric helical CT: image quality, radiation dose, and usefulness for evaluation of bronchiectasis. Invest Radiol 2000;35:557–63.

[46] Huda W, Scalzetti EM, Roskopf M. Effective doses to patients undergoing thoracic CT examinations. Med Phys 2000;27:838–43.

[47] Barnes NA, Pilling DW. Bronchopulmonary foregut malformations: embryology, radiology and quandary. Eur Radiol 2003;13:2659–73.

[48] Berrocal T, Madrid C, Novo S, et al. Congenital anomalies of the tracheobronchial tree, lung, and mediastinum: embryology, radiology, and pathology. Radiographics 2004;24:e17.

[49] Chen SJ, Lee WJ, Wang JK, et al. Usefulness of three-dimensional electron beam computed tomography for

evaluating tracheobronchial anomalies in children with congenital heart disease. Am J Cardiol 2003;92: 483–6.

[50] McNamara VM, Crabbe DC. Tracheomalacia. Paediatr Respir Rev 2004;5:147–54.

[51] Austin J, Ali T. Tracheomalacia and bronchomalacia in children: pathophysiology, assessment, treatment and anaesthesia management. Paediatr Anaesth 2003; 13:3–11.

[52] Shell R, Allen E, Mutabagani K, et al. Compression of the trachea by the innominate artery in a 2-month-old child. Pediatr Pulmonol 2001;31:80–5.

[53] Burden R, Shann F, Butt W, et al. Tracheobronchial malacia and stenosis in children in intensive care: bronchograms help to predict outcome. Thorax 1999; 54:511–7.

[54] Ferretti GR, Thony F, Bosson JL, et al. Benign abnormalities and carcinoid tumors of the central airways: diagnostic impact of CT bronchography. AJR Am J Roentgenol 2000;174:1307–13.

[55] Kothari NA, Kramer SS. Bronchial diseases and lung aeration in children. J Thorac Imaging 2001;16:207–23.

[56] Lynch DA, Hay T, Newell Jr JD, et al. Pediatric diffuse lung disease: diagnosis and classification using high- resolution CT. AJR Am J Roentgenol 1999; 173:713–8.

[57] Copley SJ, Coren M, Nicholson AG, et al. Diagnostic accuracy of thin-section CT and chest radiography of pediatric interstitial lung disease. AJR Am J Roentgenol 2000;174:549–54.

[58] Lau DM, Siegel MJ, Hildebolt CF, et al. Bronchiolitis obliterans syndrome: thin-section CT diagnosis of obstructive changes in infants and young children after lung transplantation. Radiology 1998;208:783–8.

[59] Jensen SP, Lynch DA, Brown KK, et al. High-resolution CT features of severe asthma and bronchiolitis obliterans. Clin Radiol 2002;57:1078–85.

[60] Kinane BT, Mansell AL, Zwerdling RG, et al. Follicular bronchitis in the pediatric population. Chest 1993;104:1183–6.

RADIOLOGIC
CLINICS
of North America

Radiol Clin N Am 43 (2005) 391 – 403

Imaging Considerations: Interstitial Lung Disease in Children

Alan S. Brody, MD[a,b,*]

[a]Thoracic Imaging, Department of Radiology, MLC-5031, Cincinnati Children's Hospital and Medical Center,
3333 Burnet Avenue, Cincinnati, OH 45229–3039, USA
[b]Radiology and Pediatrics, University of Cincinnati College of Medicine, Cincinnati, OH, USA

Strictly speaking, the term *interstitial lung disease* (ILD) describes processes that specifically affect the lung interstitium rather than the airways or air spaces. This is a pathologic distinction that is not well reflected in the imaging appearance of the lungs, even with high-resolution CT (HRCT). It has been estimated that 1 mm^3 contains approximately 170 alveoli [1]. Because of this small size, imaging cannot distinguish the alveolar and interstitial spaces. *Diffuse lung disease* is a more appropriate term and is used in this article as the primary descriptor of these diseases. Because the term *interstitial lung disease* is in wide use, it is also used. The inconsistencies caused by this usage should be understood, and the more appropriate term *diffuse lung disease* is used when possible.

A broad range of processes can be described as diffuse lung disease from an imaging standpoint. The diseases described in this article are characterized by increased parenchymal attenuation on HRCT. This article emphasizes entities that present with the clinical picture of ILD: typically an insidious or neonatal onset of tachypnea, hypoxia, and frequently crackles on lung auscultation. Although not discussed here, it should be remembered that other processes can present in this manner. Pulmonary venous obstruction, cardiac disease, and fluid over-load can all produce diffuse pulmonary abnormalities with similar clinical presentations.

Children are not small adults. This is a favorite statement of many who care for children. Children are affected by different diseases and processes than adults. Their response to various insults is different than adults. The child is still growing, and future development and current anatomy and physiology may be altered by the disease process or other insults. In the case of diffuse lung disease, these differences make it very difficult to apply information learned from imaging adults to the interpretation of imaging in the child.

The radiologist may play a number of different roles in the evaluation of children with suspected diffuse lung disease. Often the radiologist provides the first definite evidence that a diffuse lung disease is present. This frequently is followed by the need to determine the best location for biopsy. If two or more distinct appearances are seen with HRCT, obtaining more than one biopsy should be discussed. The radiologist may be able to suggest a specific diagnosis, or a short list of likely diagnoses. In this case the radiologist may be able to suggest additional tests that may be useful in making the correct diagnosis.

All of the radiologist's roles depend on the images that are obtained. This article begins with a discussion of HRCT technique. Specific entities that are seen in children are then discussed. Because adult pathologic descriptions are frequently used in pathology reports of pediatric diffuse lung disease, the adult interstitial pneumonia classification scheme is then reviewed.

* Department of Radiology, MLC-5031, Cincinnati Children's Hospital, 3333 Burnet Avenue, Cincinnati, OH 45229–3039.
E-mail address: alan.brody@cchmc.org

0033-8389/05/$ – see front matter © 2005 Elsevier Inc. All rights reserved.
doi:10.1016/j.rcl.2004.12.002

radiologic.theclinics.com

High-resolution CT technique

To best evaluate the lung parenchyma with CT scanning, thin sections are necessary to avoid the volume averaging that occurs with 5- to 10-mm sections. This volume averaging obscures fine parenchymal detail and airway abnormalities including bronchiectasis, bronchial wall thickening, and peripheral mucous plugging (Fig. 1). Image contrast is increased with the use of an edge-enhancing kernel. These kernels differ between manufacturers. The kernel used for bone imaging usually works well for pediatric HRCT. Retrospective retargeting is rarely used. Images are viewed with a window width of 1500 and a window level of −600.

HRCT is a sampling technique that uses one thin section, approximately 1 mm in thickness, at much wider intervals, usually 10 mm. This technique was developed in the 1980s to allow high-quality images of the lung parenchyma without the high dose and long imaging time that are required if contiguous thin sections are used [2]. The development of multidetector array CT, also known as *multislice CT* (especially scanners with eight or more channels) has dramatically reduced both the dose and the time required to obtain large numbers of thin sections. This allows contiguous thin section studies of the entire chest at the same dose used for 5- or 10-mm conventional CT technique. This change had reduced the need to choose between conventional and HRCT when both may provide useful information. Most current multislice scanners have the ability retrospectively to reformat the scan data to provide thin sections from studies performed as conventional 5- or 10-mm contiguous CT scans. It should be remembered that HRCT can still be performed with multislice scanners, and there is an important dose savings when only a small portion of the lung is exposed to X-rays.

Radiation dose is an important consideration when planning HRCT in children. Although there is no imaging advantage to slices thinner than 1 mm, there may be a dose savings. Whether or not the dose decreases with thinner sections depends on the CT scanner. This should be confirmed when developing an HRCT protocol. The dose characteristics of the CT scanner should also be evaluated. It has been shown that patient dose may vary by a factor of three when different CT scanners are compared [3]. Dose information should be available from acceptance testing, and relative dose comparisons between different CT scanners can be performed quickly using equipment available in most radiology departments for routine quality assurance testing [3]. These dose characteristics must be evaluated in terms of image quality so that the lowest dose for the necessary image quality can be determined. In any department with more than one model of CT scanner, this evaluation should be performed to determine which CT scanner should be used for pediatric HRCT.

For HRCT both inspiratory and expiratory images should be obtained whenever possible. In addition to detecting air trapping that cannot be identified on inspiratory images (Fig. 2), expiratory images are frequently important in assessing for the presence of ground glass opacity. This is discussed further later. At the Cincinnati Children's Hospital a slice thickness of 1.5 mm or less at intervals of 7 to 10 mm is used depending on patient size. Even in small infants I have not found additional useful information when

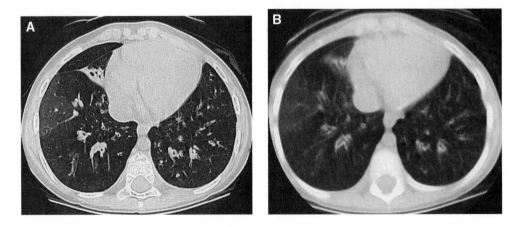

Fig. 1. Axial CT images obtained at the same location in a 5-year-old girl with bronchiolitis obliterans. Lung parenchymal detail is far better demonstrated with high-resolution technique (*A*) than with conventional 5-mm helical technique (*B*).

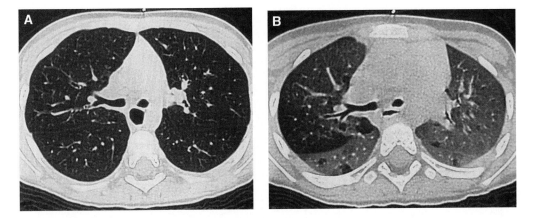

Fig. 2. Inspiratory (*A*) and expiratory (*B*) CT images in a 6-year-old girl with mild cystic fibrosis. The inspiratory image demonstrates mild bronchiectasis and bronchial wall thickening, but does not suggest the focal right upper lobe air trapping seen on the expiratory image.

decreasing the interval to 5 mm. Expiratory images should be obtained at greater intervals than the inspiratory images. For example, for clinical evaluation there is little value to obtaining expiratory images at intervals less than twice the interval used for the inspiratory series. At the Cincinnati Children's Hospital a minimum of four expiratory images is used. Images at a level just above the aortic arch, the carina, the level of the inferior pulmonary veins (or halfway between the carina and the higher hemidiaphragm), and one image 1 cm above the higher hemidiaphragm provide a sample of all lobes and of the apical, mid, and basilar zones of the lung. To localize these images correctly, an expiratory scout is required, because there is great variability in the change in lung volume between inspiratory and expiratory images.

To obtain true inspiratory and expiratory images, lung volume must be controlled. In older children voluntary cooperation can provide this control. Sufficient cooperation for high-quality inspiratory images can be obtained in many 4- or 5-year-old children, and in most 7- or 8-year-old children. Expiratory maneuvers are more challenging, and high-quality images can rarely be obtained in children less than 6 years of age. Cooperation can be increased by having a coach in the room that gives the child instructions and observes the response. The presence of a coach also allows better coordination between the patient and the CT technologist who controls when the images are obtained. Three methods have been used to control lung volume in children too young to cooperate. In order of increasing risk they are decubitus imaging, controlled volume CT, and general anesthesia.

Decubitus imaging provides images similar to inspiratory and expiratory images in the *up* lung and *down* lung, respectively. In addition, because these images are obtained during quiet respiration, there is often less motion than is seen with children who cannot cooperate fully with inspiratory and expiratory maneuvers [4]. Decubitus imaging is performed in the same manner that is used for decubitus chest radiographs. Following an initial CT scan in the supine position the patient is placed on his or her side and additional images are obtained. Whether the right or left decubitus position is used depends on the findings of the supine study (Fig. 3).

Controlled volume CT uses mask ventilation of a sedated patient. If several assisted deep breaths are given to a child, a period of 10 to 15 seconds of apnea follows. During that apneic period the lungs can again be inflated to produce an inspiratory image, and if no inspiratory pressure is administered, lung volumes decrease and allow expiratory images [5]. This technique was originally developed for infant pulmonary function tests and has been used in thousands of children. The equipment necessary for the CT technique is readily available. A sedation program must be in place, and additional training for a respiratory therapist or other health care worker to provide the mask ventilation and for the CT technologists is necessary.

General anesthesia can also be used to obtain inspiratory and expiratory images of the lungs. In this case respiration is controlled by the anesthesiologist and complete control of lung volume and respiratory motion is possible. The major imaging concern is the development of atelectasis, which can develop within a few minutes of intubation. The patient must be

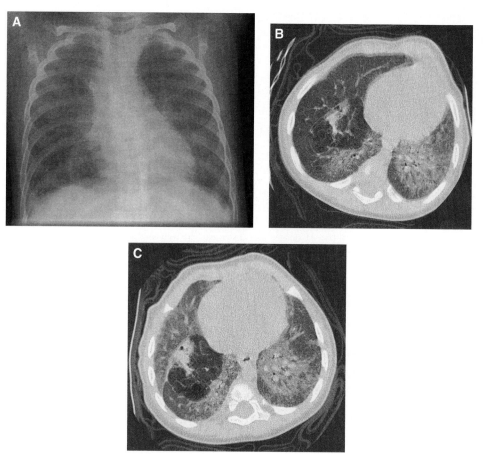

Fig. 3. Chest radiograph obtained at 5 months of age demonstrates diffusely increased attenuation, sparing part of the right lower lung (*A*). Left (*B*) and right (*C*) lateral decubitus CT images obtained without sedation demonstrate a hyperlucent area in the right lower lobe that does not change in appearance on the two images. The remaining left lung shows the normal increase in attenuation when the lung is placed in the dependent position. Left lower lobe opacity does not change with positioning, suggesting parenchymal disease rather than basilar atelectasis.

given frequent large sigh breaths and imaging should begin as soon as possible. If increased posterior opacity is seen in the lung bases, prone imaging should be considered.

Imaging findings of diffuse lung disease

Correct interpretation of HRCT images in children requires high-quality images, identification of abnormalities, description of these abnormalities, and knowledge of the associations between the HRCT and the different causes of diffuse lung disease. The identification and description of abnormalities is an area where the adult experience applies well to pediatric HRCT. Although the interpretation is frequently different, the imaging appearance of diffuse abnormalities is similar in adults and children. Such terms as *ground glass opacity, tree-in-bud, lobular air trapping, reticular opacities,* and *centrilobular nodules* can and should be used when describing findings on pediatric HRCT. A glossary of terms published by the Fleischner Society is a useful resource for this terminology [6]. Because this information is readily available in adult texts, only a few points are made here.

Ground glass opacity remains a finding that causes confusion both in identification and in interpretation [7]. Ground glass opacity describes lung that is higher in attenuation than normal lung at inspiration, but lower than the attenuation of bronchial walls and blood vessels so that these lung markings remain visible (Fig. 4). Ground glass opacity can be caused by any process that decreases

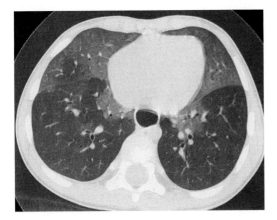

Fig. 4. Two-year-old boy with neuroendocrine cell hyperplasia of infancy. CT shows well-defined areas of ground glass opacity seen centrally and in the right middle lobe and lingula.

the relative amount of air in the lung without completely removing or replacing the air in the lung with other material. The differential diagnosis is lengthy, and includes normal lung at expiration and otherwise normal lung that is receiving greater than usual amounts of blood flow, often caused by shunting of blood from poorly ventilated lung to well-ventilated lung. In addition to normal lung, any process that partially fills the alveoli, thickens the alveolar wall or interstitium, or that results in diffuse distribution of high-attenuation material in the lung can produce this appearance. Etiologies of ground glass opacity in these categories include etiologies as diverse as pulmonary hemorrhage and infection, increased cellularity of the interstitium and pulmonary fibrosis, and pulmonary calcinosis.

The term *mosaic attenuation* is used to describe patchy areas of well-defined increased and decreased parenchymal attenuation. Etiologies for this appearance include diffuse lung disease, airway disease with air trapping, and vascular disease with areas of oligemic and plethoric lung. The interpretation of these areas can be challenging because it is often difficult to distinguish abnormal increased attenuation lung with adjacent normal lung from normal lung with adjacent air trapped lung. One reason that expiratory images are recommended for HRCT is that combined inspiratory and expiratory images can be used to make this differentiation. With expiration areas of normal lung increase in attenuation as air content is decreased, whereas areas of abnormal ground glass opacity show less increase in attenuation because the amount of air in the lung at inspiration is decreased so relatively less air can leave the lung with

expiration. In addition, air trapped lung, where decreased airway conductance limits the amount of air that can leave the lung during a brief exhalation, changes its attenuation less than normal lung.

When normal lung and air trapped lung are compared on inspiratory and expiratory images, the attenuation difference is greater on the expiratory than on the inspiratory image because the normal lung attenuation increases, whereas the air trapped area does not change. In this case the area of higher attenuation lung is normal, whereas the low-attenuation area has air trapping. When an area of abnormal lung is compared with normal lung in the same way, the normal lung shows a greater decrease in attenuation than the abnormal lung because it contains more air. The difference in attenuation between inspiration and expiration decreases, and the area of higher attenuation can be identified as abnormal. A study of HRCT scans on 70 adults found that infiltrative lung disease and airway disease were reliably distinguished, whereas vascular disease was frequently confused with one of the other etiologies of mosaic attenuation [8].

Accuracy of high-resolution CT in pediatric diffuse lung disease

Two studies have evaluated the ability of expert readers to correctly diagnose pediatric diffuse lung disease with HRCT. In one study the correct first choice diagnosis of diffuse lung disease was made in 55%, with the correct diagnosis listed in the top three diagnoses in 60% of the cases [9]. Alveolar proteinosis and idiopathic pulmonary hemosiderosis were correctly diagnosed in all cases. The correct diagnosis of lymphangiectasia was made in 83%, nonspecific or desquamative interstitial pneumonia in 50%, follicular bronchiolitis in 33%, and lymphocytic interstitial pneumonitis in 25%; one case of lymphangiomatosis was not correctly identified. Six normal patients were included in this study and were correctly identified as normal in all cases.

In a second study the correct first choice diagnosis was made in 40% with the correct diagnosis as one of the top three diagnoses in 58% [10]. This study of 20 patients included four cases of bronchiolitis obliterans that were all correctly diagnosed. All cases of bronchiolitis obliterans organizing pneumonia and hypersensitivity pneumonitis were correctly diagnosed. These studies demonstrate that the likelihood of a correct diagnosis depends on the type of diffuse lung disease, and suggests that experienced radiologists are likely correctly to identify a specific diffuse lung disease in a short differential in approximately 60% of cases.

Lung biopsy in diffuse lung disease

The diagnosis of diffuse lung diseases in children should be based on clinical and laboratory evaluation, imaging with HRCT, and often lung biopsy. In a study of 27 children with diffuse lung disease, a clear histologic diagnosis was reached in 25, and management changed in 15 of the 27 children [11]. In a second study of thoracoscopic and open lung biopsies a specific diagnosis was reached in 60% of thoracoscopic biopsies and 57% of open biopsies. Diagnostic yield did not depend on the type of biopsy, but it did increase in children over 24 months of age. The biopsies confirmed the preoperative diagnosis in only 25% [12].

Although lung biopsy remains an invasive procedure, thoracoscopic techniques have markedly decreased the morbidity of lung biopsies. In a study of 88 consecutive thoracoscopic wedge biopsies in children, the average hospital stay was 1.1 days and no complications were reported [13]. The availability of this technique and the recognition of the value of pathologic information in treating children with diffuse lung disease suggest that biopsy should be strongly considered in children with diffuse lung disease.

Specific entities in pediatric diffuse lung disease

Infantile cellular interstitial pneumonitis and pulmonary interstitial glycogenosis

These two terms likely describe the same disease. This is a rare form of diffuse lung disease that begins in early infancy. Infantile cellular interstitial pneumonitis was described in 1992 as a new form of pediatric ILD [14]. The pathology was characterized by interstitial thickening caused by oval and spindle-shaped histiocytes. Neither inflammatory nor fibrotic changes were seen. In 2002 a second report was published showing similar histologic findings, but adding that the abnormal cells in the interstitium contained large amounts of glycogen [15]. The authors of this report recognized the similarity between the histology in these series, and suggested that both might describe the same disease. These authors suggested that this entity might represent abnormal differentiation of the mesenchymal cells of the interstitium. Twelve children were included in

these two reports. Two children died; both were born prematurely and had bronchopulmonary dysplasia in addition to the findings of infantile cellular interstitial pneumonitis and pulmonary interstitial glycogenosis. Two were lost to follow-up. The remaining children have had a variable clinical course, but have shown improvement in their pulmonary symptoms over time.

Chest radiographs have been reported to show an initial ground glass appearance that progresses rapidly to a coarse interstitial pattern. Unlike surfactant deficiency, lung volumes are high. HRCT images of several children in the second group have been published and showed a varying appearance of ground glass opacity and linear opacities.

Chronic pneumonitis of infancy

Chronic pneumonitis of infancy is a very different form of pediatric diffuse lung disease despite a name similar to infantile cellular interstitial pneumonitis. In 1995 nine infants with diffuse lung disease were reported. The pathologic findings in these cases included thickened alveolar septae containing primitive mesenchymal cells, alveolar pneumocyte hyperplasia, and exudate containing macrophages and eosinophilic debris. Follow-up was available on six of these children. Two died, one had a lung transplant at 18 months of age, two had stable marked lung disease, and one had improved on chronic corticosteroids. The HRCT appearance in one case showed ground glass opacity, interlobular septal thickening, and centrilobular nodules [16].

The histologic appearance is similar to the appearance reported with surfactant protein abnormalities, and surfactant protein C (SP-C) mutation has been identified in children with a histologic diagnosis of chronic pneumonitis of infancy [17]. This much more ominous form of diffuse lung disease may result from more than one etiology; or may be caused by surfactant protein abnormalities, some of which have not yet been identified. Fig. 5 shows ground glass opacity and small cysts in a child with chronic pneumonitis of infancy.

Surfactant protein abnormalities

Genetic mutations resulting in abnormalities of surfactant structure and function have recently been shown to be an important cause of diffuse lung disease in infants and children [18–21]. There are four main surfactant proteins: SP-A, B, C, and D. SP-A and SP-D are hydrophilic, whereas SP-B and SP-C are hydrophobic. Three abnormalities have

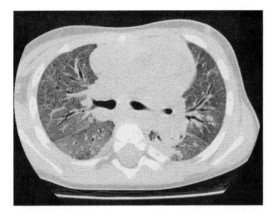

Fig. 5. HRCT image in an 11-month-old girl with a pathologic diagnosis of chronic pneumonitis of infancy shows diffuse ground glass opacity and scattered small cysts. The left lower lobe consolidation could be caused by the disease process or by atelectasis.

been identified. SP-B and SP-C mutations result in an abnormal protein structure of two of the four surfactant proteins. ATP-binding cassette transporter A3 (ABCA3) is a binding and transport protein that is found in the lamellar bodies of type II pneumocytes and results in surfactant deficiency.

Alveolar proteinosis presenting in the newborn period is now known to be caused by surfactant protein abnormality [18]. SP-B deficiency presents at birth and is fatal in the neonatal or young infancy. Cross-sectional imaging is rarely obtained in these infants because of their severe respiratory distress. Plain radiographs show diffuse hazy opacity. SP-B is an autosomal-recessive abnormality.

SP-C abnormality can present from the newborn period into childhood. Inheritance is believed to be autosomal-dominant with variable penetrance. The HRCT appearance of SP-C abnormality depends on the child's age. In infants the appearance is that of alveolar proteinosis with septal thickening and ground glass opacity. The clinical course of these patients is variable, even in families. In older children the appearance is variable, ranging from ground glass opacity to cystic changes (Fig. 6). Reticular opacities are also common. The abnormal SP-C protein that accumulates in SP-C abnormality is toxic and likely results in abnormal response to injury. In addition, disease severity is likely influenced by other lung injuries, such as episodes of pneumonia. ABCA3 mutations are more recently described, and the clinical course is not well understood. Infants frequently die in infancy (Fig. 7), although survivors into childhood have been identified (Fig. 8).

Persistent tachypnea of infancy and neuroendocrine cell hyperplasia of infancy

In 2001 Deterding et al [22] reported 16 children who presented with symptoms of ILD in the first year of life. All were born at term, none required oxygen in the neonatal period, and none had any other process identified that explained their symptoms. Lung biopsies demonstrated increased clear cells in the distal airways that demonstrated bombesin staining indicating a neuroendocrine origin for these cells. Although patients often required supplemental oxygen for months to years, their symptoms remained stable or slowly improved over time.

In a more recent publication these authors have noted that the patients' ill appearance contrasts strikingly with the mild abnormalities seen on lung biopsy. Continued follow-up continues to show slow improvement in these patients with no pulmonary deaths. Response to bronchodilators, corticosteroids, and hydroxychloroquine has been inconsistent. Because of the presence of neuroendocrine cells in the airways and aggregates of neuroendocrine cells, called neuroendocrine bodies, in the lobular parenchyma the authors suggested that neuroendocrine cell hyperplasia of infancy was a more appropriate term for this condition [23].

The HRCT appearance of neuroendocrine cell hyperplasia of infancy has not been reviewed, but a pattern of geographic ground glass opacity centrally and in the lingula and right middle lobes has been seen in many of these patients (see Fig. 4). This appearance is very similar to an appearance that has

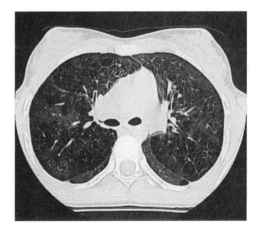

Fig. 6. HRCT in this 11-year-old with SP-C mutation shows distorted lung architecture and fine linear opacities and areas of ground glass opacity.

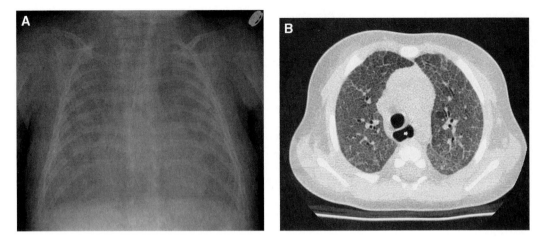

Fig. 7. (*A*) Three-month-old with an ATP-binding cassette transporter A3 surfactant mutation. Chest radiograph shows diffuse increased parenchymal opacity and normal lung volumes. (*B*) HRCT shows diffuse ground glass opacity with reticular appearance of intralobular septal thickening. This child died several weeks later.

been reported in follicular bronchiolitis (Fig. 9) [24]. Because bombesin staining is not done routinely, it is unclear whether neuroendocrine cell hyperplasia of infancy and follicular bronchiolitis are two diseases with similar pathologic and HRCT appearances, or if the subtle pathologic findings in many of these cases result in variable pathologic interpretations.

Lymphoid infiltrative disorders

Follicular bronchiolitis, also termed *follicular hyperplasia of bronchus-associated lymphoid tissue*, consists of lymphoid follicles that are distributed along the distal bronchi and bronchioles. Although

lymphocytes are commonly seen in the lung, lymphoid follicles are not. This disease is distinguished from lymphoid interstitial pneumonia by the location of the follicles along the airways, rather than diffusely throughout the interstitium. The etiology of this disorder is unknown, but it is often seen in children with abnormalities of the immune system [25]. These immunologic abnormalities may be subtle, and in-depth evaluation may be necessary to detect them. Children can present in infancy or childhood. In older children a previous history of frequent

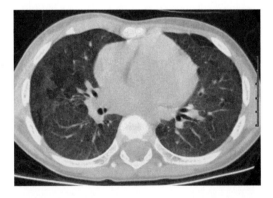

Fig. 8. Ground glass opacity in a 3-year-old with an ATP-binding cassette transporter A3 mutation is more heterogeneous than in the image shown in Fig. 6. This child underwent a lung transplant shortly after this study.

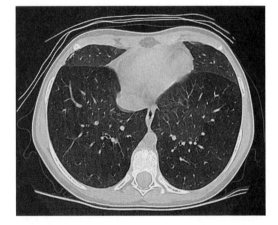

Fig. 9. HRCT images in a 9-year-old with a pathologic diagnosis of follicular bronchiolitis show a mosaic appearance of ground glass opacity. The appearance is strikingly similar to that shown in a child with neuroendocrine cell hyperplasia of infancy in Fig. 4.

pneumonias has been reported by some authors [26,27]. Two different appearances have been reported in follicular bronchiolitis. Reittner et al [26] reported centrilobular nodules with bronchial wall thickening and mild bronchiectasis. Oh et al [24] reported a very different pattern of diffuse hyperinflation with a mosaic attenuation pattern and minimal upper lobe interlobular septal thickening.

Lymphoid interstitial pneumonitis is commonly included as one of the idiopathic interstitial pneumonias. Lymphoid interstitial pneumonitis is presented here because review of lung biopsies suggests that lymphoid interstitial pneumonitis and follicular bronchiolitis are part of the spectrum of lymphoid infiltrative disorders. These diagnoses range from mild lymphocytic infiltration of the lung through large numbers of lymphoid follicles that may be diffuse or localized to the airways. Reviewing the histology may be helpful in establishing the position of one patient's disease along this spectrum (Figs. 9 and 10).

Lymphoid interstitial pneumonitis is most commonly seen in children in the setting of HIV infection, whereas in adults it is more commonly associated with autoimmune disease. Pathologic examination shows prominent diffuse interstitial infiltration of lymphocytes often accompanied by plasma cells, fibroblasts, and some macrophages [28]. Lymphoid follicles are seen in 50% or more of the patients. In an adult study of 22 patients, HRCT showed ground glass opacity and poorly defined centrilobular nodules in all cases with intralobular septal thickening in 80% [29]. One study of seven

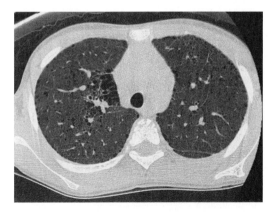

Fig. 10. Pathologically proved follicular bronchiolitis in a 9-year-old girl with juvenile rheumatoid arthritis. The CT appearance of diffuse ground glass opacity and peripheral cysts is more like the appearance described in lymphoid interstitial pneumonitis. The central area of low attenuation on the right may represent a conglomeration of cysts.

children with HIV-associated lymphoid interstitial pneumonitis found that the most common findings were 1- to 3-mm nodules [30]. A second study reported two children with lymphoid interstitial pneumonitis and HRCT findings of ground glass opacity, consolidation, and cysts [10].

Diffuse lung disease associated with systemic diseases

The most common diseases associated with diffuse lung disease are collagen vascular and storage diseases. Abnormalities on pulmonary function are common in connective tissue diseases, whereas symptomatic lung disease is less frequent. In adults a broad range of diffuse lung disease has been reported including all forms of idiopathic interstitial pneumonia and follicular bronchiolitis [31]. The frequency of symptomatic lung disease or the presence of abnormal findings on HRCT varies with the specific diagnosis. Symptomatic lung disease was found in 4% of children with juvenile rheumatoid arthritis [32]. Two of five symptomatic children had lymphoid interstitial pneumonitis. Patients with systemic lupus erythematosis have been reported to have a 5% incidence of symptomatic lung disease. Pleural disease is more common than parenchymal disease. Lupus pneumonitis is a rare condition presenting with dyspnea and associated with varying degrees of parenchymal opacity. Patients with systemic lupus erythematosis are also at risk for pulmonary hemorrhage. In children with scleroderma, 8 of 11 had diffuse lung disease on HRCT [33]. Ground glass opacity, subpleural nodules, peripheral linear opacities, and honeycombing were described (Fig. 11).

Patients with storage diseases may accumulate products of abnormal metabolism in the lung. Gaucher's disease and Niemann-Pick disease have been reported to show small nodules and septal thickening, likely representing deposition of these products in the alveoli and interstitium of the lung, respectively [34,35].

The interstitial pneumonia classification

In adults, diffuse lung disease is often classified into one of the interstitial pneumonias. These are pathologic descriptions that are characterized by interstitial inflammation with varying degrees of fibrosis. The interstitial pneumonias can be seen following an infectious or inhaled insult, but are frequently idiopathic. Although this terminology is

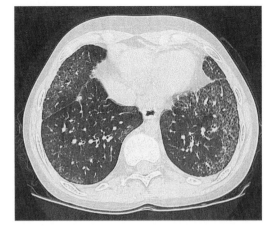

Fig. 11. Thirteen-year-old with mixed connective tissue disease. CT examination shows peripheral reticular opacities similar to the appearance seen in adults with idiopathic pulmonary fibrosis. Biopsy in this patient did not show the fibroblastic foci characteristic of idiopathic pulmonary fibrosis. She has remained stable with mild pulmonary symptoms.

used less commonly in children, it is widely used in pathology reports and in some cases suggests a likely etiology for diffuse lung disease in children. In addition, these terms can be used inappropriately in children, and this can be a source of confusion. A brief summary of the current classification of interstitial pneumonias follows.

Acute interstitial pneumonia

Acute interstitial pneumonia is unlike the remaining diseases described in this article because the onset is acute and the patients are extremely ill. Histology shows diffuse alveolar damage with hyaline membranes, interstitial edema, and fibroblast proliferation. Inflammatory changes are usually mild. The histologic appearance is the same as adult respiratory distress syndrome [36], but there is no precipitating event. The imaging appearance is also the same as adult respiratory distress syndrome, and mortality is approximately 80%. On HRCT a heterogeneous appearance of ground glass opacity is seen in nearly all cases. Although no reports of acute interstitial pneumonia in children have been published, authors have stated that this disease has been seen in children [23].

Usual interstitial pneumonia

Usual interstitial pneumonia is the histologic pattern that identifies idiopathic pulmonary fibrosis.

Idiopathic pulmonary fibrosis is a disease of adults, with a mean age of onset of 66 years [37]. Idiopathic pulmonary fibrosis is a progressive disease with a mean survival between 3 and 5 years from diagnosis [38,39]. No effective treatment is known. Although fibrosis may be present in pediatric diffuse lung disease, the clinical, imaging, and pathologic findings of idiopathic pulmonary fibrosis have not been seen to occur in children [12,23]. Reports have been published, however, describing idiopathic pulmonary fibrosis in children, but neither the pathologic findings described nor the clinical course were consistent with the diagnosis of idiopathic pulmonary fibrosis in adults [40].

The HRCT appearance of idiopathic pulmonary fibrosis is primarily patchy peripheral areas of reticular opacity. Abnormalities are usually greatest in the lung bases. Both ground glass opacity and honeycombing can be seen. HRCT is important in the diagnosis of adult idiopathic pulmonary fibrosis because the HRCT diagnosis of idiopathic pulmonary fibrosis is highly accurate with experienced observers [41] and because an atypical appearance suggests that other diagnoses should be considered [42].

A similar appearance can be seen in children with collagen vascular and autoimmune syndromes, particularly mixed connective tissue disease and scleroderma. The appearance is histologically different with less mature fibrosis, and the clinical course of these children is often one of long-term stability or very slow progression of disease.

Desquamative interstitial pneumonia

The term *desquamative interstitial pneumonia* was introduced by Liebow in 1965. The name came from the understanding that the large numbers of cells in the alveoli that characterize the pathologic appearance were desquamated alveolar cells. These cells are now known to be macrophages, which also extend diffusely into the lung parenchyma. Since its description the proper place of this entity in the understanding of diffuse lung disease has been disputed. The HRCT appearance of desquamative interstitial pneumonia is diffuse ground glass opacity that spares the upper lungs [43].

In children this pathologic appearance is rare. In a study of 25 cases reported by Sharief et al [44], children presented from 7 days to 11 years. Older children and those with mild pathologic changes had better outcomes. Sixty percent of children treated with chloroquine improved. Recently, patients with desquamative interstitial pneumonia have been found

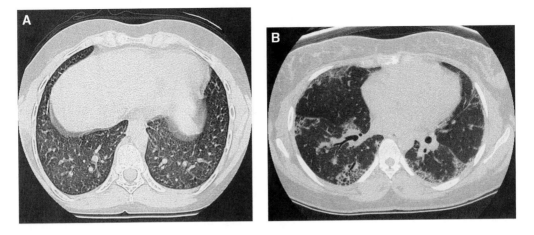

Fig. 12. Two very different appearances are seen in these images of two children with a pathologic diagnosis of nonspecific interstitial pneumonia. (*A*) Diffuse ground glass opacity is seen in a 14-year-old with dyskeratosis congenital. (*B*) A heterogeneous appearance of patchy ground glass opacity with peripheral linear and reticular opacities is seen in a previously well 18-year-old.

to have surfactant protein mutations. It seems likely that desquamative interstitial pneumonia in children represents a disease spectrum with surfactant protein mutations one of the etiologies. Evaluation for these mutations should be considered when this appearance is seen in children.

Nonspecific interstitial pneumonia

The term *nonspecific interstitial pneumonia* was introduced in 1994 to describe cases of interstitial pneumonia that could not be classified as usual interstitial pneumonia, desquamative interstitial pneumonia, or acute interstitial pneumonia. Nonspecific interstitial pneumonia is poorly named, because it is associated with a specific histologic appearance, and is associated with several specific conditions. In children, the diagnosis of nonspecific interstitial pneumonia suggests either an associated systemic disease, such as collagen vascular or autoimmune disease, or a surfactant protein abnormality.

The pathology is characterized by a greater inflammatory infiltrate that is seen with the other interstitial pneumonias. Inflammation and fibrosis vary in degree, but are temporally uniform, unlike usual interstitial pneumonia. There is a broad age range with nonspecific interstitial pneumonia reported in children as young as 9 years of age [25].

Ground glass opacity is the most common abnormality on HRCT. Areas of consolidation in addition to ground glass opacity occur in up to one third of patients. Peripheral linear opacities are common. Other findings that have been reported include

nodules and dilation of bronchi within areas of consolidation [45] (Fig. 12).

Summary

The understanding of diffuse lung disease in children has changed dramatically in the last few years with the identification of surfactant mutations and improvements in the understanding of several specific types of diffuse lung disease. Efforts are now underway to review larger numbers of children with these disorders to improve the ability to classify them both by histopathology and by imaging. Imaging, and particularly HRCT, will likely take an increasing role in the diagnosis and care of these children as new knowledge allows clinicians to offer greater insights into these rare and important diseases.

References

[1] Ochs M, Nyengaard JR, Jung A, et al. The number of alveoli in the human lung. Am J Respir Crit Care Med 2004;169:120–4.
[2] Mayo JR, Jackson SA, Muller NL. High-resolution CT of the chest: radiation dose. AJR Am J Roentgenol 1993;160:479–81.
[3] Cassese JA, Brody AS, Thomas SR. Utility of simple radiation dose measurements in the evaluation of different CT scanners used for high-resolution CT. J Thorac Imaging 2003;18:242–5.
[4] Choi SJ, Choi BK, Kim HJ, et al. Lateral decubitus HRCT: a simple technique to replace expiratory CT

in children with air trapping. Pediatr Radiol 2002;32: 179–82.

[5] Long FR, Castile RG, Brody AS, et al. Lungs in infants and young children: improved thin-section CT with a noninvasive controlled-ventilation technique: initial experience. Radiology 1999;212:588–93.

[6] Austin JH, Muller NL, Friedman PJ, et al. Glossary of terms for CT of the lungs: recommendations of the Nomenclature Committee of the Fleischner Society. Radiology 1996;200:327–31.

[7] Collins J, Stern EJ. Ground-glass opacity at CT: the ABCs. AJR Am J Roentgenol 1997;169:355–67.

[8] Worthy SA, Muller NL, Hartman TE, et al. Mosaic attenuation pattern on thin-section CT scans of the lung: differentiation among infiltrative lung, airway, and vascular diseases as a cause. Radiology 1997;205: 465–70.

[9] Copley SJ, Coren M, Nicholson AG, et al. Diagnostic accuracy of thin-section CT and chest radiography of pediatric interstitial lung disease. AJR Am J Roentgenol 2000;174:549–54.

[10] Lynch DA, Hay T, Newell Jr JD, et al. Pediatric diffuse lung disease: diagnosis and classification using high-resolution CT. AJR Am J Roentgenol 1999;173: 713–8.

[11] Coren ME, Nicholson AG, Goldstraw P, et al. Open lung biopsy for diffuse interstitial lung disease in children. Eur Respir J 1999;14:817–21.

[12] Fan LL, Kozinetz CA, Wojtczak HA, et al. Diagnostic value of transbronchial, thoracoscopic, and open lung biopsy in immunocompetent children with chronic interstitial lung disease. J Pediatr 1997;131:565–9.

[13] Rothenberg SS. Thoracoscopic lung resection in children. J Pediatr Surg 2000;35:271–4 [discussion: 274–5].

[14] Schroeder SA, Shannon DC, Mark EJ. Cellular interstitial pneumonitis in infants: a clinicopathologic study. Chest 1992;101:1065–9.

[15] Canakis AM, Cutz E, Manson D, et al. Pulmonary interstitial glycogenosis: a new variant of neonatal interstitial lung disease. Am J Respir Crit Care Med 2002;165:1557–65.

[16] Olsen EO, Sebire NJ, Jaffe A, et al. Chronic pneumonitis of infancy: high-resolution CT findings. Pediatr Radiol 2004;34:86–8.

[17] Fan LL, Langston C. Pediatric interstitial lung disease: children are not small adults. Am J Respir Crit Care Med 2002;165:1466–7.

[18] Nogee LM, de Mello DE, Dehner LP, et al. Brief report: deficiency of pulmonary surfactant protein B in congenital alveolar proteinosis. N Engl J Med 1993; 328:406–10.

[19] Nogee LM, Dunbar III AE, Wert SE, et al. A mutation in the surfactant protein C gene associated with familial interstitial lung disease. N Engl J Med 2001; 344:573–9.

[20] Shulenin S, Nogee LM, Annilo T, et al. ABCA3 gene mutations in newborns with fatal surfactant deficiency. N Engl J Med 2004;350:1296–303.

[21] Hamvas A, Nogee LM, White FV, et al. Progressive lung disease and surfactant dysfunction with a deletion in surfactant protein C gene. Am J Respir Cell Mol Biol 2004;30:771–6.

[22] Deterding RR, Fan LL, Morton R, et al. Persistent tachypnea of infancy (PTI): a new entity. Pediatr Pulmonol 2001;23:72–3.

[23] Fan LL, Deterding RR, Langston C. Pediatric interstitial lung disease revisited. Pediatr Pulmonol 2004; 38:369–78.

[24] Oh YW, Effmann EL, Redding GJ, et al. Follicular hyperplasia of bronchus-associated lymphoid tissue causing severe air trapping. AJR Am J Roentgenol 1999;172:745–7.

[25] Nicholson AG, Kim H, Corrin B, et al. The value of classifying interstitial pneumonitis in childhood according to defined histological patterns. Histopathology 1998;33:203–11.

[26] Reittner P, Fotter R, Lindbichler F, et al. HRCT features in a 5-year-old child with follicular bronchiolitis. Pediatr Radiol 1997;27:877–9.

[27] Benesch M, Kurz H, Eber E, et al. Clinical and histopathological findings in two Turkish children with follicular bronchiolitis. Eur J Pediatr 2001;160:223–6.

[28] Fishback N, Koss M. Update on lymphoid interstitial pneumonitis. Curr Opin Pulm Med 1996;2:429–33.

[29] Johkoh T, Muller NL, Pickford HA, et al. Lymphocytic interstitial pneumonia: thin-section CT findings in 22 patients. Radiology 1999;212:567–72.

[30] Becciolini V, Gudinchet F, Cheseaux JJ, et al. Lymphocytic interstitial pneumonia in children with AIDS: high-resolution CT findings. Eur Radiol 2001; 11:1015–20.

[31] Tanaka N, Newell JD, Brown KK, et al. Collagen vascular disease-related lung disease: high-resolution computed tomography findings based on the pathologic classification. J Comput Assist Tomogr 2004;28: 351–60.

[32] Athreya BH, Doughty RA, Bookspan M, et al. Pulmonary manifestations of juvenile rheumatoid arthritis: a report of eight cases and review. Clin Chest Med 1980;1:361–74.

[33] Seely JM, Effmann EL, Muller NL. High-resolution CT of pediatric lung disease: imaging findings. AJR Am J Roentgenol 1997;168:1269–75.

[34] Yassa NA, Wilcox AG. High-resolution CT pulmonary findings in adults with Gaucher's disease. Clin Imaging 1998;22:339–42.

[35] Rodrigues R, Marchiori E, Muller NL. Niemann-Pick disease: high-resolution CT findings in two siblings. J Comput Assist Tomogr 2004;28:52–4.

[36] Katzenstein AL, Myers JL, Mazur MT. Acute interstitial pneumonia: a clinicopathologic, ultrastructural, and cell kinetic study. Am J Surg Pathol 1986;10: 256–67.

[37] Johnston ID, Prescott RJ, Chalmers JC, et al. British Thoracic Society study of cryptogenic fibrosing alveolitis: current presentation and initial management. Fibrosing Alveolitis Subcommittee of the Research

Committee of the British Thoracic Society. Thorax 1997;52:38–44.

[38] Panos RJ, Mortenson RL, Niccoli SA, et al. Clinical deterioration in patients with idiopathic pulmonary fibrosis: causes and assessment. Am J Med 1990;88: 396–404.

[39] Schwartz DA, Van Fossen DS, Davis CS, et al. Determinants of progression in idiopathic pulmonary fibrosis. Am J Respir Crit Care Med 1994;149(2 Pt 1): 444–9.

[40] Hacking D, Smyth R, Shaw N, et al. Idiopathic pulmonary fibrosis in infants: good prognosis with conservative management. Arch Dis Child 2000;83: 152–7.

[41] Lynch DA, Newell JD, Logan PM, et al. Can CT distinguish hypersensitivity pneumonitis from idio-

pathic pulmonary fibrosis? AJR Am J Roentgenol 1995;165:807–11.

[42] ATS and Society-ERS, ER. Idiopathic pulmonary fibrosis: diagnosis and treatment. International Consensus Statement. Am J Crit Care Med 2000;161: 646–64.

[43] Hartman TE, Primack SL, Swensen SJ, et al. Desquamative interstitial pneumonia: thin-section CT findings in 22 patients. Radiology 1993;187:787–90.

[44] Sharief N, Crawford OF, Dinwiddie R. Fibrosing alveolitis and desquamative interstitial pneumonitis. Pediatr Pulmonol 1994;17:359–65.

[45] Kim TS, Lee KS, Chung MP, et al. Nonspecific interstitial pneumonia with fibrosis: high-resolution CT and pathologic findings. AJR Am J Roentgenol 1998; 171:1645–50.

ELSEVIER
SAUNDERS

Radiol Clin N Am 43 (2005) 405 – 418

RADIOLOGIC
CLINICS
of North America

Pediatric Chest Ultrasound

Brian D. Coley, MD[a,b,*]

[a]*Section of Ultrasound, Department of Radiology, Columbus Children's Hospital,
700 Children's Drive, Columbus, OH 43205, USA*
[b]*Radiology and Pediatrics, Ohio State University School of Medicine and Public Health, Columbus, OH, USA*

After conventional radiography, CT and MR imaging are the dominant modalities for imaging the pediatric chest, as reflected by the other issues in this volume. With acoustic limitations imposed by bone and air, the thorax at first seems to be an unforgiving place to perform ultrasonography (US). Many diseases and pathologic conditions allow an acoustic window into the chest, however, and the unique anatomy of the pediatric chest provides other imaging windows for the creative sonologist. US will never replace CT and MR imaging, but it can provide very useful and important (and at times superior) information, without the need for sedation or exposure to radiation.

Technique

All patients undergoing sonographic examination of the chest should have a preceding conventional radiographic examination [1,2]. This helps to focus the US study and to improve diagnostic utility. As with sonography elsewhere in the body, the appropriate transducers and frequencies vary with the size of the patient and the structure being examined. Small infants and neonates are easily examined with high-frequency linear transducers, whereas older children and adolescents require lower-frequency transducers. Smaller footprint sector or vector transducers are needed to insonate between ribs, below the dia-

phragm, or from the suprasternal notch. Linear transducers are valuable for examining chest wall lesions.

Useful acoustic windows are depicted in Fig. 1. The relatively unossified thorax of the neonate and infant, along with the presence of a relatively large thymus, allows imaging of the anterior chest and mediastinum through sternal and costochondral cartilages. Suprasternal or supraclavicular approaches may also be useful in examining the anterior mediastinum and thoracic vessels. Intercostal scanning allows imaging of the lung and pleura throughout the thorax, and of the posterior mediastinum [2–8]. Using the liver, spleen, or fluid-filled stomach as acoustic windows allows examination of the inferior thoracic cavity [9].

Indications

The most common indication for chest sonography is an opaque hemithorax on a chest radiograph [2,3,5]. US can readily differentiate whether parenchymal or pleural disease (or both) is to blame (Fig. 2) [10,11], and may help to guide the appropriate direction of therapy and possible thoracic intervention [12]. Focal masses can be imaged to determine location and whether they are solid or cystic. Abnormal mediastinal contours in infants are usually caused by an unusually sized or shaped thymus, which can be easily shown by US [4], avoiding radiation exposure with CT. Palpable chest wall lesions are best initially imaged with US, because nonpainful pediatric chest wall masses are typically benign and require no further investigation. Although CT and MR angiographic techniques can produce

---
* Section of Ultrasound, Department of Radiology, Columbus Children's Hospital, 700 Children's Drive, Columbus, OH 43205.

E-mail address: bcoley@chi.osu.edu

0033-8389/05/$ – see front matter © 2005 Elsevier Inc. All rights reserved.
doi:10.1016/j.rcl.2004.12.003

radiologic.theclinics.com

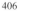

Fig. 1. Acoustic windows for thoracic sonography: (1) supraclavicular, (2) suprasternal, (3) parasternal, (4) transsternal, (5) intercostals, (6) subxyphoid, (7) subdiaphragmatic, and (8) posterior paraspinal. (*Adapted from* Kim O, Kim W, Min J, et al. US in the diagnosis of pediatric chest disease. Radiographics 2000;20:653–71; with permission.)

exquisite vascular images, US is often the first and only necessary study for examination of suspected thromboses and other abnormalities of thoracic vasculature.

Normal anatomy

Unossified costochondral and sternal cartilage appears hypoechoic on US. The shape of costochondral cartilage is often varied, and may produce irregular chest wall "masses" [13]. With aging, these cartilages gradually ossify, diminishing acoustic access to the thorax. The thymus is physically largest during adolescence, but is relatively largest compared with the rest of the thorax during the first few years of life. Usually confined to the anterior mediastinum, the thymus may extend into the neck or middle and posterior mediastinum, which may produce concern for pathology [14]. Fortunately, the thymus has a characteristic echotexture, with regular linear and punctate echogenicities that allows its confident recognition and differentiation from mediastinal pathology (Fig. 3) [4,15]. Although the normal pleural space contains a tiny amount of fluid, this is not normally seen with US. The acoustic interface of the chest wall with normal aerated lung provides a strong reflective surface, and produces a characteristic reverberation within the US image (Fig. 4), although the thinner chest wall of infants and small children may not demonstrate this artifact. Aerated lung is also seen to move along the parietal pleural surface with respiration, termed the "gliding sign" [6,12,16]. Deviations from this normal appearance provide clues to pleural and parenchymal disease.

The pleural space

Being superficial to normally echogenic aerated lung, the pleural space is well visualized by US. Although pleural fluid collections are often suspected from chest radiographs, US is much more sensitive in detecting pleural fluid [17], particularly in critically ill patients in whom upright or decubitus radiographs are not possible. The sonographic appearance of

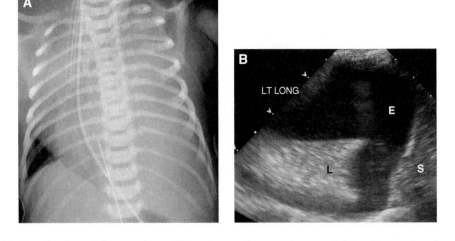

Fig. 2. (*A*) Frontal radiograph in a newborn with respiratory distress and opaque left hemithorax of unclear etiology. (*B*) Longitudinal parasternal sonogram shows a large anechoic effusion (E) and consolidated left lung (L). The diaphragm is partially everted, displacing the spleen (S). Aspiration revealed a chylothorax.

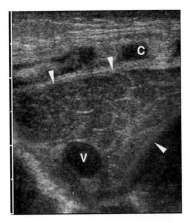

Fig. 3. Normal thymic ultrasound examination. Right parasternal longitudinal view shows a normal triangular-shaped right thymic lobe (*arrowheads*) with characteristic linear and punctate echogenicities conforming to the contours of the brachiocephalic vein (V). Note the hypoechoic costochondral cartilages (C) allowing imaging through the chest wall.

pleural fluid depends on its composition [18] and may range from completely anechoic in the case of simple transudative collections, to collections with mobile echogenic debris in cases of infection and hemorrhage, to septated and more solid-appearing collections with empyema and organizing infection (Fig. 5). Simple nonloculated collections can be seen to change shape with patient breathing or change in position. The distinction of echogenic but still fluid collections from more solid collections can be aided by the "fluid color sign" in which mobile debris produces color signal with color Doppler, whereas nonmobile solid material does not [19,20].

As infected collections progress and organize, fibrinous strands begin to form within pleural collections. Initially thin and mobile, these fibrin strands thicken and increase, creating multiple loculations that produce a honeycomb-like pleural space in which fluid no longer changes with patient position or respiration. The parietal and visceral pleura may be thickened, as is often seen with CT. Infected pleural collections may progress to solidify into a homogenous echogenic gelatinous mass encasing the underlying lung, eventually producing a fibrothorax.

US is superior to CT in characterizing the nature of pleural fluid collections [7,21], and can help to guide percutaneous drainage [12,22,23]. Simple fluid collections are amenable to percutaneous aspiration, and are most safely performed with US guidance (Fig. 6) [24,25]. Because 50% of pediatric parapneumonic effusions recur after aspiration, however,

it is often more prudent to leave a drainage catheter in place, even if only for a short time [26]. The US detection of fibrinous strands and even honeycombing of the pleural space is not necessarily a contraindication to percutaneous drainage, but it does mean that fibrinolytic therapy is required to clear the collections and should be started promptly to achieve proper drainage (Fig. 7) [27–29]. In the setting of continued fevers after pleural drainage, radiographs may not adequately assess whether undrained pleural collections or underlying parenchymal infection are to blame. Although US can adequately assess the pleural space and portions of the underlying lung, CT generally gives a more global evaluation in complicated cases.

Metastatic disease to the pleural space is much less common in children than in adults, but can occur with Wilms' tumor, neuroblastoma, and sarcomas. Pleural metastases are often accompanied by large effusions with hemorrhage, which appears as echogenic debris-filled fluid at sonography. The presence of pleural fluid aids in detection of solid masses adherent to the parietal or visceral pleura (Fig. 8). If visible sonographically, pleural masses readily undergo biopsy with US guidance [12,30,31], allowing confirmatory histologic diagnoses.

The normal strong acoustic interface between pleura and aerated lung produces posterior reverberation, and one can see the normal sliding motion of the lung during respiration. When air is introduced into the pleural space the normal tension between the pleural layers is lost, and a gap is created between the parietal and visceral pleura disrupting the normal acoustic interface. The sliding of the underlying lung

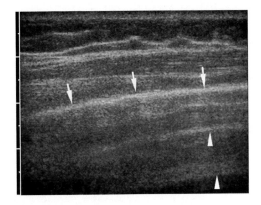

Fig. 4. Normal chest wall–lung interface. Intercostal sonogram using a linear transducer shows the strong echogenic surface of the aerated lung (*arrows*) and the reverberation artifacts projected within the deeper lung parenchyma (*arrowheads*).

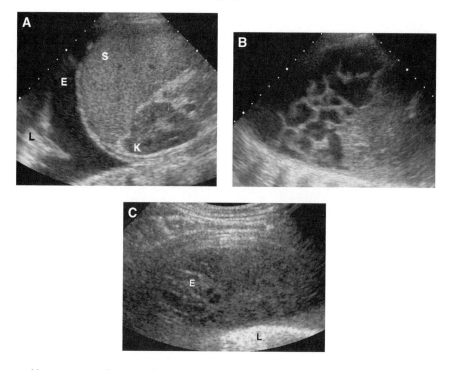

Fig. 5. Sonographic appearances of pleural collections. (*A*) Subdiaphragmatic longitudinal sonogram shows a mostly anechoic left pleural effusion (E) along with consolidated lung (L). The spleen (S) and kidney (K) help to provide acoustic windows into the inferior chest. (*B*) Empyema with moderate septations forming. (*C*) Well-organized solid-appearing empyema (E) adjacent to aerated lung (L).

can no longer be seen, and the normal reverberation is replaced by a static homogeneous posterior acoustic shadowing. Some reports indicate that that US is superior to plain radiographs in pneumothorax detection, and may be useful in monitoring procedural complications and assessing critically ill and trauma patients [32–35]. Similarly, the "curtain sign" has been described in hydropneumothorax where the normal pleural gliding is lost and mobile air-fluid levels are visualized [36].

Lung parenchyma

Radiography usually suffices for the evaluation of parenchymal lung disease, but unclear cases may

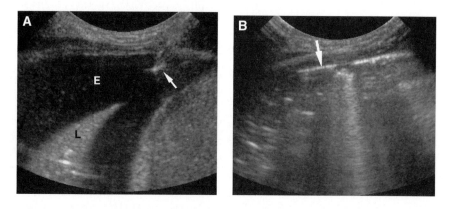

Fig. 6. Pleural effusion aspiration. (*A*) Right pleural effusion (E) and consolidated lung (L), with entry of aspiration catheter (*arrow*). (*B*) Complete aspiration of effusion through catheter (*arrow*) with partial aeration of underlying lung.

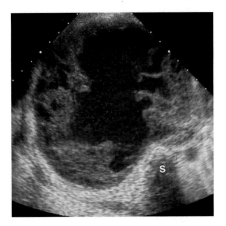

Fig. 7. Transverse sonogram of a large septated empyema with mediastinal shift. This collection responded well to interventional drainage and lytic therapy. S, spine.

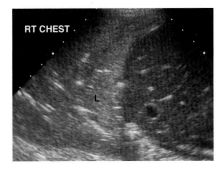

Fig. 9. Consolidated lung. Longitudinal sonogram over the lower right chest shows consolidated lung (L) superior to the liver. Although their echogenicities differ, other internal sonographic appearance is similar.

benefit from US or CT examination. When normally aerated lung becomes atelectatic or consolidated, it becomes possible to examine the lung parenchyma with US. Airless lung appears sonographically similar to liver, so-called "hepatization" (Fig. 9). The underlying internal architecture of the lung is preserved, however, allowing differentiation from masses or other processes. Branching linear echogenicities representing air bronchograms are often seen (Fig. 10), and were first described in pediatric patients [37]. Entrapped fluid or mucoid material within bronchi in necrotizing or postobstructive pneumonias produces hypoechoic branching structures, the sonographic fluid bronchogram [8]. Pulmonary vascular flow is preserved in simple pneumonic consolidation and is readily demonstrated with color Doppler [8]. With atelectasis, vessels become crowded together and have a more parallel orientation. Their orderly linear

and branching structure is preserved, however, allowing distinction from the more irregular vasculature found in neoplasms [20].

As infections progress, pulmonary abscesses may form. Small areas of lung necrosis may appear as areas of decreased echogenicity and fluid lacking color Doppler flow contained within areas of consolidation. Larger abscesses may develop a thick wall, and air fluid levels may be seen if the abscess communicates with the bronchial tree or if there is cavitation (Fig. 11) [6,8]. Causative organisms are not always cultured from sputum or peripheral blood. If abutting the pleura, lung abscess are sonographically visible and US-guided aspiration can play an important role in diagnosis and treatment [8,38].

Primary lung neoplasms are fortunately rare in children. Pulmonary blastoma is the most common, and starts as a peripheral lesion, often attaining large size before becoming clinically apparent [4]. Other less common tumors include mucoepidermoid car-

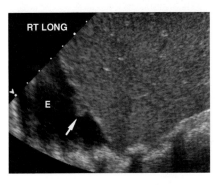

Fig. 8. Longitudinal sonogram of the right chest in a child with Wilms' tumor shows a pleural effusion (E) outlining a metastatic deposit on the diaphragmatic parietal pleura (*arrow*).

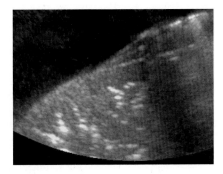

Fig. 10. Sonographic air bronchograms. Longitudinal sonogram shows pleural effusion and lower lobe consolidation with internal branching bright echogenicities representing air bronchograms. These often move with patient respiratory effort during the examination.

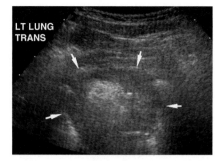

Fig. 11. Lung abscess. Transverse sonogram of the right upper chest in an immunocompromised patient with persistent chest radiographic opacity shows a thick-walled structure (*arrows*) with central echogenicity. Ultrasound-guided aspiration yielded *Aspergillus*.

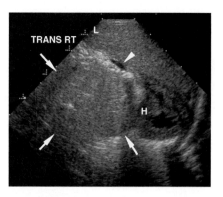

Fig. 12. Type III cystic adenomatoid malformation. Transverse sonogram through the lower chest in a newborn with cardiorespiratory distress and abnormal chest radiographs shows an echogenic mass (*arrows*) displacing the heart (H) and compressing the inferior vena cava (*arrowhead*).

cinoma, rhabdomyosarcoma, and bronchogenic tumors. Although US can confirm the presence of a mass, like other imaging modalities US cannot be histologically specific and differentiate among tumor types [39].

Congenital parenchymal masses include cystic adenomatoid malformation and sequestration. Although often regarded as separate entities, these malformations are part of a spectrum of bronchogenic foregut malformations and may have overlapping imaging and histologic features [4]. These masses may be detected prenatally by US or MR imaging, appearing as variably solid or cystic structures [40]. Postnatally, radiographs usually show the lesion, often as incidental findings or on images taken for respiratory symptoms. Cystic adenomatoid malformations are classified according to their cystic component. Type I malformations have largest cysts, greater than 2 cm in size, with types II and III having progressively smaller cystic components. The US appearance follows this histologic typing, demonstrating cysts of varying size amid echogenic parenchyma (Fig. 12) [39]. Although spontaneous regression of cystic adenomatoid malformation has been reported, most detected postnatally are still resected [41]. Superimposed infection can pose difficulties and complications for surgery. Like lung abscesses, US-guided percutaneous drainage can allow successful treatment of infected cystic adenomatoid malformations and allow a safer delayed surgical resection.

Intralobar sequestrations are most often found in the lower lobes, presenting with recurrent infections or persistent radiographic opacities. These are typically sonographically solid masses, although there may be cystic components [3]. The key diagnostic feature of sequestration is demonstrating

systemic arterial supply, usually from the descending aorta (Fig. 13) [20,42,43]. Color Doppler sonography is diagnostically reliable in this condition in the young child, although contrast-enhanced CT and MR imaging are often required in older patients. Extralobar sequestrations have a separate pleural investment and are usually found in the inferior left chest, but may even be located below the diaphragm, where they may be confused with adrenal pathology. Patients present symptomatically at a younger age than those with intralobar malformation, with cyanosis and dyspnea being more common [39]. US features are similar in both conditions, although associated anomalies are much more commonly associated with extralobar sequestrations.

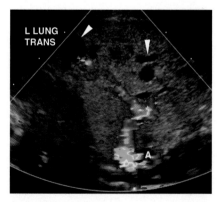

Fig. 13. Intralobar sequestration. Transverse sonogram of the inferior left chest shows an abnormal echogenic mass with arterial supply from the thoracic aorta (A). Note the cystic components (*arrowheads*), which were shown histologically to be elements of cystic adenomatoid malformation within the sequestration.

The normal chest wall and pleural interface produces a regular reverberation artifact. Occasionally, more focal ring-down artifacts are identified, thought to be caused by subpleural septal thickening or distortion by parenchymal disease [44]. Although scattered ring-down artifacts can normally be seen, multiple artifacts are associated with parenchymal lung disease. In adults, this finding has been shown with a variety of disorders, such as pulmonary fibrosis, viral pneumonias, sarcoidosis, lymphangitic carcinomatosis, and bronchiectasis [44,45]. In children, hyaline membrane disease produces a diffusely echogenic lung, which eliminates normal visualization of the diaphragm and the normal chest wall and pleural interface [46,47]. Chronic lung disease in the infant produces similar acoustic interfaces as seen in adult parenchymal disease, creating multiple ring-down artifacts (Fig. 14). The progression of US findings from surfactant deficiency to bronchopulmonary dysplasia may be useful as a predictor of the development of chronic lung disease, and may appear earlier than chest radiographic findings [47,48].

Mediastinum

The thymus is the dominant noncardiac mediastinal structure within the pediatric chest. Its appearance on chest radiography is usually recognized, although variations in size and position can occasionally be confusing and prompt further imaging. The characteristic US appearance allows confident diagnosis and obviates the need for further imaging tests (Fig. 15). Diminished thymic size is seen in infants and children subject to physiologic stress [3]. DiGeorge syndrome is a cellular immunodeficiency disorder related to hypoplasia or aplasia of the thymus. Although the associated anomalies are usually sufficient for diagnosis, failure to visualize the infant thymus by US is strongly confirmatory [3].

Primary thymic tumors are rare in children [4]. Thymomas usually occur in older children and adolescents, who often present with paraneoplastic syndromes. In this age group, mediastinal acoustic windows are more limiting, making MR imaging or CT better imaging choices. Thymomas can be heterogeneous tumors with areas of necrosis and calcification [49], whereas thymolipomas are more homogeneously echogenic because of their fatty content. Secondary neoplastic thymic infiltration occurs with leukemia, lymphoma, and even Langerhans' cell histiocytosis. In these cases, the normal sonographic thymic pattern is replaced with variably echogenic and heterogeneous soft tissue and associated abnormal lobulation of the confining fibrous thymic capsule. Small calcifications have been described with histiocytic infiltration [4,15]. An infiltrated thymus loses compliance and may be seen to displace and distort adjacent structures instead of normally conforming to their shape.

The most common benign thymic masses are lymphangiomas and thymic cysts [4]. Lymphangiomas are usually comprised of multiple loculated cysts with thin bands of intervening soft tissue. Normally hypovascular, lymphangiomas may contain hemangiomatous components that demonstrate flow with color Doppler evaluation. Cysts contents are usually anechoic, but superimposed hemorrhage or infection produces cyst contents of variable echogenicity, or even fluid-debris levels. Thymic cysts arise from remnants of the thymopharyngeal ducts [39] or from cystic degeneration of the thymus itself asso-

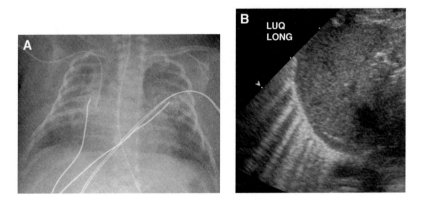

Fig. 14. Chronic lung disease. (*A*) Portable frontal chest radiograph in a former preterm infant with continued oxygen requirements shows increased interstitial markings of chronic lung disease. (*B*) Longitudinal sonogram through the left upper quadrant shows multiple comet tail artifacts from the interface with the lung, a sonographic sign of lung disease.

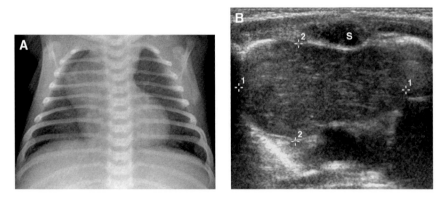

Fig. 15. Prominent thymus. (*A*) Frontal chest radiograph of a 1-year-old child with respiratory symptoms shows a prominent right-sided mediastinal contour. (*B*) Transverse sonogram of the superior chest shows a normal thymus (between cursors) to be the source of the radiographic findings. Note the hypoechoic sternal cartilage (S).

ciated with mediastinal trauma or surgery, and thymic tumors. Most congenital cases are diagnosed in childhood, presenting as slowly enlarging masses that may extend into the neck. Thymic cysts typically are unilocular with imperceptible walls and anechoic contents, and sonographic demonstration of their continuity with the thymus allows their diagnosis. Thymic cysts associated with HIV infection are more commonly multiseptated and may cause more diffuse thymic enlargement [50,51].

The anterior mediastinum is a common site for other neoplasms, particularly lymphoma. Most children with lymphoma have anterior mediastinal involvement, more frequent with Hodgkin's than with non-Hodgkin's lymphoma [3,39]. These patients may present with constitutional symptoms (fever, weight loss); respiratory complaints (cough, dyspnea); and occasionally are discovered incidentally. Sonographically, lymphoma may appear as discrete masses, nodal enlargement, or with diffuse thymic infiltration. Lymphoma tends to be hypoechoic and hypovascular compared with inflammatory processes and other neoplasms [39]. Teratomas and other germ cell tumors may also arise in the anterior mediastinum. The US appearance of germ cell tumors is more variable, ranging from purely soft tissue masses to heterogeneous masses containing fat, bone, and cystic elements seen with teratomas (Fig. 16) [3,39,52]. US can also demonstrate vascular encasement and compromise from mediastinal tumors, which can be valuable before central venous access for chemotherapy. A tissue diagnosis is required before chemotherapy, but airway compromise may make surgical biopsy unattractive. US-guided mediastinal percutaneous biopsy is an excellent alternative

in these patients, and can be done comfortably and safely, even in critically ill infants and children [6,12,31].

Middle mediastinal lesions include cystic (bronchogenic, gastrointestinal, pericardial, and lymphatic) and solid (lymphadenopathy) masses. Visualization may become more difficult with age, but the creative use of acoustic windows still makes US a valuable diagnostic modality. Lymphadenopathy arises from either neoplasia or infection, appearing abnormally enlarged and hypoechoic, often with color Doppler hyperemia. Although many papers report sonographic differences between inflammatory and neoplastic adenopathy, this distinction is not always possible. Bronchogenic cysts are usually thin walled, whereas esophageal duplication cysts may have a hypoechoic muscular rim typical of gastrointestinal duplications elsewhere in the body; this differentia-

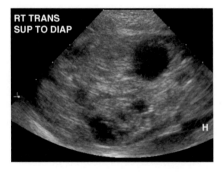

Fig. 16. Anterior mediastinal teratoma. Transverse sonogram at the level of the heart (H) in a newborn shows the complex solid and cystic mass displacing heart.

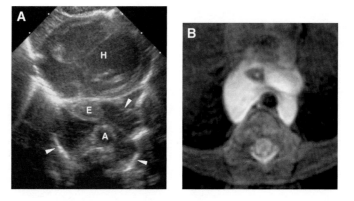

Fig. 17. Mediastinal lymphangioma. (*A*) Transverse sonogram using the heart as an acoustic window in a child with abnormal paraspinal widening on chest radiography shows a septated cystic mass (*arrowheads*) posterior to the heart (H) surrounding the aorta (A) and esophagus (E). (*B*) Transverse T2-weighted MR imaging at a similar level with the same findings.

tion may, however, be difficult. Pericardial cysts have a typical appearance on radiographs, but US can confirm their cystic nature. Lymphangiomas in the mediastinum appear similar to that elsewhere in the body (Fig. 17).

Posterior mediastinal cystic masses include lymphangiomas and neurenteric cysts, the latter often associated with vertebral body anomalies. Most pediatric posterior mediastinal masses are solid, however, and arise from neural crest cells within the sympathetic ganglion. In order of decreasing malignancy these include neuroblastoma, ganglioneuroblastoma, and ganglioneuroma. Posterior mediastinal masses can often be visualized by a posterior thoracic or subxyphoid approach. Although sometimes containing calcifications, the sonographic appearance of these tumors is nonspecific. Thoracic neuroblastomas commonly extend through neural foramina causing extradural compression of the spinal cord that may be symptomatic, and is demonstrable sonographically. US can also demonstrate neoplastic invasion of the chest wall and bony involvement, although CT and MR imaging are more commonly used.

Diaphragm

US is a valuable tool in assessing the diaphragm, allowing delineation of juxtadiaphragmatic masses, contour abnormalities and hernias, and evaluation of diaphragmatic motion [5,9,12,53,54]. Congenital diaphragmatic hernias are typically located on the left, and pose little diagnostic dilemma on plain radiographs. Sometimes radiographic findings are less clear, however, especially with right-sided hernias, and US becomes a useful modality. Sagittal and

coronal scanning using the liver and spleen as acoustic windows allows depiction of the diaphragm and assessment of its integrity. Discontinuity of the diaphragm is readily seen, and the herniated viscera evaluated (Fig. 18). Eventration of the diaphragm results from a congenital weakness or thinness of the central tendon or muscle [39]. Patients may present with respiratory difficulties, but the radiographic findings are often incidental. Although further imaging may not be required, ultrasound can confirm the diagnosis by demonstrating an intact hemidiaphragm, helping to exclude contained hernias or masses.

Elevation of a hemidiaphragm after surgery raises the question of diaphragmatic paralysis. US provides a portable method for evaluating diaphragmatic motion without the use of radiation. Sagittal or coronal imaging provides information on that particular diaphragm, whereas transverse imaging allows comparison of both hemidiaphragms and evaluation for paradoxical motion with unilateral paralysis [12]. With M-mode recording, US and can provide quantitative information about diaphragmatic excursion [53].

Chest wall

Abnormalities of the pediatric chest wall are particularly amenable to high-resolution sonography. Nonpainful soft tissue masses are usually benign, and sonography often provides a definitive diagnosis. Cystic and vascular masses are more often benign than solid masses [39]. US accurately assess the extent and depth of lesions, important if surgical resection is considered. Doppler evaluation can help characterize the type of vascular malformation, which

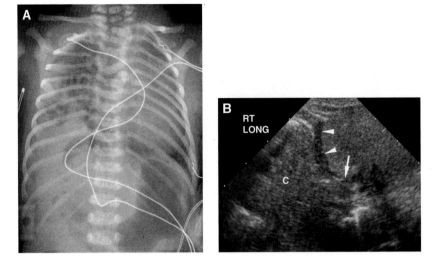

Fig. 18. Right-sided congenital diaphragmatic hernia. (*A*) Frontal chest radiograph in an infant with respiratory distress and right lower chest opacity of unclear etiology. (*B*) Sagittal sonogram through the inferior right chest shows a defect (*arrow*) in the muscular right hemidiaphragm (*arrowheads*) with herniation of abdominal contents into the chest (C).

can be useful in determining an efficacious treatment [55,56]. Common benign chest wall masses include vascular malformations, lymphangiomas, lipomas, and lymph nodes.

Hemangiomas and other vascular lesions usually have discoloration of the overlying skin, providing the first clue to diagnosis. On gray-scale imaging hemangiomas are variably echogenic depending on the amount of fatty stroma, and are typically well circumscribed. Hemangiomas usually have high Doppler frequency shifts and high color Doppler vessel density, whereas other vascular malformations do not [55]. Lymphangiomas have variably sized cystic components whose echogenicity depends on whether there has been infection or hemorrhage into the normally anechoic cyst fluid. They may be found anywhere in the chest, but are most common in the axilla. Extension and infiltration into the mediastinum is common and may necessitate other imaging, such as MR imaging, for complete evaluation. Treatment may be surgical excision, although less invasive percutaneous sclerotherapy shows great promise. Lipomas are generally well-circumscribed masses usually located within the subcutaneous tissues, typically echogenic because of their fat content [39]. Color Doppler flow to lipomas is minimal. Lymph nodes are usually recognizable by their echogenic fatty hila containing the central nodal blood supply, although inflamed and infiltrated nodes may have distorted internal architecture and color Doppler flow.

Firm, nontender masses may be secondary to bony or cartilaginous anomalies [13,57]. Bony ab-

normalities are often detectable by radiography, but US can clarify and confirm findings. Anomalous rib ends can be diagnosed, and osteochondromas and their cartilaginous components assessed and followed. Anterior chest wall irregularities are often caused by asymmetric cartilaginous costochondral junctions [57], readily visible sonographically. Traumatic separation of the costochondral cartilage from rib ends has been reported in child abuse [58], a finding visible sonographically but not with radiographs. Rib fractures are common after trauma, but radiographic detection may be difficult if there is little fragment displacement. Sonography easily shows the disruption of the cortical surface of the rib, and there may be an adjacent hematoma or callous formation depending on the age of the injury (Fig. 19)

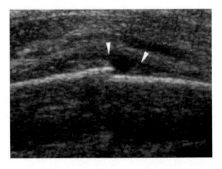

Fig. 19. Rib fracture. Longitudinal sonogram along a painful rib after a football injury shows cortical discontinuity and a small associated hematoma (*arrowheads*) of a radiographically occult rib fracture.

[12,59,60]. Sternal fractures are also readily detected with US [60,61].

Malignant chest wall lesions are uncommon in children, but include Askin's tumor and rhabdomyosarcoma. Echogenicity is variable, and lesion margins may be distinct or infiltrative; color Doppler flow is usually increased [39]. Chest wall and rib invasion can be detected as interruption of the normal muscular layers of the chest wall and loss of the normally smooth bony cortical surface [12]. As with most other imaging, US is not histologically specific, and some benign lesions (eg, abscesses and hematomas) may have aggressive sonographic appearances [39]. Tissue sampling (often by US-guided biopsy) is usually needed for diagnosis.

Vessels

Advances in contrast MR imaging and CT angiography allow beautiful depiction of the thoracic vasculature. Deep structures, such as the superior vena cava and thoracic aorta, are difficult to evaluate sonographically in the older pediatric patient, but US still remains a principle method of investigation of vascular disease particularly within the subclavian and brachiocephalic vessels. The most common indication for vascular US is the evaluation of suspected venous thrombosis [62]. Acute thrombosis often occurs in association with an indwelling vascular catheter, and appears as hypoechoic material expanding the vessel lumen. Because compression of the thoracic veins is not possible, color and pulsed Doppler are important in confirming thrombosis. Depending on patient size and anatomy, it may be difficult directly to interrogate medial portions of the subclavian and brachiocephalic veins, and one may have to rely on indirect Doppler findings of venous stenosis or occlusion. Having no valves, the central thoracic veins show the effects of cardiac and respiratory activity, with marked phasicity and even reversal of flow with atrial systole [63]. With central venous occlusion or stenosis, this phasicity is lost or dampened, and interrogation of more lateral segments of the subclavian vein can indicate a more central problem (Fig. 20) [64,65]. Investigation of both sides is often helpful in uncovering subtle flow differences that may indicate abnormalities [63]. With chronic occlusion, collaterals may become quite large and give the appearance of normal native vessels. Doppler flow seldom appears normal, however, and typically is dampened and more monophasic in collateral vessels [65].

Arterial stenoses and aneurysms may occur from vascular access misadventures or from one of the arteritides. Inadvertent arterial puncture during line placement can lead to vessel injury or rarely arteriovenous fistula formation. Doppler can detect the abnormal high diastolic arterial flow in arteriovenous fistulas and the elevated and turbulent venous flow.

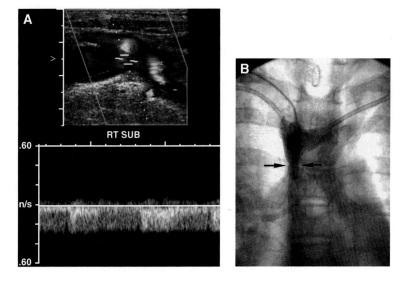

Fig. 20. Superior vena cava stenosis. (*A*) Duplex Doppler sonogram of the medial right subclavian vein in a sickle-cell patient with bilateral central venous ports and intermittent upper body swelling shows a patent vessel with loss of normal transmitted cardiac pulsations. (*B*) Venogram shows stenosis of the superior vena cava at the level of the central lines (*arrows*) with poor distal flow. The stenosis was successfully treated with angioplasty and the symptoms resolved.

Thoracic arterial stenoses, like those elsewhere in the body, are detectable by elevation of peak systolic flow, and delayed systolic upstroke and elevated flow in diastole if very severe.

Thoracic outlet syndrome produces neurologic or vascular symptoms from compression of neurovascular structures in the upper chest. Anomalous cervical or first thoracic ribs, the anterior scalene muscle, and vascular variants may all contribute. Duplex US provides important anatomic and physiologic information by demonstrating alterations in arterial or venous flow, especially during reproduction of the position in which symptoms occur. Arterial flow may show acceleration or dampening of flow, depending how close one is to the stenotic segment [66]. Venous flow is similarly affected, and there may be engorgement of the lateral subclavian and axillary veins and loss of transmitted cardiac waveforms [63,67]. Thrombosis may complicate repetitive venous compression (Paget-Schroetter syndrome), which should be readily diagnosable by US.

Summary

Many pediatric thoracic diseases are adequately evaluated with plain radiographs, but further imaging is often required. The beautiful images provided by current CT and MR imaging techniques are aesthetically seductive, but it should be remembered that US often provides the clinically needed information at lesser cost, without sedation or radiation exposure. If US cannot provide all the required information in a given case, it may help direct which additional imaging modality is most definitive or clinically relevant [11,54,68]. Tissue sampling or fluid drainage is often best performed under US guidance, speeding diagnosis and recovery. US of the pediatric chest does require more physician involvement than other modalities to maximize its yield, but even a small amount of effort can prove very rewarding.

References

[1] Stein S, Cox J, Hernanz-Schulma M, et al. Pediatric chest disease: evaluation by computerized tomography, magnetic resonance imaging, and ultrasonography. South Med J 1992;85:735–42.

[2] Rosenberg H. The complementary roles of ultrasound and plain film radiography in differentiating pediatric chest abnormalities. Radiographics 1986;6:427–45.

[3] Ben-Ami T, O'Donovan J, Yousefzadeh D. Sonog-

raphy of the chest in children. Radiol Clin North Am 1993;31:517–31.

[4] Kim O, Kim W, Min J, et al. US in the diagnosis of pediatric chest disease. Radiographics 2000;20: 653–71.

[5] Haller J, Schneider M, Kassner E, et al. Sonographic evaluation of the chest in infants and children. AJR Am J Roentgenol 1980;134:1019–27.

[6] Koh D, Burke S, Davies N, et al. Transthoracic US of the chest: clinical uses and applications. Radiographics 2002;22:1e. Available at: http://radiographics. rsnajnls.org/cgi/collection/ultrasound?page=3.

[7] Krejci C, Trent E, Dubinsky T. Thoracic sonography. Respir Care 2001;46:932–9.

[8] Mathis G. Thoraxsonography - Part II: peripheral pulmonary consolidation. Ultrasound Med Biol 1997; 23:1141–53.

[9] Baron R, Lee J, Melson G. Sonographic evaluation of right juxtadiaphragmatic masses in children using transhepatic approach. J Clin Ultrasound 1980;8: 156–9.

[10] Acunas B, Celik L, Acunas A. Chest sonography: differentiation of pulmonary consolidation from pleural disease. Acta Radiol 1989;30:273–5.

[11] Glasier C, Leithiser R, Williamson S, et al. Extracardiac chest ultrasonography in infants and children: radiographic and clinical implications. J Pediatr 1989; 114:540–4.

[12] Sistrom C, Wallace K, Gay S. Thoracic sonography for diagnosis and intervention. Curr Probl Diagn Radiol 1997;26:2–49.

[13] Donnelly L, Taylor C, Emery K, et al. Asymptomatic, palpable, anterior chest wall lesions in children: is cross-sectional imaging necessary? Radiology 1997; 202:829–31.

[14] Han B, Yoon H, Suh Y. Thymic ultrasound: II. Diagnosis of aberrant cervical thymus. Pediatr Radiol 2001;31:480–7.

[15] Han B, Suh Y, Yoon H. Thymic ultrasound: I. Intrathymic anatomy in infants. Pediatr Radiol 2001;31: 474–9.

[16] Targhetta R, Chavagneux R, Bourgeois J, et al. Sonographic approach to diagnosing pulmonary consolidation. J Ultrasound Med 1992;11:667–72.

[17] Kocijancic I, Vidmar K, Ivanovi-Herceg Z. Chest sonography versus lateral decubitus radiography in the diagnosis of small pleural effusions. J Clin Ultrasound 2003;31:69–74.

[18] Yang P, Luh K, Chang D, et al. Value of sonography in determining the nature of pleural effusion: analysis of 320 cases. AJR Am J Roentgenol 1992;159:29–33.

[19] Wu R, Yang P, Kuo S, et al. Fluid color sign: a useful indicator for discrimination between pleural thickening and pleural effusion. J Ultrasound Med 1995;14:767–9.

[20] Yang P. Applications of colour Doppler ultrasound in the diagnosis of chest diseases. Respirology 1997;2: 231–8.

[21] Lin F, Chou C, Chang S. Usefulness of the suspended

microbubble sign in differentiating empyemic and nonempyemic hydropneumothorax. J Ultrasound Med 2001;20:1341–5.

[22] Lichtenstein D, Hulot J, Rabiller A, et al. Feasibility and safety of ultrasound-aided thoracentesis in mechanically ventilated patients. Intensive Care Med 1999;25:955–8.

[23] Coley B. Ultrasound-guided interventional procedures. In: Siegel M, editor. Pediatric sonography. 3rd edition. Philadelphia: Lippincott Williams & Wilkins; 2002. p. 699–725.

[24] Raptopoulos V, Davis L, Lee G, et al. Factors affecting the development of pneumothorax associated with thoracentesis. AJR Am J Roentgenol 1991;156:917–20.

[25] Grogan D, Irwin R, Channick R, et al. Complications associated with thoracentesis: a prospective, randomized study comparing three different methods. Arch Intern Med 1990;150:873–7.

[26] Mitri R, Brown S, Zurakowski D, et al. Outcomes of primary image-guided drainage of parapneumonic effusions in children. Pediatrics 2002;110:37–42.

[27] Feola G, Shaw L, Coburn L. Management of complicated parapneumonic effusions in children. Tech Vasc Interv Radiol 2003;6:197–204.

[28] Wells R, Havens P. Intrapleural fibrinolysis for parapneumonic effusion and empyema in children. Radiology 2003;228:370–8.

[29] Chen K, Liaw Y, Wang H, et al. Sonographic septation: a useful prognostic indicator of acute thoracic empyema. J Ultrasound Med 2000;19:837–43.

[30] Chandrasekhar A, Reynes C, Churchill R. Ultrasonically guided percutaneous biopsy of peripheral pulmonary masses. Chest 1976;70:627–30.

[31] Sheth S, Hamper U, Stanley D, et al. US guidance for thoracic biopsy: a valuable alternative to CT. Radiographics 1999;210:721–6.

[32] McGahan J, Richards J, Fogata M. Emergency ultrasound in trauma patients. Radiol Clin North Am 2004;42:417–25.

[33] Lichtenstein D, Meziere G, Biderman P, et al. The "lung point": an ultrasound sign specific to pneumothorax. Intensive Care Med 2000;26:1434–40.

[34] Dulchavsky S, Schwarz K, Kirkpatrick A, et al. Prospective evaluation of thoracic ultrasound in the detection of pneumothorax. J Trauma 2001;50:201–5.

[35] Rowan K, Kirkpatrick A, Liu D, et al. Traumatic pneumothorax detection with thoracic US: correlation with chest radiography and CT—initial experience. Radiology 2002;225:210–4.

[36] Targhetta R, Bourgeois J, Chavagneux R, et al. Ultrasonographic approach to diagnosing hydropneumothorax. Chest 1992;101:931–4.

[37] Weinberg B, Diakoumakis E, Kass E, et al. The air bronchogram: sonographic demonstration. AJR Am J Roentgenol 1986;147:593–5.

[38] Yang P, Luh K, Lee Y. Lung abscesses: ultrasonography and ultrasound-guided transthoracic aspiration. Radiology 1991;180:171–5.

[39] Siegel M. Chest. In: Siegel M, editor. Pediatric sonography. 3rd edition. Philadelphia: Lippincott Williams & Wilkins; 2002. p. 167–211.

[40] Dhingsa R, Coakley F, Albanese C, et al. Prenatal sonography and MR imaging of pulmonary sequestration. AJR Am J Roentgenol 2003;180:433–7.

[41] Khosa J, Leong S, Borzi P. Congenital cystic adenomatoid malformation of the lung: indications and timing of surgery. Pediatr Surg Int 2004;20:505–8.

[42] Hang J, Guo Q, Chen C, et al. Imaging approach to the diagnosis of pulmonary sequestration. Acta Radiol 1996;37:883–8.

[43] Schlesinger A, DiPietro M, Statter M, et al. Utility of sonography in the diagnosis of bronchopulmonary sequestration. J Pediatr Surg 1994;29:52–5.

[44] Lim J, Lee K, Kim T, et al. Ring-down artifacts posterior to the right hemidiaphragm on abdominal sonography: sign of pulmonary parenchymal abnormalities. J Ultrasound Med 1999;18:403–10.

[45] Reissig A, Kroegel C. Transthoracic sonography of diffuse parenchymal lung disease: the role of comet tail artifacts. J Ultrasound Med 2003;22:173–80.

[46] Avni E, Braude P, Pardou A, et al. Hyaline membrane disease in the newborn: diagnosis by US. Pediatr Radiol 1990;20:143–6.

[47] Avni E, Cassart M, de Maertelaer V, et al. Sonographic prediction of chronic lung disease in the premature undergoing mechanical ventilation. Pediatr Radiol 1996;26:463–9.

[48] Pieper C, Smith J, Brand E. The value of ultrasound examination of the lungs in predicting bronchopulmonary dysplasia. Pediatr Radiol 2004;34:227–31.

[49] Sakai F, Sone S, Kawai T, et al. Ultrasonography of thymoma with pathologic correlation. Acta Radiol 1994;35:25–9.

[50] Kontny H, Sleasman J, Kingma D, et al. Multilocular thymic cysts in children with human immunodeficiency virus infection: clinical and pathologic aspects. J Pediatr 1997;131:264–70.

[51] Leonidas J, Berdon W, Valderrama E, et al. Human immunodeficiency virus infection and multilocular thymic cysts. Radiology 1996;198:377–9.

[52] Wu T, Wang H, Chang Y, et al. Mature mediastinal teratoma: sonographic imaging patterns and pathologic correlation. J Ultrasound Med 2002;21:759–65.

[53] Gerscovich E, Cronan M, McGahan J, et al. Ultrasonographic evaluation of diaphragmatic motion. J Ultrasound Med 2001;20:597–604.

[54] Riccabona M. Thoraxsonographie im neugeborenen: und kindesalter. Radiologe 2003;43:1075–89.

[55] Dubois J, Patriquin H, Garel L, et al. Soft-tissue hemangiomas in infants and children: diagnosis using color Doppler sonography. AJR Am J Roentgenol 1998;171:247–52.

[56] Dubois J, Garel L, David M, et al. Vascular soft-tissue tumors in infancy: distinguishing features on Doppler sonography. AJR Am J Roentgenol 2002;178:1541–5.

[57] Donnelly L, Frush D. Abnormalities of the chest

wall in pediatric patients. AJR Am J Roentgenol 1999;173:1595–601.

[58] Smeets A, Robben S, Meradji M. Sonographically detected costo-chondral dislocation in an abused child: a new sonographic sign to the radiological spectrum of child abuse. Pediatr Radiol 1990;20:566–7.

[59] Mathis G. Thoraxsonography - Part I: chest wall and pleura. Ultrasound Med Biol 1997;23:1131–9.

[60] Bitschnau R, Gehmacher O, Kopf A, et al. Ultrasound in the diagnosis of rib and sternal fracture. Ultraschall Med 1997;18:158–61.

[61] Fenkl R, Carrel T, Knaipler H. Diagnosis of sternal fractures with ultrasound. Unfallchirurg 1992;95:375–9.

[62] Babcock D. Sonographic evaluation of suspected pediatric vascular diseases. Pediatr Radiol 1991;21:486–9.

[63] Beidle T, Letourneau J. Arm swelling. In: Bluth E, Arger P, Benson C, et al, editors. Ultrasound: a practical approach to clinical problems. New York: Thieme; 2000. p. 566–82.

[64] Patel M, Berman L, Moss H, et al. Subclavian and internal jugular veins at Doppler US: abnormal cardiac pulsatility and respiratory phasicity as a predictor of complete occlusion. Radiology 1999;211:579–83.

[65] Nazarian G, Foshager M. Color Doppler sonography of the thoracic inlet veins. Radiographics 1995;15:1357–71.

[66] Rose S. Noninvasive vascular laboratory for evaluation of peripheral arterial occlusive disease. Part III. Clinical applications: nonatherosclerotic lower extremity arterial conditions and upper extremity arterial disease. J Vasc Interv Radiol 1991;12:11–8.

[67] Longley D, Yedlicka J, Molina E, et al. Thoracic outlet syndrome: evaluation of the subclavian vessels by color duplex sonography. AJR Am J Roentgenol 1992;158:623–30.

[68] Durand C, Garel C, Nugues F, et al. L'echographie dans la pathologie thoracique de l'enfant. J Radiol 2001;82:729–37.

ELSEVIER
SAUNDERS

Radiol Clin N Am 43 (2005) 419–433

RADIOLOGIC
CLINICS
of North America

Technique of Pediatric Thoracic CT Angiography

Donald P. Frush, MD

Division of Pediatric Radiology, Department of Radiology, Duke University Health System,
1905 McGovern-Davison Children's Health Center, Box 3808, Erwin Road, Durham, NC 27710, USA

One of the principle applications derived from the evolution of multidetector row CT (MDCT), initially seen with 16-slice and currently up to 64-slice CT, is CT angiography. The ease, safety, and quality of the examinations compared with traditional angiography were quickly recognized, and the value of CT angiography firmly established. For a variety of reasons, the earliest MDCT angiography with single-slice technology was problematic for the pediatric population [1–4]. Some of these problems included breathing artifact in children who could not hold their breath, small volumes of contrast material, relatively slow and inconsistent rates of injection, and small cardiovascular structures [4]. Although these same issues currently exist with pediatric CT angiography, much faster scanning and isotropic display with submillimeter image thickness have, to a large extent, minimized the impact of these factors. Nevertheless, it is still important to understand the special considerations with pediatric CT angiography [5]. In trying to make a potentially complex technique relatively simple and practical, the following material is divided into two parts: study preparation and study performance. The format is essentially step-by-step (Box 1), with the supporting technical information either cited or included in tables. Despite the fact this material somewhat betrays the traditional academic format, a greater benefit is served: excellent CT angiography is possible in even the most problematic of pediatric cases.

E-mail address: frush943@mc.duke.edu

Planning the pediatric CT angiogram

Determine that CT angiography is the appropriate examination

In addition to CT angiography, considerations for thoracic cardiovascular structural and functional assessment include echocardiography, MR angiography and venography, and conventional angiography. CT angiography is advantageous in that it provides a more global assessment of cardiovascular structures and adjacent structures, such as the lung and airway. The examination is also relatively quick to perform, with times that can approach 1 second given 64-slice technology. Sedation is rarely necessary compared with MR imaging and echocardiography, and the examination quality is more consistent (operator independent). CT angiography is a relatively non-invasive procedure, compared with angiography. In addition, monitoring and direct observation of the patient are easier with CT angiography than with MR imaging. Contraindications for MR imaging vascular assessment including pacemakers and recent surgical procedures with some metallic materials are not present with CT angiography. Moreover, metal artifact is much less an issue with CT angiography than with MR angiography. For a more in-depth discussion of the relative merits and disadvantages with CT angiography and MR angiography, the reader is referred to a recent series of reviews [5–8].

There are disadvantages with CT angiography. CT angiography requires administration of intravenous (IV) contrast media. Adverse reactions, however, are singularly unusual in children. In addition, nephrotoxicity from contrast media in children is much less

Box 1. Example of step-by-step method for performing pediatric CT angiography

History: otherwise healthy 4-week-old boy with congenital stridor and echocardiogram suggesting a vascular ring.

Planning the CT angiogram

- Determine that CT angiography is the appropriate examination: echocardiography was inconclusive; MR imaging requires sedation. CT angiography 1-day turnaround. MR imaging study a 2- to 3-week wait for sedation slot.
- Define question to be answered: aortic arch and airway. High detail examination (eg, small vessels) not necessary. There is no need to image below the mid to lower thoracic aorta (decreases the radiation dose).
- Understand the anatomy: aortic rings, including inominate compression; pulmonary sling does not present with true stridor.
- Patient limitations: essentially none. Will feed immediately before CT angiography but after intravenous line is in place.

Performing the CT angiogram

Intravenous contrast material
- Type: nonionic, 300 mgI/mL
- Dose: total volume of 6 mL (4 kg × 1.5 mL/kg)
- Rate and route: 24-gauge angiocatheter in hand vein. Manual administration as fast as possible.
- Onset of scanning: determined with test bolus of 0.6 mL of 300 mgI/mL in TB syringe. Short extension tubing. Start monitoring images at 2-second intervals and begin push of test bolus when first monitoring image appears. Contrast reaches right ventricle in 5 seconds and left in 6 to 7 seconds. Six-scan delay selected for examination.

Select scan parameters
- 16-detector row
- FOV: small. Note $CTDI_{vol}$ 1.65 mGy and DLP 10.59 mGy·cm for small FOV. Large FOV reads $CTDI_{vol}$ 0.71 mGy and DLP 4.54 mGy·cm (less than half of small FOV), more appropriate dose estimates for a large patient.
- Detector thickness: 16 × 0.625, anticipating multiplanar and three-dimensional reconstruction especially for airway depiction (were not necessary in the end)
- Slice thickness and interval for axial review: 2.5 mm at 2.5-mm reconstruction interval
- Milliampere: 60
- Kilovolt (peak): 80
- Gantry cycle time: 0.5 seconds (30 mAs)
- Pitch: 1.375

Abbreviations: CTDI, CT dose index; DLP, dose length product; FOV, field of view.

an issue than it is with adults. The radiation dose from CT angiography and angiography should be considered [9]. CT angiographic techniques can be used that reduce the amount of radiation (see later). Nevertheless, whenever echocardiography or MR imaging provide the same information with similar or less risk (eg, without sedation; see Box 1), these modalities should be the first considerations. Obviously, when physiologic parameters, such as chamber pressures, gradients, or oxygen saturation, are requisite, then conventional angiography should be the initial consideration. Compared with echocardiography, CT is not portable. In addition, real-time information afforded by echocardiography is lacking with CT angiography.

Define the questions to be answered

Before performing pediatric thoracic CT angiography, the radiologist must be familiar with the questions that need to be addressed [5]. Direct communication with a referring service or clinician is optimal. This allows the examination to be designed to provide the highest yield. For example, identification of the status of pulmonary veins requires slightly different technique than assessing for an aortic arch abnormality, particularly in the smallest children. This approach implies that CT angiography in children is less protocol driven than in adult CT angiography.

Understand the anatomy

This is a critical point in designing the study. This is necessary both for optimizing diagnostic information and the safety of the child. With respect to this latter point, certain admixture lesions or right-to-left shunts are at risk for embolization with improper flushing of the catheter or injection of contrast media. That is, thrombus or air, which is not usually much of an issue with normal anatomy, can potentially have devastating complications. With respect to optimizing the examination, one must also understand the patient's cardiovascular anatomy, and the anticipated course of the contrast material. For example, with a traditional Glenn anastomosis (superior vena cava-to-right pulmonary artery), contrast only goes into the right pulmonary artery. This is not the case with a bidirectional Glenn anastomosis (superior vena cava-to-confluent pulmonary arteries). Alternatively, blood supply to a lung may be through a systemic artery to pulmonary artery anastomosis, such as with a Blalock-Taussig shunt (subclavian artery-to-pulmonary artery). In this situation, contrast first enters the systemic ventricle, aorta, and then the pulmonary artery providing slightly later than expected enhancement of the pulmonary arteries. It also may not be possible to opacify both pulmonary arteries at the same phase with a single contrast injection. For example, if the right pulmonary is connected to the superior vena cava and the left pulmonary artery to the inferior vena cava, a single upper torso injection does not provide an angiographic level of enhancement of both pulmonary arteries. In this case, depending on the clinical situation, an upper torso vein can be injected. An initial angiographic phase can be performed with a subsequent delayed (eg, portal venous phase), which potentially demonstrates the inferior vena cava-to-left pulmonary artery anastomosis, although this is not an angiographic phase.

One must also know of the location of any metal with respect to the question asked. Streak artifact off a clip may obscure a stenosis of a vessel. Stents, septal occluder devices, coils, valves, and conduits and pacing wires can also cause artifacts.

Be familiar with patient limitations

Sedation should only be rarely needed but should be anticipated [10,11]. At this time, in my practice sedation is usually limited to children between 1 and 2 years of age. The optimal CT angiographic examination is a breathhold examination. This usually only requires a 2- to 15-second breathhold (for a 16-slice scan). It is likely with 64-slice technology that subsecond CT angiography may be performed in small children, minimizing misregistration even in a breathing child. Certainly, with this faster technology, even very limited cooperation may be all that is necessary. In a child who is intubated, generally a brief pause, designing the examination for the shortest scan time, is adequate. Although various arguments can be made about whether an inspiration or expiration is optimal, I have not found that, physiologically, this has made any detectable or clinically important difference in terms of opacification and I opt for peak inspiratory hold to maximize lung parenchyma evaluation.

Performing the pediatric CT angiogram

Intravenous contrast material administration

Issues with IV contrast material administration include the type, dose, and rate of administration; route and technique of injection; and onset of diagnostic examination. The following discussion of pediatric thoracic CT angiographic technique is based on my experience with General Electric scanners. Although some of the technical factors reflect this use, minor adjustments can be made that provide techniques suited for other scanner types.

Type of contrast media

Low or isomolar contrast media is recommended for pediatric CT angiography [12]. Generally, I perform examinations with a concentration of 300 mgI/mL. An exception to this is when small test boluses are to be used or the rare circumstance when volume restriction is critically important. In these cases, a concentration of 370 mgI/mL is used and reduced doses (<1.5 mL/kg) used.

Dose of contrast media

For adult-sized children, maximum dose is 120 mL. For smaller children, a dose of 1.5 mL/kg is used for pediatric thoracic CT angiography. Empirically, this dose has provided excellent enhancement. In addition, with larger doses and 16-slice technology, the examination was often completed before a dose larger than 1.5 mL/kg was administered. For aortic evaluation, such as for rings, a smaller dose of 1 mL/kg can be considered if the rate of administration is high (>2 mL/s) and the larger detector row (16–64) scanners are used. One of the benefits of 1.5 mL/kg dose is that in the event of a missed bolus or some other need for additional contrast administration (ie, opacification of an independent circuit, such as the inferior vena cava to the left pulmonary artery), a second dose of up to 1.5 mL/kg can be used. This is certainly lower than the recommended limits for routine angiography of 5 to 6 mL/kg [5].

Rate of administration

Rates of administration through various angiocatheters can be found in Table 1. For most children under about 12 years of age, 2 mL/s is an acceptable rate. Certainly, if a larger-gauge angiocatheter (eg, 20 gauge) in a relatively large 10- or 11-year-old child is available, then rates of 3 to 4 mL/kg are an option. It should be remembered that these faster rates of administration can result in a more unpleasant and frightening experience for the child. If a child is somewhat tenuously cooperative, this may effect breathholding or cause movement, which affects image quality.

Route and technique of administration

The route of administration can be either through a peripheral angiocatheter or central venous catheter. Peripherally inserted central venous catheters do not afford sufficient rates of injection to be useful for pediatric CT angiography. In addition, I do not use butterfly needles because of the potential for vessel or other soft tissue injury with movement and the lack of sufficient access should additional IV administration be necessary. Injection can be either by manual (hand) or power injection. Power injection is always preferred given the consistency of contrast flow. Adequate CT angiography can be performed, however, with manual administration. In this institution, manual administration is reserved for angiocatheters that are in hand or feet, or which have tenuous or absent blood return. I also use manual injection with central venous catheters, although data support that

Table 1
Angiocatheter size and suggested rates of administration for pediatric CT angiography

Catheter gauge	Administration rate (mL/s)
24	1.5
22	2.0–2.5
20	3.0–4.0
18	4.0–5.0

Data from Frush DP, Herlong JR. Pediatric thoracic CT angiography. Pediatr Radiol 2004;35(1):11–25.

these can be used safely with power injection [13]. The rate with manual administration should be as fast as possible. I found that this ends up being about, on the average, about 1.5 mL/s [14].

One critical issue with IV contrast administration for pediatric CT angiography is ensuring that the total dose actually gets injected into the vein. This is problematic with small infants, such as those weighing under about 5 kg. With long extension tubing, if the tubing to the angiocatheter is not primed with contrast, a substantial portion of contrast may be left within the tubing and not available for vascular enhancement. For example, for a 3-kg infant, receiving 4.5 mL of contrast (1.5 mL/kg × 3 kg) a 1- to 2-mL connecting tubing dead space can result in a substantial portion of contrast remaining in the tubing at the end of injection and potentially insufficient vascular enhancement. Also, it is important to know the location of the angiocatheter. For example, IV injection of contrast media into a central venous catheter with the tip in the right atrium results in a much shorter time for contrast to enter the pulmonary arteries than with an angiocatheter that is in the foot. The nuances of onset of the timing of scanning are discussed in greater detail next.

Onset of diagnostic scanning

In general, there are three techniques that can be used to start diagnostic scanning for pediatric CT angiography: (1) an empiric delay, (2) bolus tracking to start the scan, and (3) a test bolus. It is important to realize that there are a number of complex factors that effect the arrival of contrast at the optimal location. The location of the catheter, injection rate (which is unknown with manual injection), cardiac output, anatomy of the lesion to be assessed, and other unknown factors conspire to make the timing of scan onset a potentially complex issue in children [4]. With small volumes of administration (ie, 5 mL or less) there is not, as with adults, a sustained or prolonged of period of enhancement [15]. This makes the timing issues in children more important to address.

For empiric delays, the onset of scanning predominantly depends on the structures being assessed and the size of the child. Overall empiric delays are from about 5 to 20 seconds after the onset of injection for younger children. For older children the delay may be longer approaching adult delays, but still should coincide with the final third of the injection duration. This depends on the volume and rate. It makes no sense to finish the examination before all the contrast is administered. For example, for a 40-kg 10-year-old, receiving 60 mL of IV contrast material at 2.5 mL/s, the total duration of injection is

24 seconds. Designing a protocol for which about 7 seconds is required to perform this CT angiography, scanning should start about 16 to 20 seconds after the start of contrast. The shorter delays are used in neonates and the longer delays are for older children and adolescents. A routine delay of about 10 to 15 seconds is generally successful in children for approximately 2 to 10 years of age at a rate of 2 to 4 mL/s. For pulmonary artery evaluation the scan should start slightly earlier than if the pulmonary vein or aorta is the focus of the examination. The difference between these is usually at most a few seconds.

Bolus tracking is a very useful and preferred method for thoracic CT angiography in children [14]. I use SmartPrep (General Electric Healthcare, Milwaukee, WI). With this technology, serial isolevel slices are obtained at a predetermined level and scanning is initiated based on the arrival of contrast at the desired location (Fig. 1). One technical tip that I found useful is to begin the bolus tracking series before the contrast injection starts [16]. This then means that every 1 to 3 seconds, depending on the interval selected, an image appears. The initial image may take longer, however, because of current hardware delays. This duration may be longer than the arrival time of the contrast and the opportunity may be missed to scan at optimal enhancement. For example, in infants it is sometimes just a few seconds from the administration of contrast through a peripheral angiocatheter (remember that the distance between the antecubital vein to the heart in infants is short, a distance more typical of a central venous catheter tip and the heart in adults). By starting the bolus tracking and contrast at the same time, I found early in my experience that the contrast was at least as far as the right side of the heart by the time the first image arrived. In addition, it takes at most a few seconds actually to begin the scanning, including moving the patient to the proper starting position. Together, these delays mean that there may be a 6- or 7-second delay from the desired start of scanning to the actual onset of scanning. Again, with small total volumes of contrast, this may mean missing optimal contrast enhancement of the desired structure. One could, with experience, anticipate this delay and begin scanning slightly earlier than the tracking indicates is ideal.

This scan initiation based on bolus tracking is generally useful for larger children and opacification of major chambers or vessels. In addition, I have not found it useful to measure enhancement (in Hounsfield units) of the vessels or chamber but simply to determine when contrast arrives at the desired location (one or two images where the chamber of vessel of interest is opacified) to start the scan. The trigger, then, is based on visual clues rather than actual metrics.

The third method that I have found very useful in small children with complex anatomy is to use a test bolus (Box 1; Fig. 1). In general, a test bolus of about 10% of the total volume administered is sufficient. This means with a total scan dose of 5 mL/kg, that a 0.5 mL test bolus can be tracked. The technique here is to administer the small test bolus in a small syringe (such as a TB syringe) being sure that, again, the contrast material is not trapped in a dead space. I begin the bolus tracking with appearance of monitoring slices and when the first image appears, the test bolus should be given as fast as possible. I count the number of seconds from the administration of the test bolus to the arrival in the desired location, such as the right ventricle or left ventricle. This, then, serves as the foundation for the delay in the diagnostic scanning. With adult CT angiography, there is a several second delay from the arrival of the test bolus that is added to this time given the dynamics of the enhancement curve of a contrast dose [15]. In children, given the small volumes, no more than one or two seconds added to the arrival of the test bolus is indicated. It should be remembered that an injection of 5 mL total dose given at 2 mL per second only lasts 2.5 seconds.

Selecting the CT scan parameters

The technical considerations when performing pediatric thoracic CT angiography include the number of detector rows; field of view ([FOV] millimeters); detector thickness (millimeters); slice thickness and interval (millimeters); tube current (milliamperes); peak kilovoltage (kVp); gantry cycle rotation time (seconds); and pitch.

Number of detector rows

If possible, the scanner or option with the greatest number of detector rows should be selected. This provides the fastest scan time, minimizing the chance of movement and optimizing scanning during what can be a quite short period of contrast enhancement.

Field of view

The FOV can be selected to provide a higher quality examination based on optimizing beam profiles using specialized filters. On the General Electric 16-slice scanner the small FOV is preferred for young children, and the large FOV for older children and adolescents. A point to remember with this 16-slice scanner is the displays of dose (dose

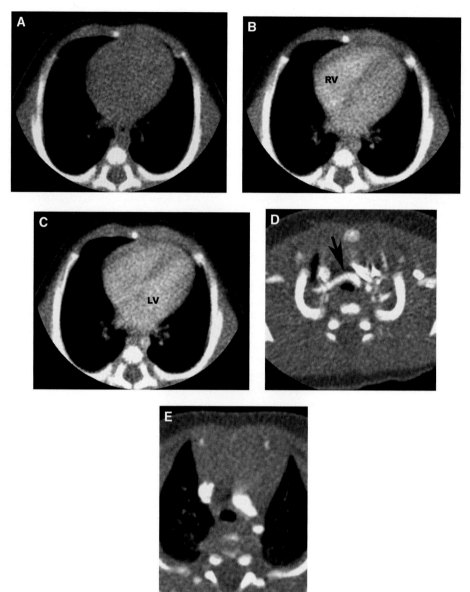

Fig. 1. Technique example for pediatric CT angiography. Four-week-old boy with congenital stridor and echocardiogram suggesting a vascular ring. Serial axial isolevel monitoring images through the mid ventricle level during test bolus demonstrate initial precontrast appearance (*A*), and the arrival of the test bolus in the right ventricle (RV) at 5 seconds (*B*) and the left ventricle (LV) and descending thoracic aorta at 6 to 7 seconds (*C*). (*D*) The trachea is narrowed at the level of the thoracic inlet to about 50% of normal anteroposterior diameter brachiocephalic artery (*arrow*). (*E*) Normal caliber trachea is seen more inferiorly, just above the carina. No aortic abnormality was present.

length product and CT dose index) depend on which of the two FOVs are selected. That is, if a large FOV is selected for an infant, the displayed CT dose index and dose length product values are lower than those if a small FOV is selected, despite the fact that the dose to the patient is the same (Box 1). This may be misleading if these indices are used as a gauge of patient dose. Although this choice may not substantially affect the scan quality, one should recognize that these scanner dose units are dependent on the FOV selected. The display FOV should also be optimized. Using a smaller display increases the pixel density, which is not the same thing as simply magnifying an image obtained on a larger FOV after the scan. If lung detail is not necessary, the FOV can be decreased to cover the central two thirds or so of the chest (Fig. 1). For dedicated cardiovascular CT, it is usually not necessary to include the lateral-most chest wall.

Detector thickness, slice thickness, and interval

Table 2 provides recommended detector and slice thickness, and reconstruction intervals. As a rule, because CT angiography review usually includes three-dimensional or multiplanar reformations, the thinnest detector option, such as 0.625 mm, should be selected to optimize image quality. The image or slice thickness depends on the size of the child and the size of the vessel or structure being evaluated. In general, for diagnostic review, slice thickness of 2.5 to 3.75 mm is usually adequate. It can be helpful with small vessels, such as the coronary arteries or collateral vessels, to review a data set composed of thinner slices (eg, 0.625–1.25 mm). This reconstructed data set should be routinely available when multiplanar reformations and three-dimensional reconstructions are expected. The reconstruction interval depends on the size of the child and the vessel or structure to be assessed. In general, reconstruction intervals of about 2.5 mm are appropriate for diagnostic review. For multiplanar reformations and three-dimensional rendering, a data set reconstructed at a slice thickness

that equals the minimum detector thickness, and at intervals at about half of the detector thickness, provide excellent rendered images. For example, an examination may be done at a 16 × 0.625 mm collimation, with 3.75-mm slice thickness and a 2.5-mm reconstruction interval. Subsequently, coronal, sagittal, and three-dimensional should be rendered from a data set of axial 0.625-mm thick slices at 0.5-mm reconstruction intervals.

Tube current

Tube current recommendations are found in Table 2. Because CT angiography diagnostic image thickness is slightly less than with routine body scanning, the tube current is increased slightly (approximately one third) over that of body imaging. Given the decrease in kilovolt (peak) (see next) afforded by CT angiography, there is still a net reduction in dose for the examination even compared with routine chest CT in children. This is caused by the fact that decreases in kilovolt (peak) result in an exponential decrease in radiation dose, whereas milliampere reduction results in a linear reduction.

Peak kilovoltage

Pediatric CT angiography offers the opportunity to use lower kilovolt (peak) than with routine body imaging at younger ages. This technique has recently found support in routine adult chest CT [17]. Lowering the kilovoltage increases contrast, increases the

Table 2
Pediatric Thoracic CT Angiography Techniques

Weight (lb)	kVp	mAs[a] SDCT	MDCT	Slice thickness (mm)[b]	Pitch: scanner single/4-slice	8-slice	16-slice	Detector thickness (mm)[c] 4- and 8-slice	16-slice	Increment (mm)
10–19	80	70	60	1.25–2.50	1.5	1.35	1.375	1.25	.625	1.0–2.5
20–39	80–100	80	70	1.25–2.50	1.5	1.35	1.375	1.25	.625	1.0–2.5
40–59	100	90	80	1.25–2.50	1.5	1.35–1.68	1.375	1.25	.625	1.0–2.5
60–79	100	120	100	1.25–2.50	1.5	1.35–1.68	1.375	1.25	.625	1.0–2.5
80–99	120	140	120	2.50–3.75	1.5	1.35–1.68	1.375	1.25	.625	1.0–2.5
100–150	120	160–180	140–160	2.50–3.75	1.5	1.35–1.68	1.375	1.25	.625	1.0–2.5
> 150	120	≥ 200	≥ 170	2.50–3.75	1.5	1.35–1.68	1.375	1.25	.625	1.0–2.5

Abbreviation: SDCT, single-detector CT.

[a] mAs slightly higher than body CT protocols. Use 0.5-second rotation time when an option.

[b] Displayed thickness. For coronal and sagittal reformats and three-dimensional reconstructions, reconstruct an axial data set at thickness of the detector (eg, 0.625 mm for 16-slice scanner) at 0.5–1.0-mm intervals. Multiplanar thickness and interval should be similar to axial. For evaluation of larger structures, especially in larger children (eg, aorta) the larger detector configuration (2.5 mm for 8-, and 1.25 mm for a 16-slice scanner) and a larger reconstructed thickness and interval can be used.

[c] For larger children, larger vessels, the highest pitch can be used for MDCT.

Data from Frush DP, Herlong JR. Pediatric thoracic CT angiography. Pediatr Radiol 2004;35(1):11–25.

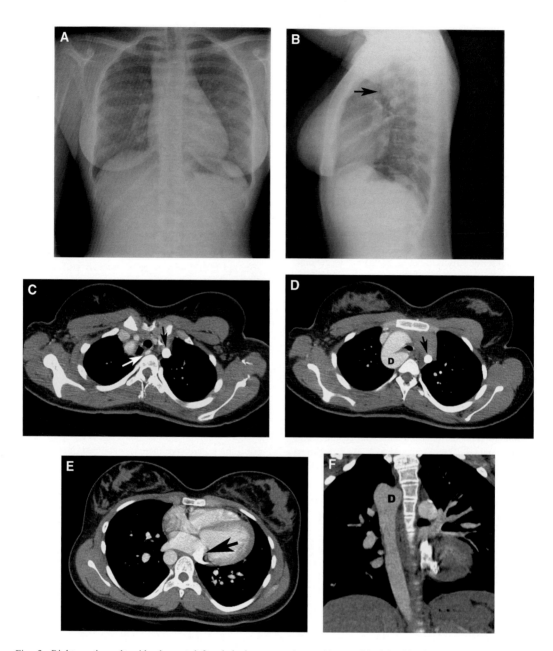

Fig. 2. Right aortic arch with aberrant left subclavian artery in an 11-year-old girl with chronic cough on exertion. (*A*) Posteroanterior chest radiograph shows a right-sided arch. (*B*) Lateral radiograph demonstrates anterior displacement (*arrow*) of the lower trachea. Axial intravenous contrast-enhanced CT angiography at the thoracic inlet shows aberrant course of the left subclavian artery (*white arrow*), associated with an aortic diverticulum (*D*) in Fig. 2D and narrowing of the airway. (*C–E*) Note also a left superior vena cava (*black arrow*), eventually connecting to the coronary sinus. (*F–H*) Coronal reformations also show right-sided arch and descending aorta, diverticulum (*D*), and the aberrant subclavian artery (*arrow*). Note dense enhancement of left superior vena cava in Fig. 2H. Three-dimensional display of trachea in the frontal (*I*) and lateral projections depict the displacement and narrowing best on the lateral views (*J*). (*K*) Volume rendering demonstrates the subclavian artery (*large arrow*) and left superior vena cava (*small arrow*).

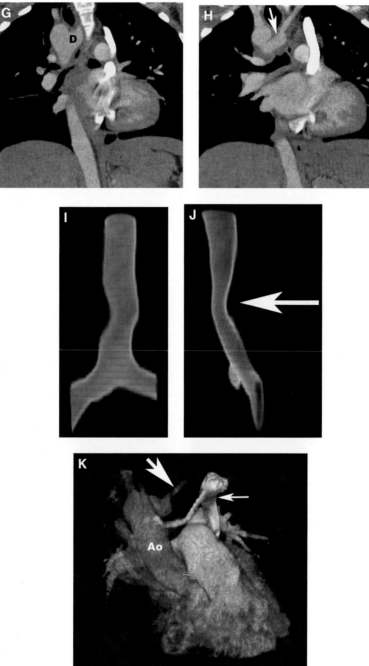

Fig. 2 (*continued*).

image noise, and lowers the radiation dose. Because of relatively high contrast of CT angiography, a lower peak kilovoltage still provides excellent image quality despite somewhat noisier images. That is, more is gained in contrast than in noise, improving the contrast-to-noise ratio. For CT angiography under about 1 year of age, I routinely use 80 kVp (Box 1; Fig. 1). Between 1 and approximately 4 years of age, 100 kVp is sufficient. After that time, 100 to 120 kVp can be used.

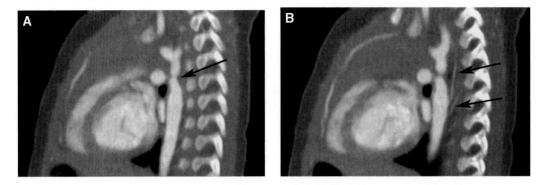

Fig. 3. Coarctation of the aorta in a 4-month-old boy. (*A*) Sagittal reformation demonstrates the location and extent of the narrowing (*arrow*). (*B*) Note large systemic collaterals (*arrows*) arising distal to the coarctation. (*From* Frush DP, Herlong JR. Pediatric thoracic CT angiography. Pediatr Radiol 2004;35(1):11–25; with permission.)

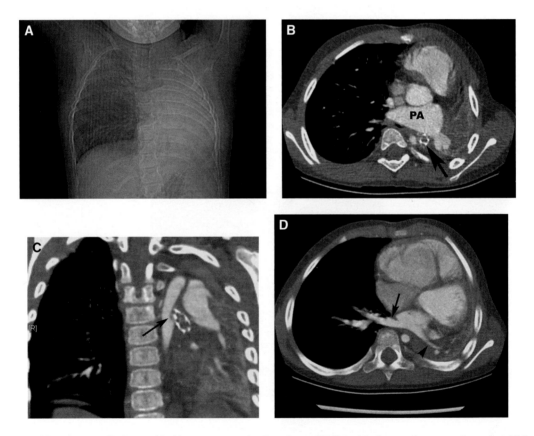

Fig. 4. CT angiogram of a 5-year-old girl status postrepair of tetralogy of Fallot with absent pulmonary valve and multiple procedures to correct left bronchial narrowing. (*A*) Frontal chest radiograph demonstrates left lung collapse and leftward shift of heart and mediastinum. (*B*) Axial image of the level of the enlarged pulmonary artery confluence (PA) demonstrates obliteration of the left bronchial lumen despite the presence of the stent (*arrow*). Note irregularity of the subjacent aorta because of mass effect from the enlarged pulmonary arteries and cardiomegaly (not shown). (*C*) Coronal depiction also demonstrates the effect on the aorta (*arrow*). (*D*) Note asymmetry in size of the inferior pulmonary veins (*arrows*) caused by shunting away from the collapsed left lung.

Gantry cycle time

As with routine body imaging, I always use the fastest gantry cycle time, such as 0.5 seconds. This is especially beneficial when the child has limited breathholding ability or there is some other reason to finish the scan as quickly as possible.

Pitch

Pitch recommendations are found in Table 2. In general, the highest or next to highest pitch options are recommended for CT angiography in children. This depends partly on the size of the vessel and the size of the child.

Applications for pediatric CT angiography

CT angiography should be performed to acquire information that one cannot obtain as well by echocardiography and MR imaging or at as low a risk. Applications of pediatric CT angiography are different from those in adults, and include predominantly evaluation of congenital defects and postoperative status of the great arteries, and other extracardiac structures [18–21].

CT has long been useful for evaluation of aortic abnormalities related to vascular rings (Figs. 1–4). This also applies to contemporary CT angiography. Disorders that are well-depicted by CT angiography include the aortic rings. These consist of right-sided aortic arch with aberrant left subclavian artery, left-sided aortic arch with aberrant subclavian artery, the associated diverticula (Fig. 2), and double aortic arch including atresia of a portion of the double arch [20,22]. Evaluation of aortic arch atresia (or interruption) and coarctation is also a routine application of CT angiography (Fig. 3). Importantly, CT angiography also provides information on the effect on the airway, not available with echocardiography (Figs. 1 and 2). In addition, systemic-to-pulmonary connections, either collateral vessels or postoperative connections (eg, Blalock-Taussig shunts), are readily amenable to CT angiographic evaluation. Assessment

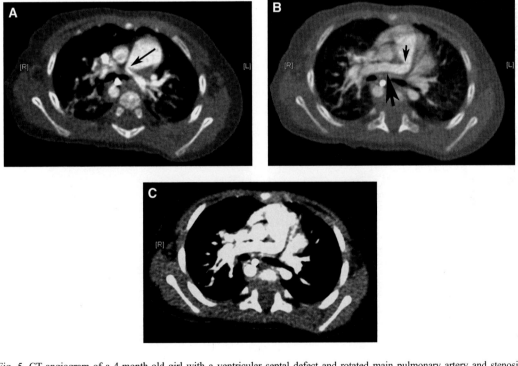

Fig. 5. CT angiogram of a 4-month-old girl with a ventricular septal defect and rotated main pulmonary artery and stenosis associated with a crisscross relationship. (*A*) Axial intravenous contrast-enhanced image at the level of the main pulmonary artery demonstrates marked narrowing of the origin of the left pulmonary artery (*arrow*). Note atypical rightward orientation compared with the right pulmonary artery (*large arrow*) in *B*. (*C*) Different window and level selection (approximate window of 350 and level of 40) obscures mild narrowing (*arrow*) of the right pulmonary artery in Fig. 5B (*small arrow*).

of posttraumatic aortic conditions, including operative complications (Fig. 4), aneurysms (ie, Marfan syndrome), and vasculitis, is also an indication for CT angiography [7].

Pediatric thoracic CT angiography is extremely valuable for pulmonary artery evaluation (Figs. 5–7). Again, echocardiography is usually excellent for intracardiac evaluation but the more distal pulmonary arteries can be difficult to visualize. Evaluation of connections, such as the Glenn or Fontan anastomoses, the patency of stents, presence of and size (including stenosis or dilation) and confluence of pulmonary arteries, and presence of systemic-to-pulmonary artery collaterals are all well assessed by

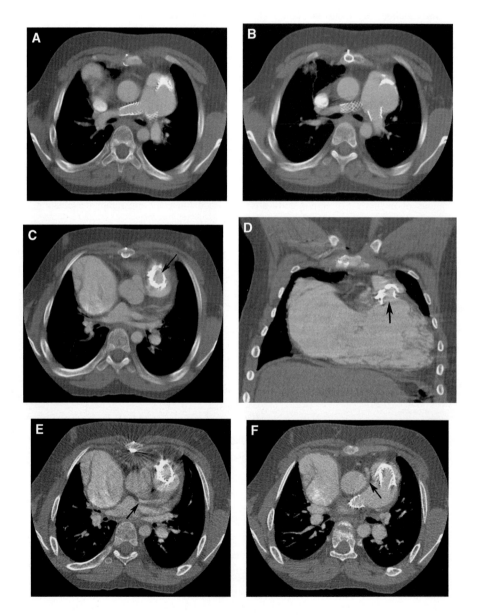

Fig. 6. CT angiogram in a 13-year-old boy following repair of tetralogy of Fallot. Axial intravenous contrasted-enhanced images at the level of the stented right pulmonary artery (*A*) and left pulmonary artery (*B*) show good caliber. (*C*) Image at the level of the main pulmonary artery shows narrowing at the stent (*arrow*), also appreciated on coronal reformation (*D*; *arrow*). Note associated marked right atrial and ventricular dilation. The left main (*E*; *arrow*) and right (*F*; *arrow*) coronary artery origins are also well depicted.

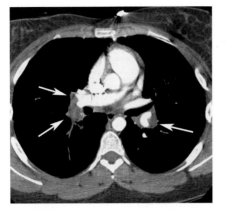

Fig. 7. CT angiogram in a 16-year-old girl with massive bilateral pulmonary thromboembolism. Axial intravenous contrast-enhanced CT image at the level of the right pulmonary artery demonstrates the thromboembolism (*arrows*). (*From* Frush DP, Herlong JR. Pediatric thoracic CT angiography. Pediatr Radiol 2004;35(1):11–25; with permission.)

CT angiography. Additional pulmonary artery evaluation includes assessment for the pulmonary sling (origin of the left from the right pulmonary artery); pulmonary thromboembolus (although relatively rare compared with adults) (Fig. 7); and assessment of arteriovenous malformations [18,19].

Thoracic venous anatomy [23], especially pulmonary veins in children, is also now possible with the current MDCT technology. Applications include evaluation of pulmonary vein stenosis or anomalous drainage (Figs. 1, 2, 4, and 8) [18–20].

Other applications of thoracic CT angiography include assessment of coronary arteries and pulmonary sequestration (Figs. 6 and 9) [24]. There has been no systematic evaluation of coronary arteries by CT angiography, partly because of the fact the echocardiography usually addresses many of the common indications, such as origin and course, and partly because of the rarity of conditions compared with the adult population. Information on compelling technology of gated CT angiography in children is

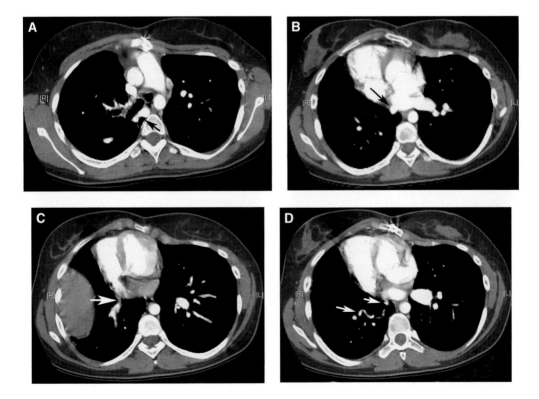

Fig. 8. CT angiogram in a 21-year-old woman with Scimitar Syndrome with possible pulmonary embolism. Intravenous contrast-enhanced axial image at the level of the main pulmonary artery (*A*) shows connection of a pulmonary vein to the azygos vein (*arrow*). (*B*) There is a venous connection into the left atrium (*arrow*). (*C*) A third connection into the right ventricle is stenotic (*arrow*). (*D*) This vein eventually ends up draining by way of a tortuous collateral (*arrows*) into the left atrium.

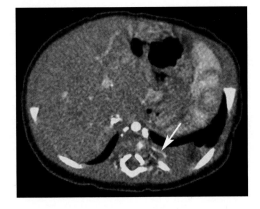

Fig. 9. Two-month-old female infant with a hybrid lesion consisting of a cystic adenomatoid malformation and pulmonary sequestration. CT angiogram clearly demonstrates the small vessel (*arrow*) supplying the sequestered component. This vessel arose from the aorta (not shown). (*From* Frush DP, Herlong JR. Pediatric thoracic CT angiography. Pediatr Radiol 2004;35(1):11–25; with permission.)

even scarcer although some data are beginning to emerge, with a cautionary note based on the potential radiation dose delivered [25]. In addition, vascular applications include the evaluation of the systemic arterial supply to pulmonary sequestration, emphasizing the MDCT benefits of multiplanar reformations and three-dimensional reconstructions [26,27].

Summary

Thoracic CT angiography is possible even in the most challenging cases. Familiarity with the appropriate technique, including patient preparation, IV contrast administration, and selection of appropriate CT parameters, is fundamental in obtaining diagnostic pediatric thoracic CT angiography. CT angiography can be performed in a step-by-step fashion. This includes understanding the specific clinical questions, nature of the anatomy and patient requirements, and providing the safest examination for the child. With this pragmatic approach, CT angiography can be a flexible and reliable tool for a broad range of thoracic vascular structures, especially the aorta, pulmonary arteries, and pulmonary veins. Familiarity with the appropriate technique also implies that other modalities, such as MR angiography or echocardiography, will supplant CT angiography when these are more appropriate.

References

[1] Arnould V, Worms AM, Galloy MA, et al. Diagnosis using x-ray computed angiotomography of an iliac artery aneurysm in an infant [in French]. Can Assoc Radiol J 1996;47:260–4.

[2] Brochhagen HA, Benz-Bohm G, Mennicken U, et al. Spiral CT angiography in an infant with severe hypoplasia of a long segment of the descending aorta. Pediatr Radiol 1997;27:181–3.

[3] Hopkins KL, Patrick LE, Simoneaux SF, et al. Pediatric great vessel anomalies: initial clinical experience with spiral CT angiography. Radiology 1996; 200:811–5.

[4] Cohen RA, Frush DP, Donnelly LF. Data acquisition for pediatric CT angiography: problems and solutions. Pediatr Radiol 2000;30:813–22.

[5] Frush DP, Herlong JR. Pediatric thoracic CT angiography. Pediatr Radiol 2004;35(1):11–29.

[6] Grist TM, Thornton FJ. Magnetic resonance angiography in children: technique, indications, and imaging findings. Pediatr Radiol 2004;35(1):26–39.

[7] Chan FP, Rubin GD. MDCT angiography of pediatric vascular diseases of the abdomen, pelvis, and extremities. Pediatr Radiol 2004;35(1):40–53.

[8] Chung T. Magnetic resonance angiography of the body in pediatric patients: experience with contrast-enhanced time-resolved technique. Pediatr Radiol 2004;35(1):3–10.

[9] Li LB, Kai M, Kusama T. Radiation exposure to patients during pediatric cardiac catheterization. Radiat Prot Dosimetry 2001;94:323–7.

[10] Pappas JN, Donnelly LF, Frush DP. Marked reduction in the frequency of sedation of children using new multislice helical CT. Radiology 2000;215:897–9.

[11] Frush DP, Bisset GS, Hall SC. Pediatric sedation: the practice of safe sleep. AJR Am J Roentgenol 1996; 167:1381–7.

[12] Cohen MD, Smith JA. Intravenous use of ionic and nonionic contrast agents in children. Radiology 1994; 191:793–4.

[13] Herts BR, O'Malley CM, Wirth SL, et al. Power injection of contrast media using central venous catheters: feasibility, safety and efficacy. AJR Am J Roentgenol 2001;176:447–53.

[14] Frush DP, Spencer EB, Donnelly LF, et al. Optimizing contrast-enhanced abdominal CT in infants and children using bolus tracking. AJR Am J Roentgenol 1999;172:1007–13.

[15] Fleischmann D. Use of high-concentration contrast media in multiple-detector-row CT: principles and rationale. Eur Radiol 2003;13(Suppl 5):M14–20.

[16] Denecke T, Frush DP, Li J. Eight-channel CT: multidetector CT: unique potential for pediatric chest. J Thorac Imaging 2002;17:306–9.

[17] Sigal-Cinqualbre AB, Hennequin R, Abada HT, et al. Low-kilovoltage multi–detector row chest CT in adults: feasibility and effect on image quality and iodine dose. Radiology 2004;231:169–74.

[18] Gilkeson RC, Ciancidello L, Zahka K. Multidetector CT evaluation of congenital heart disease in pediatric and adult patients. AJR Am J Roentgenol 2003;180: 973–80.

[19] Goo HW, Park I-S, Ko FK, et al. CT of congenital heart disease: normal anatomy and typical pathologic conditions. Radiographics 2003;23:S147–65.

[20] Siegel MJ. Multiplanar and three-dimensional multidetector row CT of thoracic vessels and airways in the pediatric population. Radiology 2003;229:641–50.

[21] Donnelly LF, Frush DP. Pediatric multidetector body CT. Radiol Clin North Am 2003;41:637–55.

[22] Lee EY, Siegel MJ, Hildebolt CF. MDCT evaluation of thoracic aortic anomalies in pediatric patients and young adults: comparison of axial, multiplanar, and 3D images. AJR Am J Roentgenol 2004;182: 777–84.

[23] Lawler LP, Corl FM, Fishman EK. Multi-detector row and volume-rendered CT of the normal and accessory flow pathways of the thoracic systemic and pulmonary veins. Radiographics 2002;22:S45–60.

[24] Desjardins B, Kazerooni EA. ECG-gated cardiac CT. AJR Am J Roentgenol 2004;182:993–1010.

[25] Hollingsworth CL, Chan FP, Yoshizumi TT, et al. Pediatric gated cardiac CT angiography: What is the radiation dose. Presented at the RSNA 90th Scientific Convention. Chicago, Illinois, November 29, 2004.

[26] Frush DP, Donnelly LF. Pulmonary sequestration spectrum a new spin with helical CT. AJR Am J Roentgenol 1997;169:679–82.

[27] Lee EY, Siegel MJ, Sierra LM, et al. Evaluation of angioarchitecture of pulmonary sequestration in pediatric patients using 3D MDCT angiography. AJR Am J Roentgenol 2004;183:183–8.

ELSEVIER
SAUNDERS

Radiol Clin N Am 43 (2005) 435 – 447

RADIOLOGIC
CLINICS
of North America

Thoracic Disorders in the Immunocompromised Child

Caroline L. Hollingsworth, MD

Division of Pediatric Radiology, Department of Radiology, Duke University Health System,
1905 McGovern-Davison Children's Health Center, Box 3808, Erwin Road, Durham, NC 27710, USA

The population of children afflicted with primary or secondary immunodeficiencies is in evolution. The primary immunocompromised host was first defined over 50 years ago when Bruton [1] discovered X-linked agammaglobulinemia (XLA), a congenitally acquired humoral immunodeficiency. Delineation and description of over 100 other primary immunodeficiency syndromes has ensued, which includes a diverse group of conditions caused by abnormalities in antibody production, cell-mediated immunity, or the phagocyte and complement activity. Although the number of children afflicted with primary immunodeficiencies remains relatively small, the impact of such diseases on each child is considerable. Secondary immunodeficiencies in childhood may result from infection with HIV or can be caused by chemotherapy, radiotherapy, or immunosuppressive therapy aimed at treating childhood malignancies; transplant rejection; rheumatologic disorders or inflammatory or infectious diseases; and any state of debilitation. Moreover, the development and success of many aggressive cytotoxic regiments and immunosuppressive therapies for children with cancer or autoimmune disorders and the increasing use of stem cell or bone marrow transplantation (BMT) have increased the number of immunocompromised children. This complex and varied population of immunocompromised children is at high risk for pulmonary complications related to both their underlying disease state and to various treatment regimes. Although infections obviously account for many complications, immunocompromised children are also at high risk for development of many other types of thoracic complications. These include primary and secondary thoracic malignancies and nonmalignant lymphoid proliferation, noninfectious pneumonias, bronchiolitis obliterans, pulmonary edema, graft-versus-host disease (GVHD), radiation injury, and pulmonary thromboembolism.

Specific thoracic complications vary according to the child's underlying immune status and specific treatment protocols. As such, the type of infection or other disease states encountered depends on the child's type of immunologic abnormality, severity of immunologic deficit, therapeutic interventions, and environmental exposures [2]. Although this discussion does not include all immunodeficiencies, the common primary immunodeficiencies and secondary immunocompromised states of childhood are addressed with emphasis on the mechanism of the disorder; imaging features of thoracic complications; and, where appropriate, imaging surveillance strategies.

Primary immunodeficiencies

Humoral immunodeficiencies

Humoral immunodeficiencies are the most commonly encountered type of primary immunodeficiency, accounting for over 70% of all primary immunodeficiencies [3–5]. This diverse group of disorders is characterized by defective antibody production causing increased susceptibility of affected individuals to recurrent pyogenic infections, particularly caused by encapsulated bacteria, such as *Haemophilus influenzae*, *Streptococcus pneumoniae*, and *Staphylococci*. Typical manifestations include

E-mail address: holli016@mc.duke.edu

radiologic.theclinics.com

recurrent pneumonia, otitis media, sinusitis, and sepsis. Most patients with humoral immunodeficiencies are able to recover from viral infections caused by normal T-cell production and activity. Humeral deficiencies include XLA, IgA deficiency, and common variable immunodeficiency. Children with XLA are nearly completely lacking all serum immunoglobulins and all isotypes of antibodies. These children are also deficient in germinal centers within their lymphoid tissue, which results in small tonsillar tissue and scarce lymph nodes. This disorder is caused by a mutation on the X chromosome, which encodes for Bruton's tyrosine kinase, an essential regulator of B-cell maturation [6,7]. Individuals with XLA have normal T-cell function and thymic tissue. Although the incidence is not known, it is regarded as less common than either IgA deficiency or common variable immunodeficiency (CVID). Children with XLA are generally protected from infections during the first 6 to 9 months of life because of maternal IgG antibodies. Increased susceptibility to pyogenic infections occurs as levels of these antibodies decline. Recurrent sinopulmonary infections are common, often eventually resulting in bronchiectasis. Although onset of symptoms in infancy is characteristic of this immunodeficiency, approximately 20% of affected children present later, between the ages of 3 to 5 years, possibly because of the widespread use of antibiotics. Consequently, these children can develop widespread structural lung damage before diagnosis [4]. Other less common sequellae include chronic conjunctivitis, giardiasis, malabsorbtion syndromes, and chronic meningoencephalitis [8]. Therapy consists of treatment with intravenous immunoglobulin and use of various antibiotics to treat recurrent infections.

Radiographically, children with XLA classically demonstrate thoracic abnormalities related to recurrent pulmonary infections including bronchiectasis, bronchial wall thickening, and atelectasis (Fig. 1). Bronchiectasis is commonly located in the middle and lower lobes with an upper lobe distribution being unusual [9]. Splenomegaly is not part of the disease spectrum and lymph node tissue including tonsils and adenoids are sparse. If infection of the central nervous system occurs, there may be diffuse leptomeningeal enhancement or thickening and findings that support encephalitis.

IgA deficiency is the most common primary immunodeficiency disorder with an estimated incidence of 1:333 to 1:700 in whites [4]. Asians and African Americans are much less frequently affected [10]. Although some children with IgA deficiency are clinically healthy, others are susceptible to recurrent

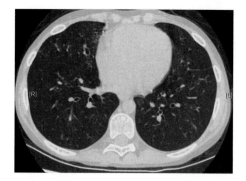

Fig. 1. A 4-year-old girl with X-linked agammaglobulinemia. Axial chest CT shows right middle lobe bronchiectasis with bilateral bronchial wall thickening evident elsewhere.

pulmonary and gastrointestinal infections, allergies, autoimmune disorders, and malignancies. Imaging findings are predominately caused by bacterial pneumonias, which account for most pulmonary complications. In contrast to XLA, bronchiectasis is not a common complication in IgA-deficient children because of properly functioning IgG antibodies. Standard treatment includes administration of antibiotics for specific infections.

CVID comprises a varied group of disorders thought to represent several different genetic defects [11]. CVID is characterized by defective antibody production in all major classes with an incidence estimated at 1:10,000 [12,13]. Although children with this disorder have normal absolute numbers of circulating B cells, serum immunoglobulins are either low or absent. After antigen stimulation B-cell proliferation does occur, but there is lack of differentiation into antibody-secreting plasma cells. These children demonstrate varied T-cell abnormalities with abnormal T-cell function present in up to 60% [13]. Onset of symptoms varies from early childhood to adulthood. In many cases inheritance has been shown to be autosomal-dominant with incomplete penetrance [5]. From a clinical perspective CVID and XLA share several common features including recurrent sinopulmonary infections, bronchiectasis, gastrointestinal disorders, and chronic meningoencephalitis [14]. Children with CVID, however, have normal amounts of tonsillar and adenoidal tissue and the development of lymphadenopathy and splenomegaly is seen in up to 25% [5]. Patients with this disorder may develop lymphoid interstitial pneumonia as part of a generalized lymphoproliferative process and have an increased propensity for the development of cancers, particularly from the lymphoreticular system. Autoimmune diseases are seen

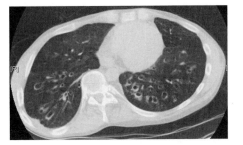

Fig. 2. A 15-year-old child with common variable immunodeficiency. Axial chest CT demonstrates bilateral lower lobe bronchiectasis. The substantial scoliosis is an unrelated finding.

in up to 20% of patients with CVID [15]. Radiographically, children with CVID may demonstrate recurrent infections, atelectasis, and bronchiectasis or bronchial wall thickening (Fig. 2). These patients can be differentiated from children with XLA because of the presence of normal to increased amounts of lymphoid tissue possibly with lymphadenopathy or splenomegaly. In contrast to children with XLA who invariably present in early childhood, the diagnosis of CVID may be made in early or late childhood or as an adult.

Cellular and combined immunodeficiencies

Patients with cellular immunodeficiencies have increased susceptibility to disseminated viral and opportunistic infections. Progressive pneumonia often occurs because of respiratory syncytial virus, parainfluenza 3 virus, *Pneumocystis carinii*, varicella, or cytomegalovirus. Patients with cellular immunodeficiencies may also develop infections with the high-grade pathogens that plague patients with humoral immunodeficiencies because B-cell production is T-cell dependent. Disorders include DiGeorge syndrome and severe combined immunodeficiency (SCID).

DiGeorge syndrome, also known as *thymic hypoplasia* or *aplasia*, is a classic example of a primary T-cell deficiency. This immunodeficiency most often results from a genetic defect on chromosome 22 resulting in abnormal development of the third and fourth pharyngeal pouches. This leads to abnormal development of the organs originating from these structures including the thymus, parathyroid glands, and heart and accounts for the constellation of clinical presentations. Most commonly children with DiGeorge have variably severe T-cell dysfunction secondary to aplasia or hypoplasia of the thymus. Infants may present with hypocalcemic tetany caused by hypoparathyroidism and congenital cardiovascular anomalies. Typical dysmorphic facial features include micrognathia, low-set ears, and hypertelorism [16]. Although circulating B cells are normal in number, antibody response to antigen may be impaired, particularly if the T-cell abnormality is severe. In fact, children with severe forms of this disease may have a similar clinical course as children with SCID. As with all children with a cellular immunodeficiency, patients with DiGeorge have increased susceptibility to opportunistic organisms. As such, viruses and *P carinii* are common pathogens. These children are also highly susceptible to GVHD from nonirradiated blood or blood products [14]. Aside from infectious sequelae, chest radiographs may demonstrate narrow upper mediastinal contour and retrosternal lucency caused by absence of thymic tissue (Fig. 3). Cardiovascular anomalies including right-sided aortic arch, interrupted aortic arch, truncus arteriosus, tetralogy of Fallot, and septal defects are

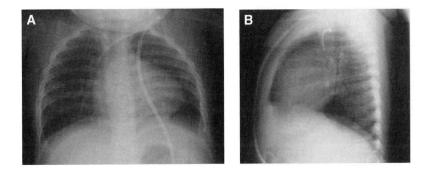

Fig. 3. A 6-month-old boy with DiGeorge syndrome. Frontal (*A*) and lateral (*B*) chest radiographs demonstrate narrow appearance to the superior mediastinum caused by thymic aplasia.

common [17]. Treatment depends of the severity of disease. Immunologic support is usually unnecessary in the partial form of DiGeorge; however, thymic epithelial transplant or HLA-identical sibling BMT is recommended for children with complete DiGeorge syndrome [17].

SCID syndrome is characterized by the absence of both T- and B-cell function. Occasionally, natural killer cell function is also absent. There are many cytokine and enzymatic defects identified that lead to this clinical spectrum, although most commonly inheritance patterns are autosomal-recessive or X-linked. The X-linked type is responsible for approximately 46% of all children with SCID [18]. Clinical and histologic features of this disease are similar despite different types of inheritance and different cytokine or enzymatic defects. Children with SCID syndrome commonly present with severe infections with opportunistic organisms in early infancy. Pulmonary complications include recurrent pneumonias cause by *P carinii*, parainfluenza, respiratory syncytial virus, adenovirus, cytomegalovirus, or bacterial organisms. *Pneumocystis* pneumonia typically manifests as diffuse interstitial infiltrates, which may progress to alveolar infiltrates (Fig. 4). Viral pneumonias may be indistinguishable from *P carinii* pneumonia (PCP). Importantly, in contrast to immunocompetent children or children with other types of immunodeficiencies, children with SCID have an absent thymic shadow. Adenosine deaminase–deficient children with SCID are noteworthy in that they typically have more profound lymphopenia than other children with SCID and also

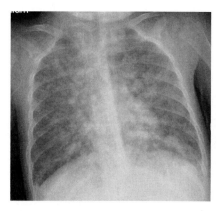

Fig. 4. Infant with severe combined immunodeficiency and respiratory distress. Frontal chest radiograph reveals diffuse interstitial and nodular alveolar opacities from fulminate cytomegalovirus infection.

may present with abnormalities of the axial skeleton including costochondral and metaphyseal abnormalities, increased separation of the rib head and vertebral body, and *bone-in-bone* appearance of the vertebral bodies [18]. SCID is universally fatal without immune reconstitution. Current treatment is by BMT, although gene therapy for X-linked SCID has been performed in a handful of children [19].

Partial combined immunodeficiency syndromes

Partial combined immunodeficiency syndromes encompass a spectrum of disorders with varied clinical manifestations. These diseases include Wiskott-Aldrich syndrome, cartilage-hair hypoplasia, ataxia-telangiectasia, purine-nucleoside phosphorylase deficiency, and X-linked lymphoproliferative disease. Although the clinical courses of these immunodeficiencies differ, children with partial combined immunodeficiencies have increased susceptibility to recurrent sinopulmonary infections. In addition, children afflicted with Wiskott-Aldrich syndrome and ataxia-telangiectasia have the highest malignancy rates of all primary immunodeficiencies. Patients with ataxia-telangiectasia are highly susceptible to radiation-induced malignancies and use of ionizing radiation for evaluation of these children should be performed judiciously [20].

Disorders of phagocytic cells and adhesion molecules

Chronic granulomatous disease is the most common phagocytic disorder, occurring in approximately 1 in 125,000 live births [21]. This disorder is most commonly inherited in an X-linked fashion, although several forms of autosomal-recessive chronic granulomatous disease have been described [4]. Not surprisingly, this disorder is seen most commonly in males. Chronic granulomatous disease is a combination of several molecular defects that result in defective NAPDH oxidase activity in leukocytes [22]. Children with chronic granulomatous disease develop recurrent infections, commonly with catalase-positive bacteria, such as *Staphylococcus aureus* or fungi including *Aspergillus,* caused by defective intracellular killing by neutrophils [23]. This disease usually presents before 1 year of age with pulmonary infections occurring most frequently. Other sites of involvement include lymph nodes, skin, liver, gastrointestinal tract, and bones [3]. Bacterial infections occur more frequently than fungal infections but up to 20% of children develop fungal disease. *Aspergillus* occurs more commonly than other fungal infections, such as *Candida* [24]. Chest radiographs or chest CT typically demonstrate lymphadenopathy, recurrent pneumonia, and pleural thickening (Fig. 5) [25]. The radiographic manifestations of *Aspergillus* vary but segmental or lobar infiltrates, nodular opacities, and cavitation are typical [24]. Although recurrent pneumonias and pulmonary abscesses are common, other thoracic manifestations include lymphadenitis, osteomyelitis, and chest wall abscesses. Esophageal strictures can also be a complication of chronic granulomatous disease.

Leukocyte adhesion deficiency results from a defect in the gene encoding CD18, a component of three different types of leukocyte adhesion molecules required for effective cell adhesion and migration [2]. This defect results in faulty phagocyte migration and ultimately increased host susceptibility to pyogenic infections. Severity of symptoms varies greatly, but these patients typically present with recurrent bacterial pneumonias and other severe and repetitive bacterial infections.

Other primary immunodeficiencies

Hyperimmunoglobulinemia E syndrome typically is associated with widespread staphylococcal abscesses of the skin, lungs, viscera, and other sites. Onset of symptoms characteristically occurs in infancy in association with markedly elevated serum IgE levels [26]. Pulmonary sequellae include recurrent staphylococcal pneumonias, which typically result in pneumatocele formation (Fig. 6). The most striking radiographic manifestation of this disease is persistent single or multiple, often large, pneumatoceles. These pulmonary air cysts may persist, expand, or become superinfected. Not infrequently, surgical

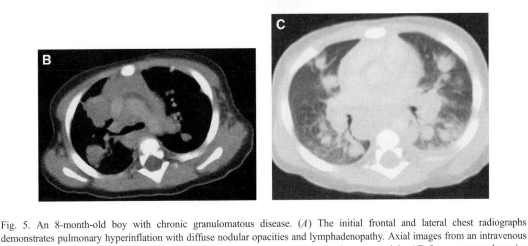

Fig. 5. An 8-month-old boy with chronic granulomatous disease. (*A*) The initial frontal and lateral chest radiographs demonstrates pulmonary hyperinflation with diffuse nodular opacities and lymphadenopathy. Axial images from an intravenous contrast-enhanced chest scan better delineate the extensive adenopathy (*B*) and pulmonary nodules (*C*) from an unusual species of gram-negative bacteria.

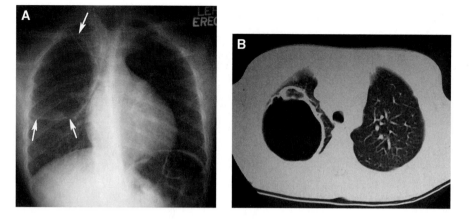

Fig. 6. An 8-year-old boy with hyper IgE syndrome. (*A*) Frontal chest radiograph shows a large right upper lobe pneumatocele (*arrows*). (*B*) Axial image from chest CT better delineates the postinfectious right upper lobe pneumatocele.

excision is needed (Fig. 7). Osteopenia and scoliosis are additional thoracic abnormalities seen in these patients [27]. The mechanisms underlying these skeletal changes have not been identified.

Secondary (acquired) immunodeficiencies

AIDS

AIDS in children (13 years or younger at diagnosis) accounts for approximately 2% of all cases of the disease. Most of these cases are acquired through vertical transmission from HIV-positive mothers [28]. HIV binds to the CD4 surface antigen on T4 lymphocytes, monocytes, and macrophages. This interaction leads to abnormal cell function and death. The resulting immunodeficiency is widespread because the impaired cellular immunity causes abnormal induction of B-cell–mediated antibody response to antigen. Children with AIDS have increased susceptibility to bacterial, viral, fungal, and protozoal infections.

Pulmonary infections are a major source of morbidity and mortality in children with AIDS. Fifty percent of children who die from AIDS do so as a result of complications from pulmonary disease [29]. Although these children are at risk for many opportunistic infections, such as PCP and mycobacterial pneumonia, acute bacterial pneumonias are common. Typical childhood viral and bacterial infections in children with AIDS include *S pneumoniae*, *H influenzae*, respiratory syncytial virus, and adenovirus [3]. Other thoracic manifestations include

edema from AIDS-related cardiomyopathy and thoracic tumors (B-cell lymphoma, leiomyoma, and leiomyosarcoma). Interestingly, cytomegalovirus infection and Kaposi's sarcoma, although common in the adult AIDS population, are unusual in childhood AIDS [28]. PCP deserves special consideration because it is the most common opportunistic pulmonary pathogen in children with HIV. Nearly half of all children with AIDS develop PCP. The initial infection leads to a terminal event in approximately 40% of the children with AIDS and PCP. Half of the children who survive their initial infection with PCP develop recurrent PCP infections [30]. PCP typically occurs in young children with a peak incidence between 3 and 7 months. In some children their initial infection with PCP is at presentation and serves as an AIDS-defining illness. In many instances PCP occurs in children known to be HIV-positive with a breakthrough infection on prophylaxis. The typical radiographic appearance of PCP includes increased interstitial markings, which spread from an initial perihilar distribution to the periphery. Alveolar opacities often accompany progression of interstitial disease (Fig. 8). Pneumatoceles and pneumothoraces are not uncommon (Fig. 9). Lobar consolidation may occur, but is not typical. Adenopathy and pleural effusions are rarely seen in association with PCP. Chest CT in children with PCP typically demonstrates peribronchial cuffing, patchy consolidation, ground glass opacity, and parenchymal cysts [31].

Lymphocytic interstitial pneumonia results from abnormal proliferation of bronchus-associated lymphoid tissue. If the pattern is more nodular than interstitial the term *pulmonary lymphoid hyperplasia* is often used. Lymphocytic interstitial pneumonia is

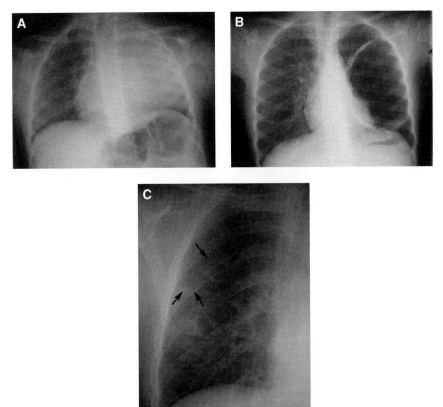

Fig. 7. Hyper IgE syndrome. (*A*) At 5 years of age, frontal chest radiograph demonstrates left upper lobe pneumonia. (*B*) After resolution of the left upper lobe pneumonia the child developed a large left upper lobe pneumatocele. This was surgically excised. (*C*) Frontal chest radiograph 8 years later shows the same patient has developed several smaller right mid-lung pneumatoceles (*arrows*).

thought to be the sequelae of an exaggerated response of the immune system in response to an infection. A causative organism has not yet been identified, although some speculate that Epstein-Barr virus infection is the culprit [3]. Lymphocytic interstitial pneumonia is much more commonly seen in children with AIDS than in the adult AIDS population. Children typically present after 1 year of age with increased interstitial markings, reticulonodular opacities, and mediastinal adenopathy (Fig. 10). Bronchiectasis is also seen in up to one third of pediatric patients with lymphocytic interstitial pneumonia [31]. Occasionally, cystic lesions in the lung develop causing the radiographic findings to resemble those small cystic changes seen with Langerhans' cell histiocytosis [32]. The development of lymphocytic interstitial pneumonia in a child with AIDS is a good prognostic indicator, with these children having a better outcome than children with AIDS who do not

develop lymphocytic interstitial pneumonia. Conversely, with improvement in the radiographic appearance, children often demonstrate clinical decline because of decreasing CD4 counts [33].

Children with AIDS are also susceptible to mycobacterial infections, although the incidence is less common than in the adult population with AIDS. The radiographic appearance mimics that seen in immunocompetent children with hilar adenopathy and lobar collapse or consolidation. *Mycobacterium avium-intracellulare* is also encountered in children with AIDS and cannot be distinguished based on imaging findings from other forms of mycobacterial infections. Miliary tuberculosis in children with AIDS, however, is distinctly unusual [3].

The wide availability of highly active antiretroviral therapy since 1997 has led to a dramatic reduction in morbidity, hospitalization, and mortality from HIV-related infections in the pediatric popula-

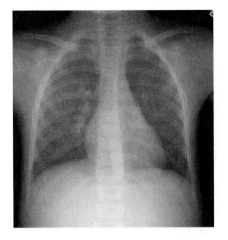

Fig. 8. An 8-year-old boy with AIDS. Frontal chest radiograph demonstrates subtle diffuse interstitial opacities caused by *Pneumocystis carinii* pneumonia.

tion. Twenty-five percent of children with AIDS are now reaching teenage years and chronic lung disease secondary to early childhood infections is increasingly common [34].

Bone marrow and stem cell transplantation

BMT and stem cell transplantation have an expanding role in the pediatric population for treatment of hematologic malignancies, solid tumors, select immunodeficiencies, and other disorders. In contrast to solid organ transplantation where immunosuppression is aimed at preventing rejection, BMT requires complete eradication of the immune system.

The temporal sequence of events after BMT is predictable with initial profound neutropenia lasting from 2 to 4 weeks. Recovery of absolute lymphocyte counts lags behind return of normal neutrophil numbers, taking up to 3 months. Even with return of normal numbers of lymphocytes, both cellular and humoral immunity remain impaired for up to 1 year. Local lung defense mechanisms are also impaired after BMT for up to 12 months [35]. The development of GVHD requiring further immunosuppression results in delay of immunologic recovery and carries an increased risk of pulmonary complications [3].

Early infectious complications after BMT are most frequently caused by bacteria and fungi, most commonly gram-negative organisms and *Aspergillus*. Bacterial pneumonias may be seen in up to 10% of children in the pre-engraftment stage and are particularly ominous. The classic bacterial pneumonias are caused by gram-negative organisms, such as *Pseudomonas* and *Klebsiella* (Fig. 11). Widespread use of

long-term in-dwelling catheters has led to an increased incidence of both *S aureus* and α-hemolytic streptococcal pneumonias, however, and has been associated with increased incidence of septic emboli (Fig. 12). Chest radiographs may show a classic focal or lobar consolidation, although atypical features are not uncommon. Anaerobic infections are atypical [36]. Children are also at increased risk of viral infections, most importantly respiratory syncytial virus, herpes simplex virus, adenovirus, and varicella (Fig. 13). Respiratory syncytial virus infection usually occurs early in the posttransplant period and carries 50% mortality. Radiographic findings are nonspecific but may include marked pulmonary hyperinflation and bilateral perihilar opacities, which coalesce into diffuse airspace disease [37]. Infection with cytomegalovirus is also an important contributor to morbidity and mortality, usually occurring 50 to 60 days post-BMT (Fig. 14) [3]. Fungal pneumonias in children who have undergone BMT are typically caused by *Aspergillus* or *Candida* species. Angioinvasive pulmonary aspergillosis is reported to occur in approximately 4% of children after BMT. The absence of neutrophils allows the hyphae of *Aspergillus* to proliferate and invade the pulmonary parenchyma and blood vessels causing thrombosis and hemorrhagic infarction of lung tissue. Prolonged episodes of profound or refractory neutropenia and sequellae of treatment for GVHD increase the likelihood of angioinvasive pulmonary aspergillosis, which carries a particularly grave prognosis and high mortality rate [38].

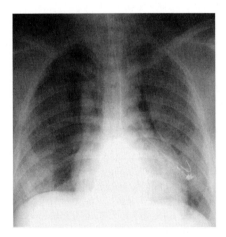

Fig. 9. Adolescent boy with AIDS and *Pneumocystis carinii* pneumonia. Frontal chest radiograph demonstrates diffuse bilateral interstitial opacities and bilateral, predominantly medial pneumothoraces.

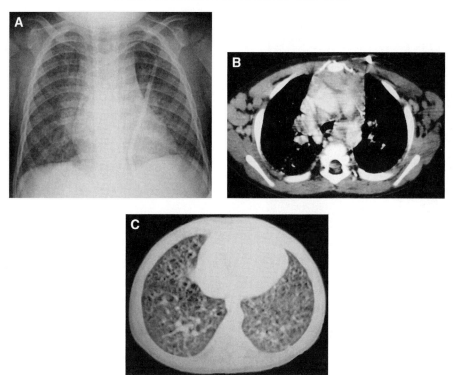

Fig. 10. A 29-month-old girl with AIDS and lymphocytic interstitial pneumonia. (*A*) Frontal chest radiograph demonstrates diffuse bilateral reticulonodular opacities and mediastinal fullness. (*B*) Axial image from intravenous contrast-enhanced chest CT demonstrates axillary and mediastinal lymphadenopathy. (*C*) Axial image from the same chest CT is in (*B*), lung algorithm, shows diffuse interstitial and reticulonodular opacities and small cysts. (Courtesy Edward F. Patz, Jr., MD, Durham, NC.)

Early noninfectious pulmonary complications of BMT include idiopathic pneumonia syndrome, pulmonary edema, pulmonary hemorrhage, and recurrence of the primary malignancy. Idiopathic pneumonia syndrome usually occurs approximately 45 days after transplantation. Both GVHD and radiation injury play a causative role in its patho-

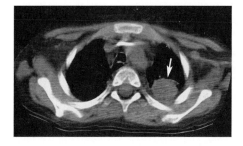

Fig. 11. Adolescent boy who developed persistent fevers after bone marrow transplant. Axial image from a noncontrast chest CT, soft-tissue algorithm, demonstrates a left upper lobe lung abscess (*arrow*). Ultrasound-guided percutaneous aspiration of the fluid collection yielded *Legionella*.

genesis [39]. Radiographic features are variable and may include diffuse airspace disease or interstitial opacities with or without a nodular component. Diffuse alveolar hemorrhage occurs in up to 10% of children undergoing allogenic BMT and typically develops at the time of engraftment. Pulmonary hemorrhage is often associated with other pulmonary pathology, particularly infection, and carries a high mortality rate. If the patient survives the initial event, rapid clearing may be seen over several days [40].

Late sequelae of BMT differ from the complications encountered early in the posttransplant period and include infections and bronchiolitis obliterans, diffuse alveolar damage, lymphocytic interstitial pneumonitis, and relapse of the underlying disease. Even after the engraftment period children continue to be at increased risk for bacterial infections caused by persistent abnormal humoral immunity. Encapsulated organisms, such as *S pneumoniae* and *H influenzae*, are the most frequent perpetrators. *P carinii*, cytomegalovirus, and adenovirus are also common [36]. The pathogenesis of chronic pulmonary fibrosis, bronchiolitis obliterans, and other types

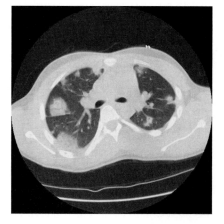

Fig. 12. Axial image from a chest CT in an immunosuppressed adolescent with a central venous catheter demonstrates multiple cavitary pulmonary nodules from septic emboli from *Staphylococcus aureus* sepsis.

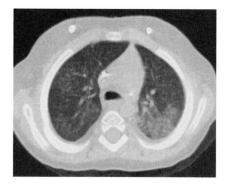

Fig. 14. A 9-month-old girl status post–bone marrow transplant with cytomegalovirus pneumonia. Axial image, lung algorithm, from a CT examination through the upper chest demonstrates scattered bilateral ground glass and interstitial opacities.

of noninfectious lung injury after BMT is poorly defined [39].

Bronchiolitis obliterans, also known as *constrictive bronchiolitis*, results from submucosal and peribronchial inflammation, which leads to restricted airflow in medium-sized airways [41]. Chest radiographs may demonstrate bronchial wall thickening or dilation, but are often normal. High-resolution chest CT improves diagnostic detection and may demonstrate subtle regions of lung lucency correlating with a decrease in the number and size of vessels along with bronchial dilation and wall thickening.

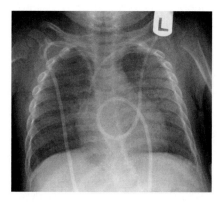

Fig. 13. A 4-year-old girl with Hurler's syndrome status post–bone marrow transplant with bilateral subtle interstitial opacities from cytomegalovirus pneumonia. Note broad ribs and undertubulation of the humeri caused by marrow packing from Hurler's syndrome.

Solid organ transplantation

Infection is a significant threat to the pediatric transplant recipient after solid organ transplantation, second only to allograft rejection. The thorax is a common site of infectious complications in this subset of the pediatric population (Fig. 15). Long-term immunosuppressive therapy increases the risk of infection and the risk of neoplasms including various lymphoproliferative disorders. Although there is significant overlap in incidence of infections caused by common drug-related effects of immunosuppression, different types of solid organ transplantation are predisposed to specific infections. In all transplant recipients viral infections can become life-threatening, particularly when treatment requires a decrease in immunosuppressive therapy, which increases the risk of graft rejection.

Children who have undergone renal transplantation are highly susceptible to infection with cytomegalovirus. Disease typically develops in the fourth to sixth week after transplantation and may occur in seronegative or seropositive recipients. These children are at even greater risk if OKT3 levels are increased to battle rejection [35]. PCP and *Aspergillus* infection are also common infections after renal transplantation. After liver transplantation children are at increased risk for development of infection with gram-negative bacteria and fungi, particularly *Candida* and *Aspergillus*. Children are especially susceptible in the first 30 days posttransplantation. PCP is also commonly encountered in liver transplant recipients but tends to occur later, typically 3 to 5 months after transplantation [35]. Children who have undergone lung transplantation are at increased

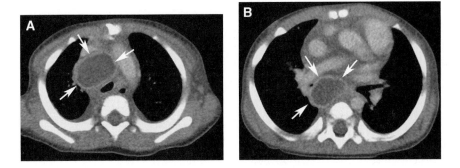

Fig. 15. A 10-month-old girl status post–heart transplant. Axial images from an intravenous contrast-enhanced chest CT, soft-tissue algorithm, at the level of the aortic arch (*A*) and main pulmonary artery (*B*) show two large mediastinal abscesses (*arrows*), which were surgically drained revealing *Mycobacterium tuberculosis*. This child also had multiple small pulmonary nodules (not shown).

risk of infections stemming from blood products or donor-to-recipient transmission, particularly in the first 6 months after transplantation. Reactivation of latent viruses or opportunistic infections constitutes the primary pathogens. Infection rates are high in these children secondary to decreased cough reflex, continued exposure of the transplanted organ to the environment, denervation, dysfunctional mucocilliary clearance, and immunosuppression [42]. Common infectious agents include cytomegalovirus, *P carinii*, and Epstein-Barr virus if either the recipient or donor is seropositive.

Patients with cancer

Children undergoing chemotherapy and radiation therapy for malignancy are also at increased risk for pulmonary complications. Of note, relative increased susceptibility to bacterial pneumonias depends on the specific immunologic impairment. As such, children with leukemia are at increased risk for infection with *S pneumoniae*, *H influenzae*, and gram-negative bacilli. Children who are predominately neutropenic as a result of chemotherapy are at risk for gram-negative infections, such as *Pseudomonas aeruginosa* and *Klebsiella* species, and gram-positive infections with such organisms as *S aureus*. Children with T-cell defects related to high-dose corticosteroid treatment or Hodgkin's disease are more likely to develop viral or fungal infections [43]. Pulmonary edema is not uncommon in children after solid organ transplantation or BMT and may also complicate recovery after chemotherapy or radiation treatment. After lung transplantation lymphatic drainage is impaired; this can lead to development of pulmonary edema. Cardiac or renal dysfunction resulting from

transplantation of heart, lung, kidney, or bone marrow may also cause pulmonary edema [35,44].

Lymphoproliperative disorders in the immunocompromised child

Many types of immunodeficiencies, whether congenital, acquired, or iatrogenic, are associated with an increased risk of both abnormal lymphoid proliferation and neoplasm [2]. Most cases are related to Epstein-Barr virus with a clinical spectrum of severity ranging from polyclonal lymphoid hyperplasia to monoclonal lymphoma [45,46]. In children, post-transplant lymphoproliferative disorder is most common when an initially seronegative patient develops

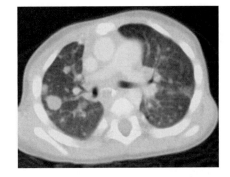

Fig. 16. Axial images from an intravenous contrast-enhanced chest CT in an 11-month-old girl status post–heart transplant and treatment for pulmonary and mediastinal tuberculosis. Lung algorithm shows multiple pulmonary nodules, which were a manifestation of graft-versus-host-disease (biopsy proved). Note calcification (*arrows*) in the mediastinum from prior *Mycobacterium tuberculosis* infection, soft-tissue algorithm.

a primary infection with Epstein-Barr virus after transplantation. The risk of posttransplant lymphoproliferative disorder rises with increasing use of high-dose corticosteroids and cyclosporine [3]. The incidence varies between 1% in renal transplant recipients and 10% in heart and heart-lung transplant recipients [45]. Posttransplant lymphoproliferative disorder may manifest early in the posttransplant period or may develop as late as several years after transplantation. Radiographically the findings associated with lymphoproliferative disorders in the chest are variable and nonspecific. Children may develop solitary or multiple parenchymal nodules, diffuse or focal reticulonodular opacities, or consolidation with or without mediastinal adenopathy. Pleural effusions or pericardial masses may also be seen (Fig. 16) [47]. The varied imaging appearance and clinical presentation often lead to biopsy for definitive diagnosis.

Summary

Thoracic complications are frequent in children with all types of immunodeficiencies and may be serious or potentially life-threatening. Infectious complications are the most common; however, sequelae of rejection and therapeutic regimes also pose a serious threat to the immunocompromised child. Many children with immunodeficiencies are at increased risk for neoplasia, particularly the development of lymphoproliferative disorders in which the thorax is a frequent site of involvement. The imaging characteristics of many thoracic diseases in the immunocompromised host overlap. It is necessary to be familiar with the type and mechanism of the immune disorder when interpreting imaging findings.

References

[1] Bruton OC. Agammaglobulinemia. Pediatrics 1952; 9:722–8.

[2] Buckley R. Pulmonary complications of primary immunodeficiencies. Paediatr Respir Rev 2004; 5(Suppl A):S225–33.

[3] Pennington DJ. Pulmonary disease in the immunocompromised child. J Thorac Imaging 1999;14:37–50.

[4] Primary immunodeficiency diseases. Report of an IUIS Scientific Committee. International Union of Immunological Societies. Clin Exp Immunol 1999; 118(Suppl 1):1–28.

[5] Buckley RH. Primary immunodeficiency diseases. In: Paul WE, editor. Fundamental immunology. Philadelphia: Lippincott-Raven; 1999. p. 1427–53.

[6] Vetrie D, Vorechovsky I, Sideras P, et al. The gene involved in X-linked agammaglobulinemia is a member of the src family of protein-tyrosine kinases. Nature 1993;361:226–33.

[7] Tsukada S, Saffran DC, Rawlings DJ, et al. Deficient expression of a B cell cytoplasmic kinase in human X-linked agammaglobulinemia. Cell 1993;72:279–90.

[8] Wilfert CM, Buckley RH, Rosen FS, et al. Persistent enterovirus infections in agammaglobulinemia. In: Schessinger D, editor. Microbiology. Washington: ASM; 1977. p. 488.

[9] Curtin JJ, Webster AD, Farrant J, et al. Bronchiectasis in hypogammaglobulinaemia: computed tomography assessment. Clin Radiol 1991;44:82–4.

[10] Schaffer FM, Monteiro RC, Volanakis JE, et al. IgA deficiency. Immunodeficiency 1991;3:15–44.

[11] Cunningham-Rundles C, Bodian C. Common variable immunodeficiency: clinical and immunological features of 248 patients. Clin Immunol 1999;92:34–48.

[12] Primary immunodeficiency diseases. Report of an IUIS Scientific Committee. International Union of Immunological Societies. Clin Exp Immunol 1999; 118(Suppl 1):1–28.

[13] Sneller MC, Strober W, Eisenstain E, et al. New insights into common variable immunodeficiency. Ann Intern Med 1993;118:720–30.

[14] McKinney RE, Katz SL, Wilfert CM. Chronic enteroviral meningoencephalitis in agammaglobulinemic patients. Rev Infect Dis 1987;9:334–56.

[15] Heraszewsli RA, Webster ADB. Primary hypogammaglobulinemia: a survey of clinical manifestations and complications. Q J Med 1993;86:31–42.

[16] Demuczick S, Aurias A. DiGeorge syndrome and related syndromes associated with 22q11.2 deletions: a review. Ann Genet 1995;38:59–76.

[17] Markert ML, Boeck A, Hale LP, et al. Thymus transplantation in complete DiGeorge syndrome. N Engl J Med 1999;341:1180–9.

[18] Buckley RH, Schiff RI, Schiff SE, et al. Human severe combined immunodeficiency (SCID): genetic, phenotypic and functional diversity in 108 infants. J Pediatr 1997;130:378–87.

[19] Broome CB, Graham ML, Saulsbury FT, et al. Correction of purine nucleoside phosphorylase deficiency by transplantation of allogeneic bone marrow from a sibling. J Pediatr 1996;128:373–6.

[20] Yin EZ, Frush DP, Donnelly LF, et al. Primary immunodeficiency disorders in pediatric patients. AJR Am J Roentgenol 2001;176:1541–52.

[21] Etzioni A. Adhesion molecule deficiencies and their clinical significance. Cell Adhes Commun 1994;2: 257–60.

[22] Kishimoto TK, Springer TA. Human leukocyte adhesion deficiency: molecular basis for a defective immune response to infections of the skin. Curr Probl Dermatol 1989;18:106.

[23] Malech HL, Nauseef WM. Primary inherited defects in neutrophil function: etiology and treatment. Semin Hematol 1997;34:279–90.

[24] Chusid MJ, Sty JR, Wells RG. Pulmonary aspergillo-

sis appearing as chronic nodular disease in chronic granulomatous disease. Pediatr Radiol 1998;18:232–4.

[25] Gold RH, Douglas SD, Peger L, et al. Roetgenographic features of the neutrophil dysfunction syndromes. Radiology 1969;92:1045–54.

[26] Grimbacher B, Holland SM, Gallin JI, et al. Hyper-IgE syndrome with recurrent infections: an autosomal dominant multisystem disorder. N Engl J Med 1999; 340:692–702.

[27] Kirchner SG, Sivit CJ, Wright PF. Hyperimmuno-globulinemia E syndrome: association with osteoporosis and recurrent fractures. Radiology 1985;156:362.

[28] AIDS among children—United States, 1996. MMWR Morb Mortal Wkly Rep 1996;45(46):1005–10.

[29] Marolda J, Paca B, Bonforte RJ, et al. Pulmonary manifestations of HIV infection in children. Pediatr Pulmonol 1991;10:231–5.

[30] Sivit CJ, Miller CR, Rakusan TA, et al. Spectrum of chest radiographic abnormalities in children with AIDS and *Pneumocystis carinii* pneumonia. Pediatr Radiol 1995;25:389–92.

[31] Haller JO, Cohen HL. Pediatric HIV infection: an imaging update. Pediatr Radiol 1994;24:224–30.

[32] Berdon WE, Mellins RB, Abramson SJ, et al. Pediatric HIV infection in its second decade: the changing pattern of lung involvement. Radiol Clin North Am 1993; 31:453–63.

[33] Prosper M, Omene JA, Ledlie S, et al. Clinical significance of resolution of chest X-ray findings in HIV-infected children with lymphocytic interstitial pneumonitis (LIP). Pediatr Radiol 1995;25:243–6.

[34] Morris A, Lundgren JD, Masur H, et al. Current epidemiology of *Pneumocystis* pneumonia. Emerg Infect Dis 2004;10:1713–20.

[35] Ettinger NA, Turlock EP. Pulmonary considerations of organ transplantation. Part 2. Ann Rev Respir Dis 1991;144:213–23.

[36] Jeanes AC, Owens CM. Chest imaging in the immunocompromised child. Paediatr Respir Rev 2002; 3:59–69.

[37] Englund JA, Sullivan JC, Jordan MC. Respiratory syncytial virus infection in immunocompromised patients. Ann Intern Med 1988;109:203.

[38] McWhinney PHM, Kibbler CC, Hamon MD. Progress in the diagnosis and management of *Aspergillus* in bone marrow transplantation: 13 years experience. Clin Infect Dis 1993;17:397.

[39] Stokes DC. Pulmonary complications of tissue transplantation in children. Curr Opin Pediatr 1994;6: 272–9.

[40] Palmas A, Tefferi A, Myers JL. Late-onset non-infectious pulmonary complications after allogeneic bone marrow transplantation. Br J Haematol 1998; 100:680–7.

[41] Kaplan EB, Wodell RA, Wilmott RW, et al. Chronic graft-versus-host disease and pulmonary function. Pediatr Pulmonol 1992;14:141–8.

[42] Kurlund G, Orenstein DM. Complications of pediatric lung and heart transplantation. Curr Opin Pediatr 1994;6:262–71.

[43] Stover DE, Kaner RJ. Pulmonary complications in cancer patients. CA Cancer J Clin 1996;46:303–20.

[44] Ettinger NA, Turlock EP. Pulmonary considerations of organ transplantation. Part 3. Ann Rev Respir Dis 1991;144:213–23.

[45] Knowles DM. Immunodeficiency-associated lympho-proliferative disorders. Mod Pathol 1999;12:200–17.

[46] Bragg DG, Chor PJ, Murray KA, et al. Lymphoproliferative disorders of the lung: histopathology, clinical manifestations, and imaging features. AJR Am J Roentgenol 1994;163:273–81.

[47] Ettinger NA, Turlock EP. Pulmonary considerations of organ transplantation. Part 1. Ann Rev Respir Dis 1991;143:1386–405.

ELSEVIER
SAUNDERS

Radiol Clin N Am 43 (2005) 449–457

RADIOLOGIC
CLINICS
of North America

Index

Note: Page numbers of article titles are in **boldface** type.

radiologic.theclinics.com